AF881130

**Series Title:** **Frontiers in Cancer Immunology**

**Volume Title:** **Cancer Immunotherapy: Mechanisms of Cancer Immunity, Engineering Immune-Based Therapies and Developing Clinical Trials**

**Editor**


**Jianxun Song**

*Department of Microbiology and Immunology*
*The Pennsylvania State University College of Medicine*
*Hershey, PA 17033*
*USA*

# CONTENTS

# FOREWORD

It is a privilege to write the Foreword for this book which is an outstanding review of cutting edge cancer immunotherapy. Despite early promises in some cancers, immunotherapy had generally failed to achieve consistent success. This scenario has changed drastically in the past few years. Indeed, Science Magazine hailed the advances in cancer immunotherapy as the number one breakthrough in all scientific disciplines for 2013.

The chapters of the book encompass all the different aspects of cancer immunotherapy and are authored by worldwide authorities in this field. There is a nice introductory chapter by the editor J. Song who provides a broad overview of the field. All chapters have a focus on clinical application and translational medicine. Individual chapters discuss the basic immunology of cytotoxic T cells, NK cells, dendritic cells, and regulatory T cells. Cancer vaccines draw attention in the dendritic cell chapter as well as in a focused separate chapter near the end of the book. Cytokines are also discussed extensively with a chapter discussing the role of IFNα as a vaccine adjuvant. Potential therapeutic roles for cytokines of the IL-12 family are the basis of another chapter.

Extensive consideration of technological advances is a focus of the book. These methodologies include genetic engineering of T cells, targeting of T cell co-stimulation, and antibody engineering. Adoption of such technologies has shown marked clinical responses in a variety of cancers. A limitation of the field of adoptive T cell therapy has been the challenge in generally sufficient numbers of antigen- specific T cells. The generation of such antigen - specific CTL using iPSC technology then is a fascinating potential solution as proposed in Chapter 10.

I would like to congratulate the editor, J. Song for bringing together a stellar group from around the world to summarize the current state of the art in the reinvigorated field of cancer immunotherapy.

***Thomas P. Loughran***
F. Palmer Weber-Smithfield Foods
Professor in Oncology Research
University of Virginia
USA

# PREFACE

Battling cancer is an all-time endeavor of both clinicians and scientists in the past several decades; however, the patient outcomes have not been significantly improved with those efforts, which urge people to find new strategies to change the *status quo*. In recent years, in the awareness that the human immune system has its intrinsic mechanism to control microbial pathogens and dysfunctioned self-tissues, therefore, people started to conceive the idea of treating cancer by using the immune mechanism that shortly has become a major research field coined as cancer immunotherapy. After gaining solid evidences in recent years that immunotherapy has critically enhanced the prognoses of cancer patients, it acclaimed a wider recognition from the society, for instances, it has been named the 2013 *Science's* Breakthrough of the Year. Of note, at this cheerful moment, it is a great pleasure and honor for us to provide our understandings and perspectives in cancer immunotherapy by presenting this book to our respected audiences. We hope this book will help audiences comprehend the concept and mechanistic studies involved in this emerging but booming subject of cancer immunotherapy.

The key feature of this book is it attempts to summarize different approaches have been studied and used in cancer immunotherapy based on the different components of human immune system. The book lists the major immune system components which have been demonstrated involving in limiting or killing tumor and their relevant applications in treating cancer patients. In addition, general introductions of engineered as well as targeted cancer immunotherapies are also included in this book to further broad the scope of our audiences. In summary, this book serves as a big map trying to picture all major branches in cancer immunotherapy; meanwhile, it also tries to pull different information together to give our audiences a general impression of utilizing components of the immune system in treating cancer.

In terms of the organization of this book, first of all, in the opening section of this book, it briefly summarizes the major features of different components of human immune system then introduces the relationships and interactions between tumor and the immune system. Later on, it focuses on the immunity of different immune components that against tumor and their relevant applications in clinics. The second section emphasizes on the cancer immunotherapy by using engineered components of the immune system to treat cancer, such as engineered antibodies, T cell receptors and cytokines. Following this, the concluding section of this book puts some outlooks on the emerging studies in designing of potential new cancer therapies, for example, targeting costimulatory signals in controlling T cell function; applying stem cell as a novel source of T cells in treating cancer; restraining aberrant regulatory T cells in cancer patients, and modulating tumor microenvironment to minimize its suppressive effects on anti-cancer immunity.

Hopefully, this book series will provide an introductory description about this complex concept of cancer immunotherapy. For the best comprehension and use of the knowledge and insights this book provides, readers are highly recommended to read the references listed at the end of each chapter and browse up-to-date literatures on specific topic readers are interested in. Also, we acknowledge that it is merely possible to cover all detailed information about this fast-growing specialty of cancer immunotherapy in this book through our limited efforts, therefore, we sincerely encourage our readers to keep searching the most updated literature and we believe this is the most efficient approach to capture the essences in cancer immunotherapy.

***Jianxun Song***
Department of Microbiology and Immunology
The Pennsylvania State University College of Medicine
Hershey, PA 17033
USA

# List of Contributors


| | |
|---|---|
| **Adam W. Mailloux** | H. Lee Moffitt Cancer Center, SRB 23033, Tampa, FL 33612, USA |
| **Anatoliy Markiv** | University of Westminster, Faculty of Sciences and Technology, London, W1W 6UW, United Kingdom |
| **Carol A. Kruse** | Department of Neurosurgery, David Geffen School of Medicine, University of California, Los Angeles, CA 90095, USA |
| **Colin C. Malone** | Department of Neurosurgery, David Geffen School of Medicine, University of California, Los Angeles, CA 90095, USA |
| **Elena I. Fomchenko** | Department of Neurosurgery, David Geffen School of Medicine, University of California, Los Angeles, CA 90095, USA |
| **Fengyang Lei** | Department of Microbiology and Immunology, The Pennsylvania State University College of Medicine, Hershey, PA 17033, USA |
| **Hiroshi Kawamoto** | Department of Immunology, Institute for Frontier Medical Sciences, Kyoto University Kyoto 606-8507, Japan |
| **Ivan Shevchenko** | Skin Cancer Unit, German Cancer Research Center, Heidelberg and Department of Dermatology, Venereology and Allergology, University Medical Center Mannheim, Ruprecht-Karl University of Heidelberg, Mannheim, Heidelberg, Germany |
| **Jianxun Song** | Department of Microbiology and Immunology, The Pennsylvania State University College of Medicine, Hershey, PA 17033, USA |
| **Kate L. Erickson** | Department of Neurosurgery, David Geffen School of Medicine, University of California, Los Angeles, CA 90095, USA |
| **Kazuya Ofuji** | Division of Cancer Immunotherapy, Exploratory Oncology Research and Clinical Trial Center, National Cancer Center, Japan |
| **Kristin Fino** | Department of Microbiology and Immunology, The Pennsylvania State University College of Medicine, Hershey, PA 17033, USA |
| **Linda M. Liau** | Department of Neurosurgery, David Geffen School of Medicine, University of California, Los Angeles, CA 90095, USA |
| **Mayuko Sakai** | Division of Cancer Immunotherapy, Exploratory Oncology Research and Clinical Trial Center, National Cancer Center, Japan |
| **Megan C. Duggan** | Comprehensive Cancer Center, The Ohio State University, Columbus, OH 43210, USA |
| **Ming-Song Li** | Department of Gastroenterology, Nanfang Hospital, Southern Medical University, Guangzhou, China |
| **Mohammad Haque** | Department of Microbiology and Immunology, The Pennsylvania State University College of Medicine, Hershey, PA 17033, USA |

**Pearlie K. Epling-Burnette** H. Lee Moffitt Cancer Center, SRB 23033, Tampa, FL 33612, USA

**Richard G. Everson** Department of Neurosurgery, David Geffen School of Medicine, University of California, Los Angeles, CA 90095, USA

**Robert M. Prins** Department of Neurosurgery, David Geffen School of Medicine, University of California, Los Angeles, CA 90095, USA

**Stephen Gottschalk** Center for Cell and Gene Therapy, Texas Children's Hospital, Houston Methodist Hospital, Baylor College of Medicine, Houston, Texas, USA; Texas Children's Cancer Center, Texas Children's Hospital, Baylor College of Medicine, Houston, Texas, USA and Department of Pediatrics, and Pathology and Immunology, Baylor College of Medicine, Houston, Texas, USA

**Steven De Vleeschouwer** Experimental Neurosurgery and Neuroanatomy, Department of Neurosciences, KU Leuven, Belgium

**Tania G. Rodríguez-Cruz** Center for Cell and Gene Therapy, Texas Children's Hospital, Houston Methodist Hospital, Baylor College of Medicine, Houston, Texas, USA and Texas Children Hospital, USABaylor College of Medicine, Houston, Department of Pediatrics, Baylor college of Medicine, Houston, Texas, USA

**Tetsuya Nakatsura** Division of Cancer Immunotherapy, Exploratory Oncology Research and Clinical Trial Center, National Cancer Center, Japan

**Toshiaki Yoshikawa** Division of Cancer Immunotherapy, Exploratory Oncology Research and Clinical Trial Center, National Cancer Center, Japan

**Viktor Umansky** Skin Cancer Unit, German Cancer Research Center, Heidelberg and Department of Dermatology, Venereology and Allergology, University Medical Center Mannheim, Ruprecht-Karl University of Heidelberg, Mannheim, Heidelberg, Germany

**William E. Carson III** Comprehensive Cancer Center, The Ohio State University, Columbus, OH 43210, USA

**Xiaofang Xiong** Department of Microbiology and Immunology, The Pennsylvania State University College of Medicine, Hershey, PA 17033, USA

**Xue-Feng Bai** Department of Pathology and Comprehensive Cancer Center, The Ohio State University, Columbus, OH, USA

**Yangbing Zhao** Department of Pathology and Laboratory Medicine, Abramson Family Cancer Research Institute, Perelman School of Medicine, University of Pennsylvania, Philadelphia, PA 19104, USA

**Yu Sawada** Division of Cancer Immunotherapy, Exploratory Oncology Research and Clinical Trial Center, National Cancer Center, Japan

**Yun Shi** Department of Pathology and Comprehensive Cancer Center, The Ohio State University, Columbus, OH, USA and Department of Gastroenterology, Nanfang Hospital, Southern Medical University,

Guangzhou, China

**Zhenzhen Liu** Department of Pathology and Comprehensive Cancer Center, The Ohio State University, Columbus, OH, USA

2

**CHAPTER 1**

# Introduction: Tumor and the Host Immune System

**Fengyang Lei, Mohammad Haque, Kristin Fino, Xiaofang Xiong and Jianxun Song***

*Department of Microbiology and Immunology, The Pennsylvania State University College of Medicine, Hershey, PA 17033, USA*

**Abstract:** Cancer is not one simple disease but a group of heterogeneous diseases sharing a common feature of uncontrolled cell growth. Cancer is a leading health issue in modern society and patients succumb to the disease every day. Among many different treatment approaches, harnessing the immune system to treat cancer has gained prominence in recent years. While some of the cancer cells can evade the host immune surveillance as well as spread distally, the majority of cancer cells are removed from the host immune system in premalignant stages of the disease. Accumulating evidence indicates that the host immune system is highly involved in the elimination of cancer cells, but ultimately, cancer cells have developed their own mechanisms to subvert the immune system. A comprehensive understanding of the immune system and its interaction with cancer is crucial to develop immune-based treatments. The currently available cancer immunotherapies are developed from a systemic understanding of the human immune system. This opening chapter will serve as an introductory remark to briefly summarize the human immune system, cancer and both positive and negative interactions between the immune system and cancer.

**Keywords:** Adaptive immunity, antibody, antigen, B cell, B cell receptor, cancer, cancer-associated antigen, costimulatory molecules, cytokine, dendritic cell (DC), hematopoietic stem cell (HSC), immune system, immunoglobulin, immunotherapy, innate immunity, myeloid cells, major histocompatibility complex (MHC), natural killer (NK) cell, T cell, T cell receptor (TCR).

## INTRODUCTION

The immune system is one of the most sophisticated biological systems, especially in the mammalian kingdom. It holds the responsibility of maintaining the wellness of an individual by defending against outside intruders and disposing of internal insurgents. Any defects in this system would cause devastating

***Corresponding author Jianxun Song:** Department of Microbiology and Immunology, The Pennsylvania State University College of Medicine, Hershey, PA 17033, USA; Tel: (717) 531-0003 ext. 287768; Fax: (717) 531-4600; E-mail: jus35@psu.edu consequences such as fulminant infection and/or cancer development. Due to its complexity and limitation of current research strategies, much is still to be learned about this intriguing system. However, from the current information gained about the human immune system in past decades, many therapeutic approaches have been developed, and several have been approved for clinical use. This reflects the practical importance of the immune system in managing health. On the flip side, it also suggests the importance to keep exploring this complicated subject in order to facilitate its application in tackling human diseases.

Immunology is the study of the immune system and its associations with diseases. Cancer immunology is the study of interactions between cancer and the host immune system. Immunology is a broad term that can be used for all living organisms unless specifically indicated; the facts described in this review are obtained from studies in higher mammals such as human and mouse. In this book, immunology is discussed with a focus on cancer treatment in human beings.

In immunology, the most studied subjects are the host immune system. Generally, there are two major categories of the immune system in higher mammals: innate immunity, which makes up the first line of defense, and adaptive immunity, which is more versatile and specific in backing up the innate immunity to invading pathogens. Meanwhile, adaptive immunity is also responsible for eliminating the dysfunctional self-tissues such as tumors [1].

## INNATE IMMUNE SYSTEM

The first line of defense against microbe infection, innate immunity is defined as the natural or native immunity due to its limited pattern of antigen recognition. Innate immunity can only recognize general categories of particles or molecules expressed on the microbes, rather than being specifically targeted to a certain molecule. Because of this major limitation, currently, it is difficult to utilize the components in innate immunity in treating cancer.

The innate immune system is composed of several different layers of mechanisms mediated by cells and tissues from different systems. For example, the skin and mucosal epithelial cells compose the first physical barrier of the organism. The other components such as neutrophils, basophils, eosinophils, complement system, natural killer (NK) cells and monocyte-macrophages eliminate microbes that have penetrated the physical barrier. However, when invading microbes pass the defensive line built by innate immunity, adaptive immunity will kick into action.

As mentioned above, the innate immune system is made up of different cell types in several systems. The physical barrier built by epithelia in the skin and mucosa is beyond the scope of this book and will not be discussed. Other blood-originated innate immune cells, including neutrophils and macrophages participate in the management of infection by different mechanisms; they are incapable of specifically targeting self-derived cells, such as tumor cells, though they are essential for activating the adaptive immune cells, and for cleaning up the area after anti-tumor immunity has done its work. Two types of innate immune cells, NK cells and eosinophils, are involved in antibody dependent cell-mediated cytotoxicity (ADCC) [2], and complement system also participates in the antibody mediated killing process [3]; therefore these components of the innate immune system will be briefly discussed below.

## Macrophages and Neutrophils

After penetrating the physical barrier, microorganisms enter the tissue. When they encounter the tissue-residing phagocytes, they are likely to be recognized, ingested and killed by those phagocytes. This is the second line of innate immunity against intruding microbes. Generally, there are two major types of phagocytes, monocytes/macrophages and polymorphonuclear neutrophilic leukocytes (PMNs) or, neutrophils. These two major categories of cells play a fundamental role in eliminating invading pathogens.

Macrophages are the major tissue-residing phagocyte that comprises as the first responder to pathogen invasion [4]. Normally, macrophages mature continuously from monocytes that circulate in the blood. This is also the reason it is called the monocyte/macrophage system. After maturing from monocytes in the blood, macrophages migrate out of circulation and reside in their designated organs and tissues, such as the liver, whose specialized macrophages are called Kupffer cells [5].

After encountering microbes, macrophages engulf pathogens to form phagosomes inside of the cells. When phagosomes are formed, several different types of bactericidal agents such as superoxide, nitric oxide and lysozymes are synthesized and released into phagosomes. This transforms phagosomes into phagolysosomes, which is sufficient to degrade most phagocytosed bacteria. Meanwhile, at the time of ingesting and killing bacteria, macrophages secrete cytokines and overexpress certain costimulatory molecules to recruit other cells to the site of invasion to clean up the pathogens [6]. The neutrophil is always the first one in the circulation to respond to the call from the macrophage.

Neutrophils are a second group of phagocytes that control invading bacteria. They mainly reside in circulation, but not in tissue. Upon receiving the chemoattractant signals released from the activated macrophage, endothelium, and other cells in the inflamed region, neutrophils extravasate from blood vessels and migrate into the affected tissue. The phagocytic process in neutrophils is similar to that of the macrophage, though it also includes a wide array of enzymes that are not just released in phagosomes but also released extracellularly from their granules [7].

In addition to their role of bacteria killing, phagocytes play a second role of bridging the innate immunity to adaptive immunity through their secreted cytokines, presented antigens and expressed costimulatory molecules. When a macrophage or dendritic cell ingests and degrades bacteria, degraded bacterial components are recognized by pattern recognition receptors such as toll-like receptors (TLRs) and NOD-like receptors (NLRs), turning on signaling pathways to further activate the cell [8]. An activated macrophage secretes cytokines and chemokines to recruit both circulating and nearby phagocytes to participate in controlling infection. Also, macrophage-derived pro-inflammatory cytokines such as interleukin-1 (IL-1) and IL-6 attract circulating lymphocyte to the site of infection. In addition to secreting cytokines, activated macrophages become more effective at antigen presentation with increased expression of type II major histocompatibility complex (MHC-II) molecules and costimulatory molecules such as B7.1 (CD80) and B7.2 (CD86) to further activate the recruited lymphocytes [9].

In a two-step T cell activation mechanism, T cell receptor (TCR) engagement of MHC-loaded antigen epitope cannot activate T cells until a second costimulatory signal is received [10]. In this scenario, when a macrophage degrades ingested bacteria to small fragments of peptides, some of them are further processed and loaded on MHC-II molecule to present to those recruited T cells. Other degraded bacterial components bind and activate pattern recognition receptors to transduce activation signals into nucleus to promote the expression of costimulatory molecules and cytokines. At this point, the macrophage serves as a professional antigen-presenting cell (APC) to activate T cells, bridging innate and adaptive immunity.

### Dendritic Cells (DCs)

This innate-to-adaptive bridging property of phagocyte has been applied in the development of cancer immunotherapy. For example, activated TLR signaling pathway can upregulate the MHC II expression, costimulatory molecules, and T cell cytokines to further activate T cells for controlling tumor growth. In this category, the TLR7 agonist, imiquimod, is a very promising drug in promoting anti-cancer immunity [11]. From the study of costimulatory molecules expressed on phagocytes, other pharmaceutical agents that target costimulatory receptors on T cells have also achieved certain therapeutic effects in enhancing the cancer immunosurveillance. For example, FDA has approved anti-PD1 and anti-CTLA4 antibodies in treating different cancers [12, 13]. Mentioning macrophages and phagocytes as professional antigen-presenting cells, but there is another big group of the APCs need to be addressed that are dendritic cells (DCs) which play a more specific role of antigen presentation that connects innate immunity to adaptive immunity.

DCs are a common name of a group of different types of antigen-presenting cells, divided into myeloid DCs and plasmacytoid DCs [14]. They differentiate from myeloid progenitors in the bone marrow, but reside in different organs and tissues to act as an antigen-sensor in the immune system. After DCs uptake microorganisms, they process and present the specific antigen epitope together with their MHC-II molecules on the surface to activate CD4 T cells [15]. Mature DCs have a very high expression of MHC-II as well as other costimulatory molecules, both in infected tissue and in the lymphoid organs where T cells proliferate to activate and further enhance T cell function. As an important messenger between innate and adaptive immunity, DCs have been shown to be as promising as vaccines in cancer immunotherapy. Provenge, a DC-based vaccine against the prostate cancer antigen PAP, has been approved clinically in treating late stage prostate cancer patients [16].

## NK Cells

An important component of innate immunity that acquires potent target-killing capability is the NK cell. NK cells are developed from the bone marrow-derived common lymphoid progenitor and circulate in the blood before receiving recruiting signals. The killing mechanism of an NK cell is identical to a cytotoxic T lymphocyte (CTL), but the activation mechanism of the NK cell is different. NK cell activation is mediated by invariant receptors that recognize certain molecules expressed in the target cells. NK cells are recruited and activated by interferons and macrophage-associated cytokines. In comparison to the classical T cell activation, which needs prior immunization, NK cell activation is immunization-free [17]. Upon recruitment to the site of infection, NK cells target cells with reduced or altered MHC-I expression, which is a hallmark of many intracellular pathogens. Activated NK cells kill their target cells by either a direct cytotoxic effect or an apoptosis-inducing mechanism. In cancer immunotherapy, especially monoclonal antibody-mediated therapy targeting tumor-specific or tumor-associated antigens, a significant mechanism is antibody dependent cell-mediated cytotoxicity (ADCC). NK cell plays a central role in ADCC as its immunoglobulin receptor recognizes antigen-bound antibodies; this process is featured in Fig. **1**. In summary, NK cell activity in some degree is associated with the efficacy of a successful cancer immunotherapy.

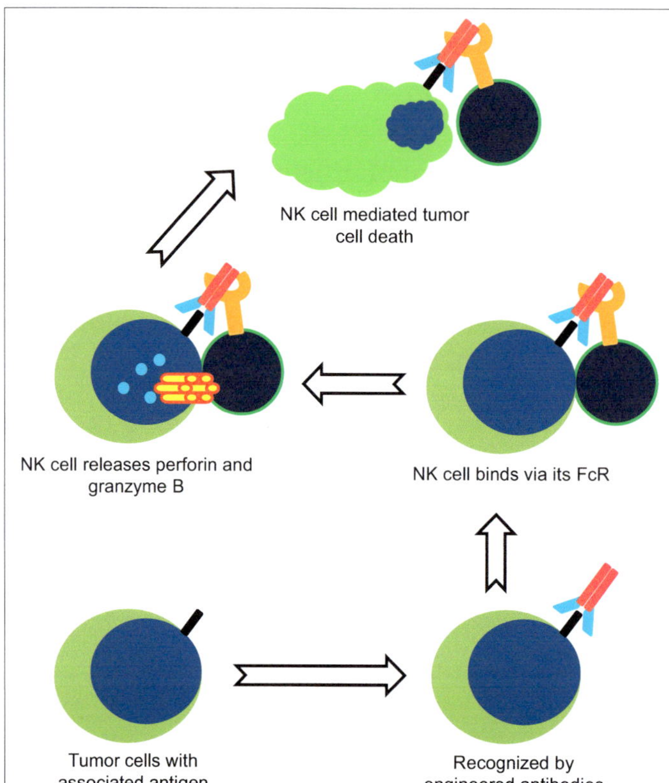


**Figure 1:** Antibody-dependent cell mediated cytotoxicity. This is a well-documented mechanism in monoclonal antibody-mediated tumor killing. Briefly, when mAbs bind to the target expressed on the tumor cell, they will recruit the surrounding NK cells to participate into the tumor killing process. The Fc receptor expressed on NK cells will bind to Fc segment on mAbs which will activate NK cells to execute cytotoxicity in target cells in terms of secreting perforin and granzyme B.

## The Complement System

The other direct target-lysing mechanism considered as part of an innate immunity is the complement system [18]. The complement system is composed by a series of small molecules that circulate in the blood. There are three complement activation pathways: the classical, alternative and mannose binding lectin-mediated pathways [19]. In short, the cascade activation of complement system eventually forms a membrane-attack complex that penetrates cell membranes and induces massive water and sodium influx to lyse the target. Meanwhile, cleaved complement components serve as chemoattractants to recruit inflammatory cells to further participate in the targeted killings of both invading cells and infected host cells. The classical complement activation pathway is particularly important for antibody-based cancer immunotherapy, because antibody binding to tumor antigens would recruit complement to complete final tumor execution. The simplified process of complement-mediated tumor killing is outlined in Fig. **2**.

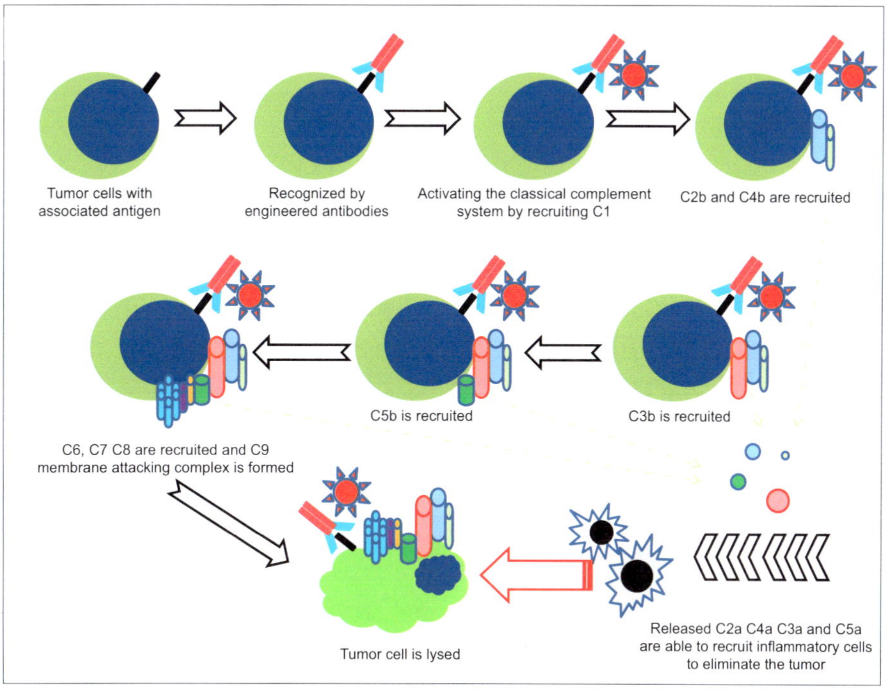


**Figure 2:** Complement mediated cytotoxicity. Complement mediated cytotoxicity requires the binding of mAbs to tumor-associated antigen first. After mAb binds to an antigen, it activates the classical activation pathway of the complement system. In short, C1 is recruited by mAb then C2 and C4 are recruited and cleaved by C1. Cleaved C2b and C4b bind to C1q but C2a and C4a, as part of the chemoattractants, are released. Following this, C3 and C5 are sequentially recruited and cleaved to form a chunky complement complex (C3b and C5b), meanwhile, C3a and C5a are released as inflammation mediators. This cascade process of complement activation is further augmented as C6, C7 and C8 joining, and finally, a membrane-attaching complex comprised by C9 will be formed to penetrate the tumor cell membrane. The tumor cells will be killed by physical property changes caused by water and sodium influx.

In addition to the above-described components of innate immunity, there are still other important members of the big innate immunity family such as eosinophils and basophils. Although their roles in the immune system are innumerable, their associations with cancer therapy are less important compared to the other components described above. Therefore, their functions will not be discussed here.

After introducing the innate immunity and its association in cancer immunotherapy, it is obvious that certain components of the innate immune system participate in killing of tumor cells. However, all of them require the prior involvement of elements from the adaptive immune system: T cells, B cells, and antibodies. To understand the complete immune response towards invading pathogens and self-tissue dysfunction, the adaptive immune system is discussed below.

## ADAPTIVE IMMUNE SYSTEM

The adaptive immunity is also called the specific or acquired immunity [20]. The adaptive immune system is composed of lymphocytes and their products such as cytokines and antibodies. While the innate immunity recognizes structurally conserved motifs of microbes, lymphocytes in the adaptive immune system specifically recognize different microbial peptide sequences by their surface-expressed receptors, namely, B cell receptor (BCR) in B cells and T cell receptor (TCR) in T cells. The molecules recognized by lymphocytes are collectively called antigens. Sometimes these immune responses go beyond foreign substances and target self-tissues; autoimmune diseases such as rheumatoid arthritis and systemic lupus erythematosus (SLE) are typically caused by lymphocytes that inappropriately target self-proteins, leading to a chronic inflammation that is unrelated to any pathogens. However, the flip side of autoimmunity is the foundation for developing cancer immunotherapy, because cancer cells are malignantly changed self-tissues and cancer antigens are often dysregulated self-antigens.

The adaptive immune system is subdivided into two categories: humoral and cellular immunity. Humoral immunity is mediated by B cells [21] and their secreted antibodies, and cellular immunity is mediated by T cells and their associated products [22]. Typically, humoral immunity plays a role in controlling extracellular microorganisms, and cellular immunity acts in eliminating viruses and other intracellular pathogens. As mentioned above, the innate and adaptive immune systems are not independent, but tightly connected and in this scenario DCs are pivotal connectors in bridging these two types of immunity.

## Humoral Immunity

In humoral immunity, B cells and antibodies are the key players. Like NK and T cells, B cells originate from the common lymphoid progenitors which develop and mature in the bone marrow. After maturation, B cells are released into circulation and migrate to secondary lymphoid organs such as spleen and lymph nodes for receiving antigen stimulation. Mature B cells that have never encountered their cognate antigen are called naive B cells. Once they encounter antigen, these mature B cells start to proliferate, and some of them become memory B cells, which are easier to activate than naïve B cells, or switch to plasma cells to secrete antibodies that specifically target the cognate antigen. There are several different isotypes of antibodies based on their presences and functions, including IgE, IgA, IgM, and IgG [23]. Engineered monoclonal antibodies are normally cloned from IgG isotypes due to their high affinity and specificity [24]. The detailed classification and description of antibody isotypes is beyond the purpose of this book since most isotypes are not useful in targeting cancers.

Antibody is the major product of activated B cells. Upon stimulation by certain antigens, B cells will differentiate into plasma cells, which produce the relevant antibody that recognizes and binds to the antigen. This mechanism plays a significant role in eliminating extracellular pathogens, but in some circumstances antibody can also recognize and bind to self-tissue. This also suggests that antibodies could be used in cancer immunotherapy, because of the self-originated nature of cancer cells. To design an ideal tumor-specific antibody, three major characters, specificity, affinity, and avidity should be considered. In searching for an efficient way to generate more potent antibodies, the production of monoclonal antibodies (mAb) [25]. A mAb is distinguished from polyclonal antibodies by the fact that each antibody molecule in the mAb preparation is an identical member of the same clone, as all have been generated not just against the same protein antigen, but also against the same epitope within the antigen. A pool of antigen-reactive antibodies is generated against a certain antigen, and the best mAb is chosen according to those three selective criteria. With an identified tumor-specific and/or tumor-associated antigen, this unique and practical property of antibodies renders them good weapons to target tumor cells.

Currently, mAbs have made a significant impact in clinical oncology. The three top-selling anti-cancer drugs on market, rituximab, trastuzumab, and bevacizumab are all mAb-based. Due to the limitations in both *in vitro* and *in vivo* testing systems, the exact antitumor mechanisms of mAbs are still vague. However, strong data support that both innate and adaptive immune responses are involved in the killing of tumor cells. Particularly, antibody-dependent cell-mediated cytotoxicity (ADCC) is the most important mechanism. In ADCC, as described in innate immune responses, after mAbs bind to the tumor cells with their Fab fragments, the Fc fragments on mAbs bind to the Fc receptor (FcR) expressed on the NK cells, which executes the tumor lysis. This phenomenon has been well recorded in the clinical administration of rituximab [26]. The other possible mechanisms observed in various studies include a combined anticancer action initiated by mAb binding, followed by activation of other members of the immune system such as DCs as well as complement system that mediates the complement-mediated cytotoxicity (CMC) towards tumor cells.

To achieve a more effective tumor cell destruction, mAbs have been further modified to increase the anti-tumor efficacy. One method is to increase Fc fragment affinity to FcR, and another involves the generation of bifunctional mAbs which could bind to tumor associated antigen and, at the same time, either recruit T cells to exert a CTL-mediated cytotoxicity or deliver anti-tumor drugs with engineered components on mAbs. Recently FDA approved drug T-DM1 (trastuzumab emtansine) is a good example of the modified bifunctional mAbs [27]. T-DM1 is constructed on the backbone of trastuzumab, which targets the HER2/neu receptor that expressed in certain breast cancer cells, by conjugating a cytotoxic agent mertansine. The conjugated mAb directly targets the HER2/neu receptor-bearing breast cancer cells and delivers the mertanisine-mediated cytotoxicity to kill the target.

Antibody mediated cancer immunotherapy requires the combined action of several components of the immune system. Any defects in the system such as NK cell anergy could prevent successful tumor cell destruction; therefore this new type of mAbs would significantly increase the anti-tumor efficacy when the direct participation of crucial components of the immune system is absent or dysfunction. However, in order to continue improving the application of mAbs in clinical oncology, extensive work is still pending to elucidate the mechanisms of action of mAb-mediated tumor cells killing.

A second category of antibodies applicable to cancer immunotherapy is the immune-modulating antibodies. As described in the section of innate immune responses, there are two groups of costimulatory molecules, stimulatory and inhibitory. Stimulatory molecules activate the T cells, but inhibitory molecules block and/or inhibit the activation of T cells. In many cancer patients, it is observed that circulating T cells have developed tolerance and/or anergy due to the insufficient presence of stimulatory molecules or the prevalence of inhibitory molecule. Boosting positive and quenching negative costimulatory signals may help mitigate tolerance. MAbs that target costimulatory molecules have been developed and applied with promising outcomes in clinical studies. For example, mAbs specifically blocking CTLA-4 ligation, an inhibitory costimulatory molecule that is highly expressed on the T cells of several cancer patients have shown initial success in treating patients with metastatic melanoma and renal cell carcinoma [28]. Studies examining the generation of other costimulatory molecules-specific mAbs are still ongoing.

## Cellular Immunity

In adaptive immune system, B cell and its associate antibodies comprise humoral immunity; T cells compose the other half, cellular immunity. Accumulating evidence has shown that T cell-mediated cellular immunity is a crucial mechanism in mammalian system to clean up both infection and dysregulated self-tissues. Any defects in T cell system would be devastating. For example, HIV patients have a great risk of acquiring opportunistic infections and develop rare forms of tumor due to their substantial losses of CD4+ T cells. In cancer immunotherapy, T cell-based therapy has been shown to be the most successful approach compared to other regimens. The cellular immune system and its application in cancer immunotherapy will be introduced.

A major player in cellular immunity is the T lymphocyte or T cell. The T cell is a common name for a group of cells with different roles, but they all originate from the common lymphoid progenitors in the bone marrow and mature in the thymus. T cells are classified based on TCR subtype, which are αβ-T cells and γδ-T cells [29]. The knowledge of γδ-T cell is still vague and its application in cancer therapy is limited, thus it will not be discussed further in this review book [30]. This chapter will focus on αβ-T cells, which comprise a majority of the T cell population. αβ-T is further divided into CD4+ and CD8+ T cell subtypes based on the surface expression of CD4 and CD8 molecules. Both CD4 and CD8 T cells develop from the same progenitor. After an intrathymic developmental process of CD4CD8 double negative (DN) and CD4CD8 double positive stages (DP), certain portions of progenitors develop into CD4 single positive (SP) T cells or CD8 SP T cells.

## CD4 T Cells

CD4 cells are also known as helper T cells or $T_H$ cells, which can differentiate into several subtypes, including $T_{H1}$, $T_{H2}$, $T_{H17}$ and other cells. During CD4 subtype differentiation, APC signaling directs T cells into particular subtypes [31]. Generally, CD4+ T cells are not directly involved in the killing process, but they are immune modulators and function to secrete cytokines and, to recruit and educate B cells and CD8+ T cells. A special fraction of regulatory T (Treg) cells is also classified as CD4+ T cells, which play an immunosuppressive role in the body. Treg cells will be introduced later as it is a major mechanism involved in the tumor-mediated immunosuppression. A more detailed description of $T_H$ cell subtypes is beyond the scope of this review and will not be discussed further.

## CD8 T Cells

The second major type of T cell is the CD8+ T cell. These cells are executors of the immune system, which directly deliver granzyme B and induce perforin mediated cytotoxicity when they get activated. This unique executor phenotype is responsible for their other name, cytotoxic T lymphocyte (CTL) [32].

For an effective CD8+ T cell-mediated immunity, the first essential step is the immunization or antigen exposure. After this initial process, when CTLs meet target cells, their TCRs quickly bind to the surface-expressed, antigen-loaded MHC-I molecule. Together with a second activating signal from costimulatory molecules, CTLs will be fully activated in terms of secreting cytokines and expressing granzyme B and perforin to make the final target execution. Through this cytotoxicity, CTLs are able to eliminate viral-infected as well as bacteria-harboring host cells by the recognition of host MHC-I loaded with foreign antigen epitopes; meanwhile, CTLs can also target abnormal self-tissues *via* a similar antigen-recognition mechanism. This important property makes CTLs ideal tools for devising novel cancer immunotherapy. And in fact, the most effective cancer immunotherapy strategies so far are CTL-based. In following paragraphs, we will briefly introduce the application of CTLs in cancer immunotherapy.

As mentioned above, CTLs are able to eliminate abnormal self-tissue by their versatile antigen recognition capability, which can serve as the basis for direct tumor-specific cancer therapy by supplementing tumor-antigen reactive CTLs. This approach is generally called adoptive T cell transfer (ACT)-based immunotherapy. The idea of carrying out ACT-based immunotherapy is partly derived from the observation that in the treatment of hematologic malignancies by allogenic stem cell transplantation (alloSCT) [33], donor T cells can target and kill leukemic cells by recognizing aberrantly expressed proteins or leukemic antigens. These effects, collectively described as the graft-*versus*-leukemia (GVL) effect, indicate that T cells are able to respond to the abnormal autoantigens on the surface of malignant cells, and this encourages us to investigate the hypothesis that CD8+ T cells can be specifically engineered and targeted to treat cancer.

## Tumor Infiltrating T Lymphocytes

A second substantial discovery supports this hypothesis is the identification of tumor infiltrating T lymphocytes (TILs) in patients with melanoma [34]. Following surgical excision and subsequent processing of melanoma tissue from patients, a group of T lymphocytes are isolated and expanded *ex vivo*. Because of their property of infiltrating into the tumor tissue, they are termed TILs. These TILs are heterogeneous populations of T cells and have varying phenotypic profiles, antigen-reactivities, and functions; however, after infusion back into the tumor-bearing patients following *ex vivo* expansion and manipulation, they control tumor growth in melanoma patients. By further modulating of the regimen, this TIL-based therapy has been documented to be an effective treatment in patients with advanced, metastatic melanoma. Modifications of TIL therapy to improve clinical outcome, includes preconditioning the patient with lymphodepletion in order to deplete immunosuppressive Treg cells and myeloid derived suppressor cells (MDSCs) and infusion of cytokines to boost the persistence of infused TILs have been tested and proven feasible. However, the use of TILs to conduct a cancer immunotherapy is limited for several reasons: TILs can only be isolated in certain types of cancer; and as recovered effector T cells, TILs have short life spans compared to naïve T cells. In order to bypass these obstacles, scientists explore other solutions to address those problems.

## CAR-T Cells

A recent approach aims at improving isolation of TILs, is called the genetic modification of T cells with antigen-reactivity to tumor associated or specific-antigens. Two major strategies to generate T cells with a specific antigen-reactivity are being explored: one is overexpression of a TCR that recognizes tumor-associated or specific-antigen and the other involves the introduction of a chimeric antigen receptor (CAR) that recognizes the tumor antigens. Both of these strategies have achieved preliminary successes in either animal models or clinical trials. The mechanism of generating modified T lymphocytes with tumor-antigen specific TCR for targeting and killing tumor cells is similar to the screening of a high-efficacy mAb. The most robust T cell clone towards antigen-stimulation is isolated to clone its recombined full length TCR gene. The selected TCR gene bearing both antigen-recognition and signal-transduction domains is introduced into peripheral blood-derived or naïve T lymphocytes to generate genetically modified T lymphocytes [35].

For CAR, the mechanism of tumor targeting and T cell activation is somewhat complicated and combines the antigen specificity of an antibody and the cytotoxic properties of a T cell. A functional CAR is a single linear structure that consists of several different components: an antigen-recognition domain, a transmembrane hinge domain and a T cell activation domain. Usually, a single chain variable fragment (scFv) of a tumor-antigen reactive mAb serves as the tumor antigen recognition domain. The intracellular signaling domains from several different T cell activation molecules are recombined to mediate T cell activation [36]. This integrated CAR gene is genetically introduced into T cells to make the CAR T cell or CAR-T. When CAR binds to antigen *via* the scFv region, it activates CAR-T through signals from the T cell activation domain on the CAR module. Activated CAR-T expresses perforin and granzyme B to lyse tumor cells [37]. An advantage of CAR is the MHC-independence, however TCR-based antigen recognition is MHC-dependent; therefore the CAR imparts an expanded targeting mechanism to CAR-Ts.

Both methods share similar principles behind generating genetically modified T cells. The identification of tumor-specific antigens and their corresponding TCR or CAR, is the most important step. This is the speed-limit step for carrying out a successful ACT-based cancer immunotherapy with genetically modified T cells. The expression profiles of the tumor-associated antigen, along with the specificities and affinities of TCR or CAR are the determining factors. The second step is to obtain a large number of T cells for the following genetic manipulation. Currently, this involves the isolation and *ex vivo* expansion of autologous T lymphocytes from the cancer patients. In the future, stem cells may provide the store of cells as some of our studies suggest [38]. Either TCR or CAR will be genetically introduced into the expanded T cells by a retroviral or lentiviral vector-mediated gene delivery. After *ex vivo* characterization, TCR-T or CAR-T will be reinfused back to patients to target tumor cells. Initially, TCR-T based ACT immunotherapy has been shown to be effective in the treatment of advanced melanoma. As documented in recent studies, this regimen has been expanded into other types of tumors, such as neuroblastoma, synovial cell sarcoma, leukemia, and lymphoma. In the context of CAR-T based ACT immunotherapy, the most important achievement is the management of B cell lymphoma by targeting CD19 molecule, a common B cell marker [39]. Based on current promising results and advancements in identifying novel tumor associated antigens in different types of cancers, additional therapeutic proposals by using either TCRs or CARs are under intensive investigation.

Although ACT-based immunotherapy with autologous T lymphocytes has produced positive results due to the nature of autologous T cell, there are several concerns. Terminally differentiated autologous T cells are short-lived compared to naïve and memory T cells, and *ex vivo* expansion by cytokines and costimulatory molecules would cause a further reduction in the cell numbers after reinfusion. Second, these T cells have already expressed an originally functional TCR on their surfaces and overexpression of an additional pair of TCR could possibly cause TCR mismatch, which might reduce their antitumor potency. Finding new sources of naïve T cells or combining with other T cell function-enhancing agents such as cytokines may help overcome these problems. The application of cancer immunotherapy by using genetically modified T cells is described in Fig. **3**.

## Cytokines

Cytokines are a group of small molecules secreted by different types of cells including T cells. Usually, they play the role of signal transduction messengers between different cells. In immunology, cytokines are pivotal elements in connecting different groups of cells. Cytokines can be immunoenhancing or immunosuppressing depend on their acting targets. For example, in the superfamily of interleukins (IL), IL-2 is an immunoenhancing cytokine, which boosts the expansion and activation of T lymphocytes. In recent clinical studies, administration of IL-2 could significantly inhibit the growth of melanoma and renal cell carcinoma by reversing the tumor-induced T cell tolerance, although global side effects are of concern [40]. In the context of boosting host immune system, other cytokines such as Interferon-alpha (IFN-$\alpha$) and Granulocyte-monocyte colony stimulating factor (GM-CSF) have also been used clinical settings in the treatment of melanoma and several hematologic malignancies [41]. In contrast, the other IL superfamily members such as IL-6 and IL-10 play the opposite function in an immunosuppressive capacity by tuning down the activated T cells. For example, IL-6 and IL-10 along with transforming growth factor-beta (TGF-$\beta$) are highly expressed in the tumor microenviroment compared to normal tissue. These cytokines can silence the tumor infiltrating lymphocytes (TIL) thus providing a mechanism for tumor cell to evade the established immune surveillance [42]. Supplementing immunoenhancing and blocking immunosuppressive cytokines could facilitate the development-improved efficacy in treating cancer patients with any immune-based, especially T cell-based therapy.

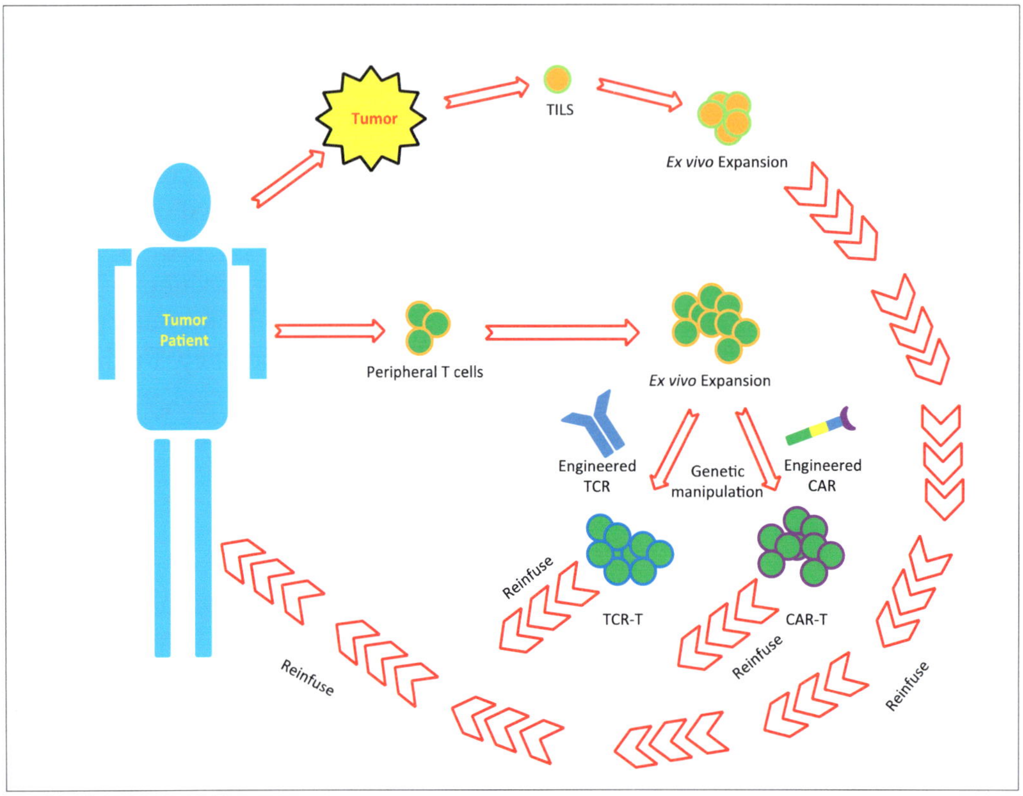


**Figure 3:** Adoptive T cell therapy for cancer. Currently, the adoptive T cell therapy for cancer falls into two major categories. One is by using tumor infiltrating T cells (TILs) and the other is by harnessing genetically modified peripheral lymphocyte. This figure briefly shows the schemes administrating ACT therapy in cancer patients. The use of TILs requires the isolation of TILs from tumor tissue first and then follows an *ex vivo* expansion in the laboratory. Expanded TILs are infused back to patients for tumor management. In the approach of using genetically modified peripheral T lymphocytes, first of all, T cells are isolated from periphery blood and expanded in the laboratory. After obtaining a significant number of T cells, either tumor antigen-specific TCR or CAR is introduced into those T cells *via* a lentiviral-mediated gene delivery strategy. At the end of *ex vivo* processing, modified T cells bearing anti-tumor targeting mechanisms are infused back to patients.

Innate immunity is the first line of defense to invading pathogens, but adaptive immunity is more specific and versatile in its ability to control both exogenous and endogenous diseases. Here, several components in the adaptive immune system together with their applications in treating cancer have been briefly described. Under ideal conditions, the adaptive immune system is able to control infection and eliminate mutated tumor cells; however, there are no ideal conditions. Invading microorganisms such as *Mycobacterium tuberculosis* are able to modulate the host immune system to survive the anti-bacterial immunity. Meanwhile, in cancer patients, it is also found that tumor cells are able to evade the attention of the immune system by various mechanisms, including the downregulation of MHC-I and costimulatory molecules, as well as inhibiting the activity of leukocytes that enter the tumor microenvironment. Much work has recently been done to establish how the tumor microenvironment contributes to the suppression of anti-tumor immunity in many cancer patients.

## TUMOR MICROENVIRONMENT AND ITS ASSOCIATION WITH IMMUNE SYSTEM

Many cancer immunotherapeutic regimens in the clinic could not achieve a sound benefit despite preclinical studies demonstrating promising results. Recently, by carefully studying the tumor itself, its surrounding tissue and secreted molecules, a new concept of tumor microenvironment has been hypothesized which plays a key role in suppressing the anti-tumor immunity. In tumor tissue, activation of the anti-tumor response, especially by T cell-mediated immunity, is significantly suppressed as observed. One possible mechanism is the accumulation of Treg cells and myeloid-derived suppressor cells (MDSCs) in the tumor microenvironment.

Treg cells are a subgroup of CD4+ T cells and are negative regulators of the immune response. These potent immunosuppressive cells express many cell surface molecules that negatively regulate the activation of effector T cells. Accumulation of Treg cells in the tumor tissue indicates that tumor cells have developed special mechanisms to evade the host anti-tumor immunity. A second group of immunosuppressive cells that have highly accumulated in tumor tissues are MDSCs. Their presences in tumors are induced by chronic inflammation in the tumor tissue [43]. These two major types of cells in the tumor tissue are key suppressors of anti-tumor immunity. Further studies have shown that inhibition of these immune suppressors could significantly reverse the suppressed anti-tumor immunity [44, 45].

Treg cells and MDSCs suppress activated immune system mainly through two approaches, first, secreting immunosuppressive cytokines such as IL-10, IL-6 and TGF-β [46, 47]; second, overexpressing certain inhibitory costimulatory molecules such as CTLA-4 and PD-L1 [48, 49]. The immunosuppressive mechanisms mediated by Treg cells and MDSCs in the tumor microenvironment are summarized in Fig. **4**.

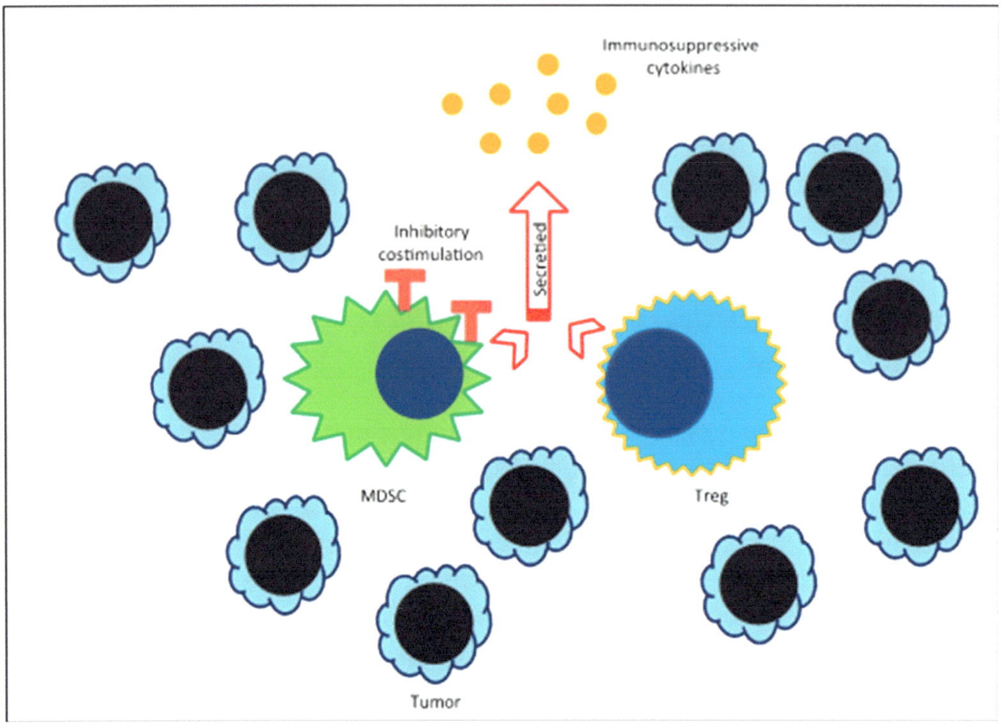


**Figure 4:** Tumor microenvironment and immune suppression. Tumor microenvironment is a complicated concept comprised of many cells, cytokines and other factors. So far, the two major immunosuppressive cell types have been well characterized in tumor microenvironment are myeloid derived suppressor cells (MDSCs) and regulatory T cells (Tregs). These two types of cells are highly accumulated in the tumor microenvironment and inhibit the activation of anti-tumor immunity by different mechanisms. To date, secreting immunosuppressive cytokines such as IL-10 and TGF-β as well as overexpressing inhibitory costimulatory ligands such as CTLA-4 are two well-studied strategies harnessed by MDSCs and Tregs in the tumor microenvironment. However, the suppression of anti-tumor immunity in tumor microenvironment is not only limited to these two mechanisms.

## CONCLUSION

The opening chapter of this book briefly summarizes the immune system as well as the relationships and applications of individual components in the development of modern cancer immunotherapy.

Although described as two separate systems, both innate and adaptive immune systems are interconnected in many aspects. To design a comprehensive cancer immunotherapy, neither innate nor adaptive immune system should be ignored. For example, it is helpful to check the NK cell and/or complement system activities before giving patients anti-cancer mAbs because the final cancer eradication requires ADCC or CMC. Also, to achieve a better result, the interactions between tumor and the immune system should also be carefully reviewed.

An understanding of the big picture of our immune system will benefit individual readers to read the following chapters, as they focus on designing or modulating unique approaches of the immune system for the rising field of cancer immunotherapy. Nevertheless, the significant progress achieved in the recent years in the field of cancer immunotherapy such as mAb-based immunotherapies and CAR therapy has made possible to the improved treatments and even cures of cancer patients [50-54].

## ACKNOWLEDGEMENT

This work is funded, in part, under grants with the National Institute of Health Grants K18CA151798 and R21AI109239, Breast Cancer Alliance, and the Pennsylvania Department of Health.

## CONFLICT OF INTEREST

The authors confirm that this chapter contents have no conflict of interest.

## REFERENCES

[1] Obermoser G, Presnell S, Domico K, Xu H, Wang Y, Anguiano E, *et al.* Systems scale interactive exploration reveals quantitative and qualitative differences in response to influenza and pneumococcal vaccines. Immunity 2013; 38(4): 831-44.

[2] Andersen BM, Pluhar GE, Seiler CE, Goulart MR, Santacruz KS, Schutten MM, *et al.* Vaccination for Invasive Canine Meningioma Induces *In Situ* Production of Antibodies Capable of Antibody-Dependent Cell-Mediated Cytotoxicity. Cancer Res 2013; 73(10): 2987-97.

[3] Simon N, Lasonder E, Scheuermayer M, Kuehn A, Tews S, Fischer R, *et al.* Malaria parasites co-opt human factor H to prevent complement-mediated lysis in the mosquito midgut. Cell Host Microbe 2013; 13(1): 29-41.

[4] Osterholzer JJ, Olszewski MA, Murdock BJ, Chen GH, Erb-Downward JR, Subbotina N, *et al.* Implicating exudate macrophages and Ly-6C(high) monocytes in CCR2-dependent lung fibrosis following gene-targeted alveolar injury. J Immunol 2013; 190(7): 3447-57.

[5] Tosello-Trampont AC, Landes SG, Nguyen V, Novobrantseva TI, Hahn YS. Kuppfer cells trigger nonalcoholic steatohepatitis development in diet-induced mouse model through tumor necrosis factor-alpha production. J Biol Chem 2012; 287(48): 40161-72.

[6] Fernandez-Arias C, Lopez JP, Hernandez-Perez JN, Bautista-Ojeda MD, Branch O, Rodriguez A. Malaria inhibits surface expression of complement receptor 1 in monocytes/macrophages, causing decreased immune complex internalization. J Immunol 2013; 190(7): 3363-72.

[7] Wu Y, Wang S, Farooq SM, Castelvetere MP, Hou Y, Gao JL, *et al.* A chemokine receptor CXCR2 macromolecular complex regulates neutrophil functions in inflammatory diseases. J Biol Chem 2012; 287(8): 5744-55.
[8] Zhao W, Wang L, Zhang M, Yuan C, Gao C. E3 ubiquitin ligase tripartite motif 38 negatively regulates TLR-mediated immune responses by proteasomal degradation of TNF receptor-associated factor 6 in macrophages. J Immunol 2012; 188(6): 2567-74.
[9] Wei J, Loke P, Zang X, Allison JP. Tissue-specific expression of B7x protects from CD4 T cell-mediated autoimmunity. J Exp Med 2011; 208(8): 1683-94.
[10] Song DG, Ye Q, Poussin M, Harms GM, Figini M, Powell DJ, Jr. CD27 costimulation augments the survival and antitumor activity of redirected human T cells *in vivo*. Blood 2012; 119(3): 696-706.
[11] Hemmi H, Kaisho T, Takeuchi O, Sato S, Sanjo H, Hoshino K, *et al.* Small anti-viral compounds activate immune cells *via* the TLR7 MyD88-dependent signaling pathway. Nat Immunol 2002; 3(2): 196-200.
[12] Ribas A. Tumor immunotherapy directed at PD-1. N Engl J Med 2012; 366(26): 2517-9.
[13] Lynch TJ, Bondarenko I, Luft A, Serwatowski P, Barlesi F, Chacko R, *et al.* Ipilimumab in combination with paclitaxel and carboplatin as first-line treatment in stage IIIB/IV non-small-cell lung cancer: results from a randomized, double-blind, multicenter phase II study. J Clin Oncol 2012; 30(17): 2046-54.
[14] Schlitzer A, McGovern N, Teo P, Zelante T, Atarashi K, Low D, *et al.* IRF4 Transcription Factor-Dependent CD11b(+) Dendritic Cells in Human and Mouse Control Mucosal IL-17 Cytokine Responses. Immunity 2013; 38(5): 970-83.
[15] Chang SY, Song JH, Guleng B, Cotoner CA, Arihiro S, Zhao Y, *et al.* Circulatory antigen processing by mucosal dendritic cells controls CD8(+) T cell activation. Immunity 2013; 38(1): 153-65.
[16] Kantoff PW, Higano CS, Shore ND, Berger ER, Small EJ, Penson DF, *et al.* Sipuleucel-T immunotherapy for castration-resistant prostate cancer. N Engl J Med 2010; 363(5): 411-22.
[17] Jahn T, Zuther M, Friedrichs B, Heuser C, Guhlke S, Abken H, *et al.* An IL12-IL2-antibody fusion protein targeting Hodgkin's lymphoma cells potentiates activation of NK and T cells for an anti-tumor attack. PLoS One 2012; 7(9): e44482.
[18] Duncan RC, Mohlin F, Taleski D, Coetzer TH, Huntington JA, Payne RJ, *et al.* Identification of a catalytic exosite for complement component C4 on the serine protease domain of C1s. J Immunol 2012; 189(5): 2365-73.
[19] Joseph K, Kulik L, Coughlin B, Kunchithapautham K, Bandyopadhyay M, Thiel S, *et al.* Oxidative Stress Sensitizes Retinal Pigmented Epithelial (RPE) Cells to Complement-mediated Injury in a Natural Antibody-, Lectin Pathway-, and Phospholipid Epitope-dependent Manner. J Biol Chem 2013; 288(18): 12753-65.
[20] Kidani Y, Elsaesser H, Hock MB, Vergnes L, Williams KJ, Argus JP, *et al.* Sterol regulatory element-binding proteins are essential for the metabolic programming of effector T cells and adaptive immunity. Nat Immunol 2013; 14(5): 489-99.
[21] Sakiani S, Olsen NJ, Kovacs WJ. Gonadal steroids and humoral immunity. Nat Rev Endocrinol 2013; 9(1): 56-62.
[22] Paley MA, Kroy DC, Odorizzi PM, Johnnidis JB, Dolfi DV, Barnett BE, *et al.* Progenitor and terminal subsets of CD8+ T cells cooperate to contain chronic viral infection. Science 2012; 338(6111): 1220-5.
[23] Hirota K, Turner JE, Villa M, Duarte JH, Demengeot J, Steinmetz OM, *et al.* Plasticity of TH17 cells in Peyer's patches is responsible for the induction of T cell-dependent IgA responses. Nat Immunol 2013; 14(4): 372-9.
[24] Schwab I, Nimmerjahn F. Intravenous immunoglobulin therapy: how does IgG modulate the immune system? Nat Rev Immunol 2013; 13(3): 176-89.
[25] Welner S, Trier NH, Houen G, Hansen PR. Identification and mapping of a linear epitope of centromere protein F using monoclonal antibodies. J Pept Sci 2013; 19(2): 95-101.
[26] Weiner GJ. Rituximab: mechanism of action. Semin Hematol 2010; 47(2): 115-23.
[27] LoRusso PM, Weiss D, Guardino E, Girish S, Sliwkowski MX. Trastuzumab emtansine: a unique antibody-drug conjugate in development for human epidermal growth factor receptor 2-positive cancer. Clin Cancer Res 2011; 17(20): 6437-47.

[28] Ribas A. Clinical development of the anti-CTLA-4 antibody tremelimumab. Semin Oncol 2010; 37(5): 450-4.

[29] Farley AM, Morris LX, Vroegindeweij E, Depreter ML, Vaidya H, Stenhouse FH, *et al.* Dynamics of thymus organogenesis and colonization in early human development. Development 2013; 140(9): 2015-26.

[30] Vantourout P, Hayday A. Six-of-the-best: unique contributions of gammadelta T cells to immunology. Nat Rev Immunol 2013; 13(2): 88-100.

[31] Adamson A, Ghoreschi K, Rittler M, Chen Q, Sun HW, Vahedi G, *et al.* Tissue inhibitor of metalloproteinase 1 is preferentially expressed in Th1 and Th17 T-helper cell subsets and is a direct STAT target gene. PLoS One 2013; 8(3): e59367.

[32] Hervas-Stubbs S, Mancheno U, Riezu-Boj JI, Larraga A, Ochoa MC, Alignani D, *et al.* CD8 T cell priming in the presence of IFN-alpha renders CTLs with improved responsiveness to homeostatic cytokines and recall antigens: important traits for adoptive T cell therapy. J Immunol 2012; 189(7): 3299-310.

[33] Horowitz MM, Gale RP, Sondel PM, Goldman JM, Kersey J, Kolb HJ, *et al.* Graft-*versus*-leukemia reactions after bone marrow transplantation. Blood 1990; 75(3): 555-62.

[34] Dudley ME, Wunderlich JR, Robbins PF, Yang JC, Hwu P, Schwartzentruber DJ, *et al.* Cancer regression and autoimmunity in patients after clonal repopulation with antitumor lymphocytes. Science 2002; 298(5594): 850-4.

[35] Morgan RA, Dudley ME, Wunderlich JR, Hughes MS, Yang JC, Sherry RM, *et al.* Cancer regression in patients after transfer of genetically engineered lymphocytes. Science 2006; 314(5796): 126-9.

[36] Gross G, Waks T, Eshhar Z. Expression of immunoglobulin-T-cell receptor chimeric molecules as functional receptors with antibody-type specificity. Proc Natl Acad Sci U S A 1989; 86(24): 10024-8.

[37] Kalos M, Levine BL, Porter DL, Katz S, Grupp SA, Bagg A, *et al.* T cells with chimeric antigen receptors have potent antitumor effects and can establish memory in patients with advanced leukemia. Sci Transl Med 2011; 3(95): 95ra73.

[38] Lei F, Zhao B, Haque R, Xiong X, Budgeon L, Christensen ND, *et al.* *In vivo* programming of tumor antigen-specific T lymphocytes from pluripotent stem cells to promote cancer immunosurveillance. Cancer research 2011; 71(14): 4742-7.

[39] Torikai H, Reik A, Liu PQ, Zhou Y, Zhang L, Maiti S, *et al.* A foundation for universal T-cell based immunotherapy: T cells engineered to express a CD19-specific chimeric-antigen-receptor and eliminate expression of endogenous TCR. Blood 2012; 119(24): 5697-705.

[40] Klapper JA, Downey SG, Smith FO, Yang JC, Hughes MS, Kammula US, *et al.* High-dose interleukin-2 for the treatment of metastatic renal cell carcinoma: a retrospective analysis of response and survival in patients treated in the surgery branch at the National Cancer Institute between 1986 and 2006. Cancer 2008; 113(2): 293-301.

[41] O'Donnell RT, Dea G, Meyers FJ. A phase II trial of concomitant interferon-alpha-2b and granulocyte-macrophage colony-stimulating factor in patients with advanced renal cell carcinoma. J Immunother Emphasis Tumor Immunol 1995; 17(1): 58-61.

[42] Disis ML. Immune regulation of cancer. J Clin Oncol 2010; 28(29): 4531-8.

[43] Meyer C, Sevko A, Ramacher M, Bazhin AV, Falk CS, Osen W, *et al.* Chronic inflammation promotes myeloid-derived suppressor cell activation blocking antitumor immunity in transgenic mouse melanoma model. Proc Natl Acad Sci USA 2011; 108(41): 17111-6.

[44] Ko JS, Zea AH, Rini BI, Ireland JL, Elson P, Cohen P, *et al.* Sunitinib mediates reversal of myeloid-derived suppressor cell accumulation in renal cell carcinoma patients. Clin Cancer Res 2009; 15(6): 2148-57.

[45] Beatty GL, Chiorean EG, Fishman MP, Saboury B, Teitelbaum UR, Sun W, *et al.* CD40 agonists alter tumor stroma and show efficacy against pancreatic carcinoma in mice and humans. Science 2011; 331(6024): 1612-6.

[46] Tanikawa T, Wilke CM, Kryczek I, Chen GY, Kao J, Nunez G, *et al.* Interleukin-10 ablation promotes tumor development, growth, and metastasis. Cancer Res 2012; 72(2): 420-9.

[47] Li H, Han Y, Guo Q, Zhang M, Cao X. Cancer-expanded myeloid-derived suppressor cells induce anergy of NK cells through membrane-bound TGF-beta 1. J Immunol 2009; 182(1): 240-9.

[48] Kalathil S, Lugade AA, Miller A, Iyer R, Thanavala Y. Higher frequencies of GARP(+)CTLA-4(+)Foxp3(+) T regulatory cells and myeloid-derived suppressor cells in hepatocellular carcinoma patients are associated with impaired T-cell functionality. Cancer Res 2013; 73(8): 2435-44.

[49] Christiansson L, Soderlund S, Svensson E, Mustjoki S, Bengtsson M, Simonsson B, *et al.* Increased level of myeloid-derived suppressor cells, programmed death receptor ligand 1/programmed death receptor 1, and soluble CD25 in Sokal high risk chronic myeloid leukemia. PLoS One 2013; 8(1): e55818.

[50] McNutt M. Cancer immunotherapy. Science 2013; 342(6165): 1417.

[51] Couzin-Frankel J. Breakthrough of the year 2013. Cancer Immunotherapy. Science 2013; 342(6165): 1432-3.

[52] Darcy PK, Ritchie DS. Editorial overview: Tumour immunology: New frontiers in cancer immunotherapy. Curr Opin Immunol 2014; 27: vii-x.

[53] Coulie PG, Van den Eynde BJ, van der Bruggen P, Boon T. Tumour antigens recognized by T lymphocytes: at the core of cancer immunotherapy. Nat Rev Cancer 2014; 14(2): 135-46.

[54] Vanneman M, Dranoff G. Combining immunotherapy and targeted therapies in cancer treatment. Nature reviews Cancer 2012; 12(4): 237-51.

**CHAPTER 2**

# T Cell-Based Immunotherapy

**Tania G. Rodríguez-Cruz[1-3] and Stephen Gottschalk[1-4,*]**

*[1]Center for Cell and Gene Therapy, Texas Children's Hospital, Houston Methodist Hospital, Baylor College of Medicine, Houston, Texas, USA; [2]Texas Children's Cancer Center, Texas Children's Hospital, Baylor College of Medicine, Houston, Texas, USA; [3]Department of Pediatrics, and [4]Pathology and Immunology, Baylor College of Medicine, Houston, Texas, USA*

**Abstract:** From its humble beginning in the 19th century, immunotherapy for cancer has emerged as a prospective curative approach in the last decade. Currently, different immunotherapies are being used in the clinic including monoclonal antibodies (MAbs), adoptively transferred T cells and cancer vaccines. Of these immunotherapies, MAbs are the most widely used, however their efficacy is restricted by their limited biodistribution, and reliance on antibody-dependent cell cytotoxicity and/or complement-mediated cell death, which can be impaired in cancer patients. In contrast, adoptively transferred T cells have the capacity to effectively traffic to tumor sites, recruit multiple cellular and humoral effector mechanisms, and persist for many years. In this chapter, we review T cell based immunotherapy for cancer, describe its current clinical impact, and discuss approaches that aim to combine T cells with other cancer-targeted therapies.

**Keywords:** Cancer, chimeric antigen receptor, clinical trial, Epstein-Barr virus, gene therapy, T cell immunotherapy, T cell receptor, tumor antigen.

## INTRODUCTION

Anton Chekhov, the Russian writer and physician, documented the first evidence supporting the role of the immune system in eradicating tumors in 1884. He and other investigators noted that the occurrence of an acute streptococcus bacterial infection in cancer patients sometimes induced spontaneous tumor regressions [1]. Based on these observations, the American surgeon William Coley developed the theory of stimulating the immune system against cancer through the use of bacterial infusions in the 1890s. Following infusion into cancer patients, the so called Coley's toxins induced high fevers and were associated with significant

***Corresponding author Stephen Gottschalk:** Center for Cell and Gene Therapy, Texas Children's Hospital, Houston Methodist Hospital, Baylor College of Medicine, Houston, Texas, USA; Texas Children's Cancer Center, Texas Children's Hospital, Baylor College of Medicine, Houston, Texas, USA; Department of Pediatrics, and Pathology and Immunology, Baylor College of Medicine, Houston, Texas, USA; Tel: (832) 824-4179; E-mail: smgottsc@txccc.org

**Jianxun Song (Ed)**

tumor regressions in some cancer patients [2]. Coley's toxins were used until the mid 1960s, but were abandoned because they usually generated mixed responses and the advent of modern chemo- and radiotherapy became favored for cancer treatment. However, the field of cancer immunotherapy resurged in the 1970s when large numbers of clinical trials explored substances like Bacillus Calmette-Guerin (BCG), Corynebacterium parvum, levamisole, and additional immune stimulators to treat patients with bladder cancer [3]. Since then, much has been learned about the cellular and molecular mechanism on how the immune system specifically recognizes and counteracts cancer. The greatest persuasive evidence for the existence of anti-tumor immunity was first demonstrated by several clinical studies performed in the 1980s. These studies showed that administration of high doses of the cytokine IL-2, which was known to be a growth factor for T cells, caused dramatic tumor regressions in some patients with metastatic melanoma or renal cell carcinoma [4, 5]. These studies led the US Food and Drug Administration to allow for the administration of IL-2 as the first FDA-approved immunotherapy method for cancer treatment in the late 1990s. Since then, immunotherapeutic strategies for cancer have 'mushroomed' due to the potential of the immune system to induce prolonged antitumor responses with minimal toxicity as compared to chemotherapy and/or radiotherapy.

To date, the most successful cancer immunotherapy strategies utilize either humoral or cellular components of the adaptive immune system, such as monoclonal antibodies (MAbs) or cytotoxic T lymphocytes (CTLs) that target unique molecules (*i.e.,* antigens) expressed by cancer cells. Although humoral responses mediated by MAbs targeting various tumor-associated antigens (TAAs) have been shown to generate significant clinical outcomes in the setting of hematologic malignancies, the clinical efficacy of such MAbs is limited for the treatment of solid tumors [6]. Cellular-mediated immune responses are crucial in the immunologic rejection of tumors, the most important being the generation of antigen-specific CTLs [7]. Therefore, the goal of most modern immunotherapeutic strategies is to generate strong CTL-mediated cellular immunity to cancer cells either through the adoptive transfer of tumor antigen-specific T cells or *via* vaccines [8].

This chapter focuses on the adoptive transfer of tumor-specific T cells, which has emerged as an effective treatment approach for cancer patients. This approach includes 1) the adoptive transfer of autologous tumor-infiltrating lymphocytes (TILs), 2) antigen-specific T cells, 3) T cells that are genetically engineered to express T cell receptors against tumor antigens, and 4) T cells that are engineered to express chimeric antigen receptors (CARs).

## ADOPTIVE CELL THERAPY USING TILS

Currently, there are different sources of T cells that can be used for adoptive T cell-based therapy. One approach takes advantage of naturally occurring TILs that have the capacity to migrate to tumor sites and eliminate cancer cells through receptor recognition of TAAs. These cells are isolated from resected tumors. A comparative study demonstrated that TILs could be isolated from a range of human tumor tissues including breast cancer, melanoma, renal-cell carcinoma and colon cancer with a success rate of 30 to 65%. The types of TILs recovered from these tumors were mostly CD4-positive T cells, except in melanoma where CD8-positive T cells predominated [9]. In order to obtain a sufficient amount of TILs required for infusion, TILs are initially expanded *ex vivo* with IL-2 followed by a rapid expansion protocol that involves CD3 MAbs in the presence of irradiated feeder cells plus IL-2. Since initial studies evaluating the effectiveness of adoptively transferred TILs reported only modest clinical responses, a lymphodepletion regimen prior to TIL infusion was developed [10-12]. Lymphodepletion prior to autologous TIL infusion was found to be critical for TIL efficacy by reducing the number of regulatory T cells and myeloid suppressor cells, and providing space for the infused TILs to proliferate [13, 14]. The intensity of the lymphodepletion regimen correlates with outcome in melanoma patients. For example, a fludarabine/cyclophosphamide (Flu/Cy) based lymphodepletion regimen resulted in an objective response rate of 49% and the response rate could be further increased to 72% with the addition of 12Gy total body irradiation. Despite these encouraging findings, studies combining conditioning regimens with TIL transfer have mostly been conducted at the National Cancer Institute. In order to determine overall clinical benefit, studies must be expanded to other centers.

## ADOPTIVE CELL THERAPY USING T CELLS DERIVED FROM PBMC

Although TILs can mediate tumor regressions in melanoma patients, TIL isolation and expansion from other tumors is difficult at best. Therefore, many groups have used T cells that were expanded from autologous peripheral blood mononuclear cells (PBMCs) for adoptive transfer. However, in contrast to TILs, these PBMCs-derived autologous T cells must be rendered antigen specific through different manipulations *ex vivo*. Autologous antigen-specific T cells can be obtained *ex vivo* using a) antigen-pulsed antigen-presenting cells (APCs) that are capable of processing and presenting the antigen/peptide of interest to T cells in a HLA-dependent manner or by b) genetic modifications utilizing viral or non-viral vectors expressing tumor-specific α/β T cell receptors (TCRs) or chimeric antigen receptors (CARs).

## Antigen-Specific T Cells Generated by APC Stimulation

Effective T-cell therapies depend on the identification of TAAs targeted by T cells as well as efficient methods to generate TAA-specific T cells *ex vivo*. One approach to activate and expand antigen-specific T cells from PBMCs is through the use of APCs, which present the antigen of interest in a MHC-dependent manner and also provide co-stimulation signals to T cells. This approach was first described in 1992, when cytomegalovirus (CMV)-specific CD8-positive T cell clones derived from healthy bone marrow donors were effectively activated and expanded following *ex vivo* co-culture with virus-infected fibroblasts. Infusion of these CMV-specific T cells clones was safe and resulted in the reconstitution of CMV-specific cellular immunity in hematopoietic stem cell transplant (HSCT) recipients [15]. Interestingly, CD8-positive CMV-specific T-cell clones only persisted if the patient recovered CD4-positive, CMV-specific T cell responses, highlighting the important role of CD4-positive T cells. Since then, many investigators have generated different antigen-specific CTLs, including Epstein-Barr Virus (EBV) and melanoma-specific CTLs through the use of APCs such as dendritic cells, autologous irradiated PBMCs, and artificial APCs (*e.g.*, K562 cells expressing co-stimulatory molecules) [16-27].

## EBV-Specific T Cells for the Treatment of EBV-Positive Malignancies

EBV is a latent herpes virus and more than 90% of the human population is EBV seropositive [28]. Moreover, EBV has been associated with a diverse group of malignancies including post transplant lymphoproliferative disease (PTLD), Hodgkin lymphoma (HL), Non Hodgkin lymphoma (NHL), and nasopharyngeal carcinoma (NPC) [29]. EBV-specific T cell therapy is being actively explored by several groups. Initial studies focused on infusing donor-derived EBV-specific T cells into HSCT recipients for the treatment and prophylaxis of PTLD. EBV-specific T cells expanded several logs, reconstituted EBV-specific cellular immunity, and prevented the development of PTLD. As therapy, EBV-specific T cells were effective in 11 of 13 PTLD patients [30]. One patient who did not respond had a deletion of several immune dominant EBV-restricted epitopes, thus highlighting that immune escape can occur if T cells with restricted specificity are infused [31]. Since then, this approach has been expanded to EBV-associated malignancies outside the transplant setting. Standard EBV-specific T cells or EBV-specific T cells enriched for specificity towards the EBV antigens LMP1 and LMP2 have produced antitumor effects in patients with EBV-positive HL, NHL, and NPC [20, 32-37]. However, their antitumor activity is lower than in PTLD patients. This lack of efficacy is most likely due to several factors including limited T cell expansion outside the transplant setting, the immunosuppressive tumor microenvironment, and the limited number of EBV antigens expressed in these malignancies in contrast to PTLD.

Some limitations of this approach have been the amount of time it takes and the use of viruses to generate the EBV-specific T cell product. The use of tissue culture devices such as G-Rexes, overlapping peptide libraries as an antigen source, and novel cytokine combinations such as IL-4 and IL-7 has reduced the production time from months to less than 4 weeks, and has eliminated the use of live viruses [38, 39]. Clinical studies with these rapidly generated EBV-specific T cells have started, and if successful, these rapid production methods should facilitate the integration of these cells into clinical practice. Using banked, partially HLA-matched EBV-specific T cells is another option to increase their accessibility. Early clinical studies for HSCT recipients with PTLD have shown promising results [40-43], and this strategy is being actively explored for patients with EBV-positive malignancies outside the transplant setting.

## Antigen-Specific T Cells for the Treatment of Malignancies

Several clinical studies of adoptive immunotherapy using antigen-specific CD8-positive T-cell clones targeting the melanoma-associated antigens MART-1 and gp100 have been conducted with no adverse toxicities [21, 44, 45]. Although the infused CTLs localized to tumor sites, the objective response rate was less than 10%. Many of the responses were mixed and durable remissions were observed in only a few select patients. The low response rates were associated with limited *in vivo* expansion and persistence of infused CTLs. Interestingly, one of the studies reported antigen-loss tumor variants in 3 out of 5 patients, which indicated immune escape mutants following the use of antigen-specific T-cell clones [21]. In an effort to increase the *in vivo* persistence of the infused CTLs, Wallen *et al.* used fludarabine to lymphodeplete patients prior to T cell infusions [46]. This strategy extended (2.9 fold increase) the *in vivo* survival of the adoptively transferred antigen-specific CD8-positive T cells. In another study, metastatic melanoma patients were infused with NY-ESO-1-specific CD4-positive T cell clones [25]. The infused CD4-positive T cell clones induced long-term responses in one patient with refractory melanoma. Although the CD4-positive T cell clones did not persist *in vivo*, an endogenous CD8-positive T cell-mediated immune response against other tumor antigens was generated [25]. This study suggested that 'epitope spreading' as reported for cancer vaccines might be critical for durable responses post T cell transfer [47, 48]. In another study, 10 metastatic melanoma patients received polyclonal tumor-specific CD4- and CD8-positive T cells, which were generated *in vitro* by repeated stimulations with irradiated, autologous tumor cells [49]. This study reported one complete regression, one partial response, and three patients with stable disease.

Adoptive transfer of autologous, antigen-specific T cells has also been used for the treatment of patients with metastatic breast cancer. In one case report, a patient with breast cancer overexpressing the human epidermal growth factor receptor 2 (HER2) was infused with HER2-specific T cell clones [50]. While infused T- cell clones were unable to penetrate the solid tumor, T cells migrated to the bone marrow and induced regression of disseminated tumor cells. This study emphasized the importance of combining T cell therapy with strategies to enhance T cell homing to solid tumors and/or targeting the tumor stroma to enhance T cell infiltration.

## Genetically Modified T Cells for the Treatment of Malignancies

The *ex vivo* generation of T cells specific for endogenous TAA is often difficult and unreliable due to low frequency and anergy of TAA-specific T cells. In addition, the autologous APCs needed for the activation and expansion of TAA-specific T cells are often limited. Genetic modification of T cells to render them tumor specific is one attractive strategy to overcome these obstacles. Two commonly used genetic modification approaches include the transfer of α/β TCRs specific for TAA or chimeric antigen receptors (CARs) (Table **1**). Genetic modification of T cells also allows the generation of T cells that have enhanced effector function, and are resistant to inhibitory molecules secreted by tumor cells.

### *T Cells Genetically Modified with αβ T-Cell Receptors*

α/β TCR chains have been isolated from T-cell clones specific for TAAs including melanoma antigens, colorectal antigens, and universal tumor antigens. Once isolated, the genes encoding α and β TCR chains are commonly subcloned into retroviral vectors to transduce mitogen-activated T cells [51, 52]. This approach allows for the rapid generation of large numbers of tumor-specific T cells for patients in which TILs cannot be generated [53].

The safety and antitumor efficacy of transgenic T cells encoding TAA-specific α/β TCRs have been evaluated in several clinical studies (Table **1**).

**Table 1:** Examples of αβ TCR and CAR T cells in clinical studies

| **Hematologic malignances** | **Clinical studies** | **References** |
|---|---|---|
| αβTCR LAGE-1 | Ongoing | [54] |
| αβTCR NY-ESO-1 | Ongoing | [54] |
| CAR-CD19 | Completed | [55-62] |
| CAR-CD20 | Completed | [62, 63] |
| **Solid tumors** | **Clinical data** | |
| αβ TCR CEA | Completed | [64] |
| αβ TCR gp100 | Completed | [65] |
| αβ TCR Mage A3 | Completed | [66, 67] |
| αβ TCR MART-1 | Completed | [23, 65] |
| αβTCR NY-ESO-1 | Completed | [68] |
| CAR-CAIX | Completed | [69] |
| CAR-CD171 | Completed | [70] |
| CAR-GD2 | Completed | [71, 72] |
| CAR-HER2 | Completed | [73, 74] |
| CAR-Mesothelin | Ongoing | [75] |

In one study, Morgan *et al.* demonstrated that the infusion of autologous polyclonal T cells encoding α/β TCRs against a melanoma antigen (MART-1) induced sustainable objective regression of disease in 2 out of 15 lymphodepleted melanoma patients [23]. In an effort to increase the response rates, the same group infused T cells encoding transgenic α/β TCRs with higher affinities against MART-1 and gp100 peptides. Although this strategy resulted in objective cancer regression in 30% (MART-1) and 19% (gp100) of melanoma patients, several patients developed side effects (skin rash, uveitis, and hearing loss) that were not associated with antitumor responses [65]. In another study, Parkhurst *et al.* adoptively transferred autologous T cells expressing a murine transgenic TCR that specifically recognized the human carcinoembryonic antigen (CEA) to 3 patients with metastatic colorectal cancer. All patients showed decreased levels of CEA in the serum and one patient had an objective regression of metastatic lesions. However, all patients developed inflammatory colitis [64]. Robbins *et al.* evaluated autologous T cells expressing a TCR directed against NY-ESO-1, a cancer/testis antigen expressed in 10% to 50% of metastatic melanomas, breast, prostate, thyroid, and ovarian cancers, as well as approximately 80% of synovial cell sarcomas [68]. NY-ESO-1 TCR T cells were infused into 11 patients with metastatic melanoma and into 6 patients with synovial cell sarcoma, all of whom had progressive disease after extensive prior standard treatment. Objective clinical responses were observed in 67% (4 out of 6) of patients with synovial cell sarcoma and 45% (5 out of 11) of patients with melanoma. Moreover, the infused T cells induced complete regressions that persisted after 1 year in 2 out of the 11 patients with melanoma. No toxicities were observed in this study, which contrasts with the side effects seen in the clinical studies with MART-1- and gp100-specific α/β TCR T cells. Similarly, an ongoing clinical study indicates that NY-ESO-1-specific α/β TCR T cells induce clinical responses in patients with multiple myeloma without off-targets effects [54]. Several α/β TCRs have been affinity matured to increase antitumor effects. This can lead to unwanted side effects, best highlighted by the recent experience with MAGE A3-specific α/β TCR T cells [66, 67]. While one study reported fatal neurotoxicity due to recognition of MAGE A12 by MAGE A3-α/β TCR T cells [66], another reported fatal cardiac toxicity due to recognition of titin [67]. Thus, clinical studies so far have not only demonstrated the potency of adoptively transferred α/β TCR-modified T cells but also their clinical limitations.

One limitation of α/β TCR gene therapy has been mispairing of endogenous TCR chains with the transgenic α/β TCRs. Such mispairings can result in the formation of TCRs with unknown antigen specificity and potential autoreactivity. One strategy to reduce mispairing with endogenous α and β chains has been to integrate a murine-derived transmembrane region in the transgenic TCR. While effective, this strategy carries the risk of inducing immune responses against the murine portion of the TCR [76]. Investigators have also introduced additional cysteines to stabilize pairing of the transgenic α and β TCR chains [77-79]. Alternatively, silencing endogenous α/β TCR gene expression [80] or selective disruption of the endogenous α/β TCR gene locus using zinc-finger nucleases (ZFNs) may prevent this problem [81, 82]. Lastly, using γδ T cells as a T cell platform can overcome mispairing [83]. Another limitation of α/β TCRs is their HLA restriction, which limits their application to patients with the appropriate HLA type. Moreover, targeting a single epitope increases the risk of immune escape.

### *T Cells Genetically Modified with Chimeric Antigen Receptors (CARs)*

Another widely used strategy to generate tumor specific T cells is genetic modification of T cells with TAA-specific CARs [84-86]. While α/β TCR T cells can recognize antigens expressed on the cell surface or inside the cells, the majority of CAR T cells can only recognize antigens expressed on the cell surface. CARs consist of an extracellular domain that is responsible for antigen recognition, a transmembrane domain and an intracellular domain that is responsible for T-cell signaling. The extracellular domain is most commonly derived from the antigen-binding portion of a specific MAb in single chain format (scFv), while the intracellular domain is usually derived from the cytoplasmic portion of the TCR/CD3ζ complex. CARs with CD3 ζ signaling domain are called first generation CARs. Second and third generation CARs incorporate additional intracellular signaling domains that provide co-stimulation, allowing T cells to pass through the multiple checkpoints that control T-cell activation, proliferation, and survival [58, 86]. CAR expression permits T cells to specifically recognize tumor antigens in a HLA-independent manner, while retaining their ability to migrate to tumor sites, proliferate *in vivo,* and recruit an array of cellular and humoral responses to eradicate tumors. Recognition of tumor antigens in a HLA-independent manner allows CAR T cells to overcome the tumor's ability to escape immune responses by downregulating HLA molecules on the surface of tumor cells. In addition, recognition in a HLA-independent manner increases the number of eligible patients and extends the types of antigens that can be recognized by T cells to include carbohydrates and glycolipids.

CAR T cells have been evaluated in preclinical [84-86] as well as clinical studies [55-63, 70, 71, 87] for the treatment of hematological malignancies and solid tumors (Table **1**). Early studies have demonstrated that T cells engineered to express first generation CARs were capable of inducing target-cell lysis, moderate amounts of IL-2 production, and antitumor responses in different mouse tumor models. However, the efficacy of first generation CARs was limited by suboptimal T cell activation leading to poor cytokine secretion and T cell proliferation, and eventual apoptosis [88, 89]. Furthermore, it was found that tumor eradication by CAR-modified T cells was dependent on the expression of co-stimulatory molecules (*e.g.,* B7.1/CD80) on the tumor cell surface. These findings led to the development of second and third generation CARs that contain additional intracellular signaling domains from co-stimulatory molecules (CD27, CD28, 41BB, OX40 or ICOS) to enhance T cell activation, cytokine secretion and effector function [90-92]. In one clinical study, investigators compared CAR. ζ and CAR.CD28. ζ T cells specific for CD19 in lymphoma patients [58]. Similar to preclinical studies, CD28 co-stimulation resulted in enhanced expansion and persistence of CAR T cells [58], however, even with CD28 co-stimulation, expansion and persistence was limited, indicating that additional CAR modifications are necessary to enhance their activity.

Several groups have reported the results of early phase clinical studies with T cells expressing CD19-specific CAR with CD28. ζ or 41BB. ζ endodomains. Impressive clinical responses have been observed in patients with CD19-positive hematological malignancies including NHL, chronic lymphocytic leukemia (CLL), and acute lympoblastic leukemia (ALL) [55-61]. Antitumor activity was dependent on significant T cell expansion *in vivo*, which was associated in several patients with a life-threatening cytokine storm. The clinical picture was reminiscent of a hemophagocytic syndrome and patients responded either to a combination of steroids, TNF-α MAb (infliximab), and IL-6 receptor MAb (tocilizumab) or monotherapy with tocilizumab, highlighting the role of IL-6.

In contrast to hematological malignancies, the experience with adoptive transfer of CAR T cells for solid tumors is limited. One clinical study has been conducted with CAR T cells specific for GD2, a disialoganglioside, for patients with advanced stage neuroblastoma, the most common extracranial tumor in children. Pule *et al.* expressed a 1st generation CAR on EBV-specific T cells and 3 of 11 children had a complete response, which was sustained in 2 patients [71, 72]. Investigators have also explored the use of HER2-specific CAR T cells in patients with advanced stage solid tumors [73, 74]. While one patient died after receiving lymphodepleting chemotherapy and $10^{10}$ T cells expressing a 3rd generation HER2-specific CAR, no dose limiting toxicities have been observed in patients receiving ~$1x10^8$ T cells expressing a 2nd generation HER2-specific CAR without a conditioning regimen. Lastly, a clinical trial targeting mesothelin with CAR T cells is in progress [75].

As with α/β TCR T-cell therapy, the limited clinical experience with CAR T cells already suggests that recognition of target antigens expressed in low levels on normal tissues might be a significant problem. Strategies to overcome this dilemma include the development of CAR T cells that only become fully activated if they recognize multiple antigens [93, 94]; while each targeted antigen might be expressed at low levels on different non-malignant cells, only cancer cells would express the entire array of antigens resulting in complete T cell activation.

### *Genetic Modifications to Enhance T Cell Function*

Besides genetic modification to render T cells tumor-specific, several groups of investigators have explored genetic modification to enhance T cell function or safety. Conceptually these can be divided into strategies to 1) increase T cell homing to tumors, 2) render T cells resistant to the immunosuppressive tumor microenvironment, 3) allow transgenic expression of cytokines, cytokine receptors, or silencing of negative regulators to enhance T cell expansion and persistence, and 4) improve T cell safety (Table **2**).

**Table 2:** Genetic modification to improve T cell therapy

| Goal | Genetic Modification | Reference |
|---|---|---|
| Improve T-cell homing to tumor sites | Chemokine receptors | [95-97] |
| Render T cells resistant to immunosuppressive tumor microenvironment | Silencing genes (*e.g.*, FAS)<br>Dominant negative receptors (*e.g.*, TGF-β)<br>Chimeric cytokine receptors (*e.g.*, IL4 Rα)<br>Cytokines (IL12, IL15) | [98-104] |
| Enhance T cell expansion and persistence | Cytokines (IL2, IL15)<br>Cytokine receptors (IL7Rα)<br>Co-stimulatory molecules<br>Anti-apoptotic genes | [92, 103, 105-107] |
| Improve Safety of T cell Therapy | Suicide genes (HSV-*tk*; inducible caspase 9)<br>Expression of antigens for which clinical grade MAb are available (*e.g.*, CD20) | [108-112] |

To increase T cell homing to tumors, investigators have expressed chemokine receptors including CXCR2, CCR4, or CCR2b [95-97]. Genetic modifications to render T cells resistant to the immunosuppressive tumor environment include making T cells resistant to TGF-β by expression of a dominant negative TGF-β receptor (TGF-β-DNR) [99, 113], silencing FAS [98] to prevent FAS-ligand induced apoptosis, or transgenic expression of cytokines such as IL-12 [100-102] or IL-15 [103]. Another approach includes the expression of chimeric cytokine receptors that convert an inhibitory signal into a positive signal. For example, one group generated a chimeric cytokine receptor consisting of the extracellular domain of the IL-4 receptor and the beta subunit of the IL-2 receptor [104]. T cells expressing this receptor proliferated in response to IL-4 and retained $T_H1$-polarization and effector function. Of the aforementioned approaches, EBV-specific T cells expressing a TGF-β-DNR are being evaluated in a clinical trial for patients with EBV-positive HL [114].

Transgenic expression of cytokines such as IL-2 and IL-15, expression of IL17Rα, or expression of anti-apoptotic proteins in T cells are other strategies aimed at improving effector function *in vivo* [92, 103, 105-107]. For example, IL-15-expressing T cells not only proliferated better than their unmodified counterparts, but also were resistant to Tregs. Similarly, expression of co-stimulatory molecules on the cell surface of CAR T cells improves their effector function [115]. While all these modification enhance the effector function of T cells, there is concern that these modifications may lead to antigen- or cytokine-independent growth [116]. Thus, it seems advisable to include 'safety switches' so that genetically modified T cells can be selectively destroyed if side effects occur. The Herpes Simplex Virus thymidine kinase (HSV-*tk*) suicide gene approach in combination with ganciclovir (GCV) has been proven to be safe and effective in humans [108, 109]. However, HSV-*tk* is an immunogenic protein and GCV is a commonly used antiviral, which cannot be used once patients have received HSV-*tk* gene-modified T cells. Several non-immunogenic suicide gene systems have been developed. Of these, the inducible caspase 9 system has been tested in humans [110]. It consists of a chimeric gene encoding a dimerizer domain and the active domain of caspase 9 [111]. Once exposed to the dimerizer, genetically modified T cells rapidly undergo apoptosis. Another approach includes the transgenic expression of CD20, rendering T cells sensitive to the clinically approved CD20 MAb rituximab [112].

## COMBINATORIAL T-CELL THERAPY

As with other cancer therapies, combinatorial regimens hold promise to improve T-cell therapy for cancer [117]. These can be divided in approaches that 1) kill tumor cells without affecting T cells, 2) enhance the expression of TAA, 3) improve T-cell expansion and persistence, and 4) reverse the inhibitory tumor microenvironment (Table **3**).

**Table 3:** Examples of combinatorial T cell therapy

| Principle | Examples | Reference |
|---|---|---|
| Concomitant tumor cell killing | Agents that are toxic to tumor cells but not T cells (*e.g.*, BRAF inhibitors for melanoma-targeted T-cell therapy) | [118, 119] |
| Increase TAA expression | Epigenetic modifiers (*e.g.*, decitabine, HDACs) | [120, 121] |
| Improve T cell expansion and persistence | Check point blockade (*e.g.*, CTLA-4 MAbs, PD-1/PD-1L MAbs); Vaccines | [122-134] |
| Reverse immunosuppressive environment | Blocking adenosine receptor signaling | [135-139] |

For example, the BRAF inhibitor vemurafenib has no adverse effects on T cell function, and combining vemurafenib with adoptive transfer of T cells enhances antitumor effects in preclinical animal models of melanoma [118, 119]. Increasing the expression of TAA in cancer cells can be achieved with epigenetic modifiers such as decitabine [120, 121].

Combining T cell therapy with blocking antibodies specific for negative regulators of T-cell responses such as the cytotoxic T-lymphocyte-associated protein (CTLA-4) and programmed cell death 1 (PD-1) is one strategy to increase their function. CTLA-4 is expressed on the cell surface of activated T cells, where it outcompetes the co-stimulatory molecule CD28 for binding to its ligands (*e.g.*, CD86). Binding of CTLA-4 to CD86 inhibits T-cell activation, expansion and effector function by interrupting CD28 co-stimulatory signals. The role of CTLA-4 as a negative regulator of T cell responses has been well demonstrated in CTLA-4-deficient mice, which die at a young age due to an aggressive lymphoproliferative disorder. Indeed, CTLA-4 antibodies were able to mediate rejection of established tumors in mice [124]. Based on these preclinical studies, an antibody to block human CTLA-4, ipilimumab, was developed, and a phase III randomized clinical trial showed that 23% of patients with metastatic melanoma survived more than 4 years following ipilimumab treatment, leading to FDA approval in March 2011 [125].

Similarly, combining T cell therapy with MAbs that block PD-1 and/or its ligands (PD-L1 and PD-L2) is another promising approach. Activated T cells express PD-1, and one of the ligands PD-L1 has been shown to be expressed on tumors, resulting in tumor-induced immune suppression that has been correlated to poor clinical outcome [126]. The role of PD-1 as a negative regulator of T cells has been shown in PD-1-deficient mice, which developed autoimmune disorders [127, 128]. In addition, blocking antibodies against PD-1 activated immune responses that resulted in reduction of tumor growth and metastasis in several experimental tumor models [129]. A recent clinical trial evaluating the safety and efficacy of a PD-L1 antibody reported encouraging objective clinical response rates in patients with advance melanoma, renal cell carcinoma and non-small-cell-lung-cancer [130]. In addition to blocking CTLA-4 and PD-1 signaling pathways, other co-inhibitory receptors expressed by activated T cells such as the B and T lymphocyte attenuator (BTLA), lymphocyte activation gene 3 (LAG3), T-cell immunoglobulin and mucin domain-containing protein 3 (TIM3) and the V-domain immunoglobulin suppressor of T cell activation (VISTA) can also be targeted [131].

The administration of cancer vaccines (*e.g.*, peptides, dendritic cells) is an attractive strategy to boost adoptively transferred T cells *in vivo*. Several groups have shown that combining peptide, dendritic cell or adenoviral vaccines augment the effectiveness of adoptive T cell therapy *in vivo* [132-134]. Besides provision of antigen, providing potent co-stimulation, and/or cytokines was critical for the observed effects. However, limited experience is available in humans except for an ongoing clinical trial in which patients are vaccinated with an autologous DC vaccine post α/β TCR T cell transfer.

Reversing the immunosuppressive tumor microenvironment is another approach to enhance the antitumor activity of adoptively transferred T cells. Tumor cells and/or its supporting stroma create a hypoxic environment, and produce a number of soluble factors that inhibit T cell effector function and promote tumor growth such as IDO (indoleamine 2,3-dioxygenase), prostaglandin E2, arginase, and TGF-β [135]. Hypoxia promotes the generation of adenosine, which has been demonstrated to induce T-cell apoptosis, and blocking of adenosine receptor signaling restores T cell function in preclinical models [136, 137].

Lastly, stromal cells, such as cancer-associated fibroblasts (CAFs) promote a highly pro-tumorigenic and immunosuppressive microenvironment that mediates therapeutic resistance [138]. Therefore, targeting CAFs as well as cancer cells represent a promising strategy to augment T cell-mediated anti-tumor responses in cancer patients. Indeed, our laboratory has demonstrated that combining T cells redirected to target CAFs together with T cells targeting lung cancer cells significantly enhanced the overall anti-tumor activity and conferred a survival advantage as compared to either type of T cell alone in a xenograft mouse model [140].

## CONCLUSION

T cell immunotherapy has shown promising results in early phase clinical studies, especially for hematological malignancies. However, formidable challenges remain, including *ex vivo* T-cell production, target antigen selection, limited *in vivo* T cell expansion and persistence, T cell trafficking to tumor sites, and the hostile tumor microenvironment. Genetic modification of T cells and combining T cell transfer with other targeted therapies holds promise to overcome some of these obstacles. Lastly, there is a critical need to develop randomized clinical studies to unequivocally assess the potential benefit of T cell therapy for cancer.

## ACKNOWLEDGEMENTS

The authors were supported by grants from the National Institutes of Health 1R01CA148748-01A1, P01CA94237, 1R01CA173750-01 and CPRIT grant RP101499.

# CONFLICT OF INTEREST

The authors confirm that this chapter contents have no conflict of interest.

# REFERENCES


[1] Gresser I. A. Chekhov, M.D., and Coley's toxins. N Engl J Med. 1987 317(7): 457.

[2] Coley WB. The treatment of malignant tumors by repeated inoculations of erysipelas. With a report of ten original cases. 1893. Clin Orthop Relat Res 1991; (262): 3-11.

[3] Lamm DL, Blumenstein BA, Crawford ED, Montie JE, Scardino P, Grossman HB, *et al.* A randomized trial of intravesical doxorubicin and immunotherapy with bacille Calmette-Guerin for transitional-cell carcinoma of the bladder. N Engl J Med 1991; 325(17): 1205-9.

[4] Morgan DA, Ruscetti FW, Gallo R. Selective *in vitro* growth of T lymphocytes from normal human bone marrows. Science 1976; 193(4257): 1007-8.

[5] Rosenberg SA, Lotze MT. Cancer immunotherapy using interleukin-2 and interleukin-2-activated lymphocytes. Annu Rev Immunol 1986; 4: 681-709.

[6] Maloney DG, Grillo-Lopez AJ, White CA, Bodkin D, Schilder RJ, Neidhart JA, *et al.* IDEC-C2B8 (Rituximab) anti-CD20 monoclonal antibody therapy in patients with relapsed low-grade non-Hodgkin's lymphoma. Blood 1997; 90(6): 2188-95.

[7] MITCHISON NA. Studies on the immunological response to foreign tumor transplants in the mouse. I. The role of lymph node cells in conferring immunity by adoptive transfer. J Exp Med 1955; 102(2): 157-77.

[8] Rosenberg SA, Yang JC, Restifo NP. Cancer immunotherapy: moving beyond current vaccines. Nat Med 2004 Sep; 10(9): 909-15.

[9] Balch CM, Riley LB, Bae YJ, Salmeron MA, Platsoucas CD, von Eschenbach A, *et al.* Patterns of human tumor-infiltrating lymphocytes in 120 human cancers. Arch Surg 1990; 125(2): 200-5.

[10] Ridolfi L, Ridolfi R, Riccobon A, De Paola F, Petrini M, Stefanelli M, *et al.* Adjuvant immunotherapy with tumor infiltrating lymphocytes and interleukin-2 in patients with resected stage III and IV melanoma. J Immunother 2003; 26(2): 156-62.

[11] Dudley ME, Yang JC, Sherry R, Hughes MS, Royal R, Kammula U, *et al.* Adoptive cell therapy for patients with metastatic melanoma: evaluation of intensive myeloablative chemoradiation preparative regimens. J Clin Oncol 2008; 26(32): 5233-9.

[12] Dudley ME, Wunderlich JR, Robbins PF, Yang JC, Hwu P, Schwartzentruber DJ, *et al.* Cancer regression and autoimmunity in patients after clonal repopulation with antitumor lymphocytes. Science 2002; 298(5594): 850-4.

[13] Antony PA, Piccirillo CA, Akpinarli A, Finkelstein SE, Speiss PJ, Surman DR, *et al.* CD8+ T cell immunity against a tumor/self-antigen is augmented by CD4+ T helper cells and hindered by naturally occurring T regulatory cells. J Immunol 2005; 174(5): 2591-601.

[14] Gattinoni L, Finkelstein SE, Klebanoff CA, Antony PA, Palmer DC, Spiess PJ, *et al.* Removal of homeostatic cytokine sinks by lymphodepletion enhances the efficacy of adoptively transferred tumor-specific CD8+ T cells. J Exp Med 2005; 202(7): 907-12.

[15] Riddell SR, Watanabe KS, Goodrich JM, Li CR, Agha ME, Greenberg PD. Restoration of viral immunity in immunodeficient humans by the adoptive transfer of T cell clones. Science 1992; 257: 238-41.

[16] Rooney CM, Smith CA, Ng CYC, Loftin SK, Sixbey JW, Gan Y-J, *et al.* Infusion of cytotoxic T cells for the prevention and treatment of Epstein-Barr virus-induced lymphoma in allogeneic transplant recipients. Blood 1998; 92(5): 1549-55.

[17] Heslop HE, Ng CYC, Li C, Smith CA, Loftin SK, Krance RA, *et al.* Long-term restoration of immunity against Epstein-Barr virus infection by adoptive transfer of gene-modified virus-specific T lymphocytes. Nat Med 1996; 2: 551-5.

[18] Savoldo B, Goss JA, Hammer MM, Zhang L, Lopez T, Gee AP, *et al.* Treatment of solid organ transplant recipients with autologous Epstein Barr virus-specific cytotoxic T lymphocytes (CTLs). Blood 2006; 108(9): 2942-9.

[19] Steinman RM. Dendritic cells and immune-based therapies. Exp Hematol 1996; 24(8): 859-62.
[20] Straathof KC, Bollard CM, Popat U, Huls MH, Lopez T, Morriss MC, *et al.* Treatment of Nasopharyngeal Carcinoma with Epstein-Barr Virus-specific T Lymphocytes. Blood 2005; 105: 1898-904.
[21] Yee C, Thompson JA, Byrd D, Riddell SR, Roche P, Celis E, *et al.* Adoptive T cell therapy using antigen-specific CD8+ T cell clones for the treatment of patients with metastatic melanoma: *in vivo* persistence, migration, and antitumor effect of transferred T cells. Proc Natl Acad Sci U S A 2002; 99(25): 16168-73.
[22] Meidenbauer N, Marienhagen J, Laumer M, Vogl S, Heymann J, Andreesen R, *et al.* Survival and tumor localization of adoptively transferred Melan-A-specific T cells in melanoma patients. J Immunol 2003; 170(4): 2161-9.
[23] Morgan RA, Dudley ME, Wunderlich JR, Hughes MS, Yang JC, Sherry RM, *et al.* Cancer regression in patients after transfer of genetically engineered lymphocytes. Science 2006; 314(5796): 126-9.
[24] Kershaw MH, Westwood JA, Parker LL, Wang G, Eshhar Z, Mavroukakis SA, *et al.* A phase I study on adoptive immunotherapy using gene-modified T cells for ovarian cancer. Clin Cancer Res 2006; 12(20 Pt 1): 6106-15.
[25] Hunder NN, Wallen H, Cao J, Hendricks DW, Reilly JZ, Rodmyre R, *et al.* Treatment of metastatic melanoma with autologous CD4+ T cells against NY-ESO-1. N Engl J Med 2008; 358(25): 2698-703.
[26] Butler MO, Lee JS, Ansen S, Neuberg D, Hodi FS, Murray AP, *et al.* Long-lived antitumor CD8+ lymphocytes for adoptive therapy generated using an artificial antigen-presenting cell. Clin Cancer Res 2007; 13(6): 1857-67.
[27] Suhoski MM, Golovina TN, Aqui NA, Tai VC, Varela-Rohena A, Milone MC, *et al.* Engineering artificial antigen-presenting cells to express a diverse array of co-stimulatory molecules. Mol Ther 2007; 15(5): 981-8.
[28] Cohen JI. Epstein-Barr virus infection. N Engl J Med 2000; 343(7): 481-92.
[29] Cohen JI, Mocarski ES, Raab-Traub N, Corey L, Nabel GJ. The need and challenges for development of an Epstein-Barr virus vaccine. Vaccine 2013; 31 Suppl 2: B194-B196.
[30] Heslop HE, Slobod KS, Pule MA, Hale GA, Rousseau A, Smith CA, *et al.* Long-term outcome of EBV-specific T-cell infusions to prevent or treat EBV-related lymphoproliferative disease in transplant recipients. Blood 2010; 115(5): 925-35.
[31] Gottschalk S, Ng CYC, Smith CA, Perez M, Sample C, Brenner MK, *et al.* An Epstein-Barr virus deletion mutant that causes fatal lymphoproliferative disease unresponsive to virus-specific T cell therapy. Blood 2001; 97(4): 835-43.
[32] Bollard CM, Aguilar L, Straathof KC, Gahn B, Huls MH, Rousseau A, *et al.* Cytotoxic T lymphocyte therapy for epstein-barr virus+ hodgkin's disease. J Exp Med 2004; 200(12): 1623-33.
[33] Bollard CM, Gottschalk S, Leen AM, Weiss H, Straathof KC, Carrum G, *et al.* Complete responses of relapsed lymphoma following genetic modification of tumor-antigen presenting cells and T-lymphocyte transfer. Blood 2007; 110(8): 2838-45.
[34] Louis CU, Straathof K, Bollard CM, Gerken C, Huls MH, Gresik MV, *et al.* Enhancing the *in vivo* expansion of adoptively transferred EBV-specific CTL with lymphodepleting CD45 monoclonal antibodies in NPC patients. Blood 2009; 113(11): 2442-50.
[35] Bollard CM, Stanojevic M, Leen AM, Lopez T, Sheehan A, Carrum G, *et al.* Complete tumor responses in lymphoma patients who receive autologous cytotoxic t lymphocytes targeting ebv latent membrane proteins. Biol Blood Marrow Transplant 2009; 15(2): 52.
[36] Louis CU, Straathof K, Bollard CM, Ennamuri S, Gerken C, Lopez TT, *et al.* Adoptive transfer of EBV-specific T cells results in sustained clinical responses in patients with locoregional nasopharyngeal carcinoma. J Immunother 2010; 33(9): 983-90.
[37] Smith C, Tsang J, Beagley L, Chua D, Lee V, Li V, *et al.* Effective treatment of metastatic forms of Epstein-Barr virus-associated nasopharyngeal carcinoma with a novel adenovirus-based adoptive immunotherapy. Cancer Res 2012; 72(5): 1116-25.
[38] Vera JF, Brenner LJ, Gerdemann U, Ngo MC, Sili U, Liu H, *et al.* Accelerated production of antigen-specific T cells for preclinical and clinical applications using gas-permeable rapid expansion cultureware (G-Rex). J Immunother 2010; 33(3): 305-15.

[39] Gerdemann U, Keirnan JM, Katari UL, Yanagisawa R, Christin AS, Huye LE, *et al.* Rapidly generated multivirus-specific cytotoxic T lymphocytes for the prophylaxis and treatment of viral infections. Mol Ther 2012; 20(8): 1622-32.

[40] Haque T, Taylor C, Wilkie GM, Murad P, Amlot PL, Beath S, *et al.* Complete regression of posttransplant lymphoproliferative disease using partially HLA-matched Epstein Barr virus-specific cytotoxic T cells. Transplantation 2001; 72(8): 1399-402.

[41] Haque T, Wilkie GM, Jones MM, Higgins CD, Urquhart G, Wingate P, *et al.* Allogeneic cytotoxic T-cell therapy for EBV-positive posttransplantation lymphoproliferative disease: results of a phase 2 multicenter clinical trial. Blood 2007; 110(4): 1123-31.

[42] Leen AM, Bollard CM, Mendizabal AM, Shpall EJ, Szabolcs P, Antin JH, *et al.* Multicenter study of banked third-party virus-specific T cells to treat severe viral infections after hematopoietic stem cell transplantation. Blood 2013; 121(26): 5113-23.

[43] Doubrovina E, Oflaz-Sozmen B, Prockop SE, Kernan NA, Abramson S, Teruya-Feldstein J, *et al.* Adoptive immunotherapy with unselected or EBV-specific T cells for biopsy-proven EBV+ lymphomas after allogeneic hematopoietic cell transplantation. Blood 2012; 119(11): 2644-56.

[44] Mackensen A, Meidenbauer N, Vogl S, Laumer M, Berger J, Andreesen R. Phase I study of adoptive T-cell therapy using antigen-specific CD8+ T cells for the treatment of patients with metastatic melanoma. J Clin Oncol 2006; 24(31): 5060-9.

[45] Mitchell MS, Darrah D, Yeung D, Halpern S, Wallace A, Voland J, *et al.* Phase I trial of adoptive immunotherapy with cytolytic T lymphocytes immunized against a tyrosinase epitope. J Clin Oncol 2002; 20(4): 1075-86.

[46] Wallen H, Thompson JA, Reilly JZ, Rodmyre RM, Cao J, Yee C. Fludarabine modulates immune response and extends *in vivo* survival of adoptively transferred CD8 T cells in patients with metastatic melanoma. PLoS One 2009; 4(3): e4749.

[47] Butterfield LH, Ribas A, Dissette VB, Amarnani SN, Vu HT, Oseguera D, *et al.* Determinant spreading associated with clinical response in dendritic cell-based immunotherapy for malignant melanoma. Clin Cancer Res 2003; 9(3): 998-1008.

[48] Disis ML, Gooley TA, Rinn K, Davis D, Piepkorn M, Cheever MA, *et al.* Generation of T-cell immunity to the HER-2/neu protein after active immunization with HER-2/neu peptide-based vaccines. J Clin Oncol 2002; 20(11): 2624-32.

[49] Verdegaal EM, Visser M, Ramwadhdoebe TH, van der Minne CE, van Steijn JA, Kapiteijn E, *et al.* Successful treatment of metastatic melanoma by adoptive transfer of blood-derived polyclonal tumor-specific CD4+ and CD8+ T cells in combination with low-dose interferon-alpha. Cancer Immunol Immunother 2011; 60(7): 953-63.

[50] Bernhard H, Neudorfer J, Gebhard K, Conrad H, Hermann C, Nahrig J, *et al.* Adoptive transfer of autologous, HER2-specific, cytotoxic T lymphocytes for the treatment of HER2-overexpressing breast cancer. Cancer Immunol Immunother 2008; 57(2): 271-80.

[51] Leisegang M, Wilde S, Spranger S, Milosevic S, Frankenberger B, Uckert W, *et al.* MHC-restricted fratricide of human lymphocytes expressing survivin-specific transgenic T cell receptors. J Clin Invest 2010; 120(11): 3869-77.

[52] Li LP, Lampert JC, Chen X, Leitao C, Popovic J, Muller W, *et al.* Transgenic mice with a diverse human T cell antigen receptor repertoire. Nat Med 2010; 16(9): 1029-34.

[53] Stauss HJ, Cesco-Gaspere M, Thomas S, Hart DP, Xue SA, Holler A, *et al.* Monoclonal T-cell receptors: new reagents for cancer therapy. Mol Ther 2007; 15(10): 1744-50.

[54] Levine BL, Rapoport AP, Stadtmauer EA, Vogl DT, Weiss B, Binder-Scholl GK, *et al.* Safety and Correlates of Clinical Response in an Early Phase Clinical Trial in Multiple Myeloma Patients Post Auto-SCT and Adoptive Immunotherapy with Engineered T Cells Expressing an HLA-A2 Restricted Affinity-Enhanced TCR for LAGE-1 and NY-ESO-1. Mol Ther 2013; 21(S1): S114.

[55] Kalos M, Levine BL, Porter DL, Katz S, Grupp SA, Bagg A, *et al.* T cells with chimeric antigen receptors have potent antitumor effects and can establish memory in patients with advanced leukemia. Sci Transl Med 2011; 3(95): 95ra73.

[56] Kochenderfer JN, Dudley ME, Feldman SA, Wilson WH, Spaner DE, Maric I, *et al.* B-cell depletion and remissions of malignancy along with cytokine-associated toxicity in a clinical trial of anti-CD19 chimeric-antigen-receptor-transduced T cells. Blood 2012; 119(12): 2709-20.

[57] Brentjens RJ, Riviere I, Park JH, Davila ML, Wang X, Stefanski J, *et al.* Safety and persistence of adoptively transferred autologous CD19-targeted T cells in patients with relapsed or chemotherapy refractory B-cell leukemias. Blood 2011; 118(18): 4817-28.

[58] Savoldo B, Ramos CA, Liu E, Mims MP, Keating MJ, Carrum G, *et al.* CD28 costimulation improves expansion and persistence of chimeric antigen receptor-modified T cells in lymphoma patients. J Clin Invest 2011; 121(5): 1822-6.

[59] Brentjens RJ, Davila ML, Riviere I, Park J, Wang X, Cowell LG, *et al.* CD19-Targeted T Cells Rapidly Induce Molecular Remissions in Adults with Chemotherapy-Refractory Acute Lymphoblastic Leukemia. Sci Transl Med 2013; 5(177): 177ra38.

[60] Grupp SA, Kalos M, Barrett D, Aplenc R, Porter DL, Rheingold SR, *et al.* Chimeric antigen receptor-modified T cells for acute lymphoid leukemia. N Engl J Med 2013; 368(16): 1509-18.

[61] Porter DL, Levine BL, Kalos M, Bagg A, June CH. Chimeric antigen receptor-modified T cells in chronic lymphoid leukemia. N Engl J Med 2011; 365(8): 725-33.

[62] Jensen MC, Popplewell L, Cooper LJ, Digiusto D, Kalos M, Ostberg JR, *et al.* Anti-Transgene Rejection Responses Contribute to Attenuated Persistence of Adoptively Transferred CD20/CD19-Specific Chimeric Antigen Receptor Re-directed T Cells in Humans. Biol Blood Marrow Transplant 2010; 16(9): 1245-56.

[63] Till BG, Jensen MC, Wang J, Chen EY, Wood BL, Greisman HA, *et al.* Adoptive immunotherapy for indolent non-Hodgkin lymphoma and mantle cell lymphoma using genetically modified autologous CD20-specific T cells. Blood 2008; 112(6): 2261-71.

[64] Parkhurst MR, Yang JC, Langan RC, Dudley ME, Nathan DA, Feldman SA, *et al.* T cells targeting carcinoembryonic antigen can mediate regression of metastatic colorectal cancer but induce severe transient colitis. Mol Ther 2011; 19(3): 620-6.

[65] Johnson LA, Morgan RA, Dudley ME, Cassard L, Yang JC, Hughes MS, *et al.* Gene therapy with human and mouse T-cell receptors mediates cancer regression and targets normal tissues expressing cognate antigen. Blood 2009; 114(3): 535-46.

[66] Morgan RA, Chinnasamy N, Abate-Daga D, Gros A, Robbins PF, Zheng Z, *et al.* Cancer regression and neurological toxicity following anti-MAGE-A3 TCR gene therapy. J Immunother 2013; 36(2): 133-51.

[67] Maus MV, Linette GP, Stadtmauer EA, Rapoport AP, Levine BL, Emery LA, *et al.* Cardiovascular Toxicity and Titin Cross-Reactivity of Affinity-Enhanced TCR-Engineered T Cells Against HLA-A1 Restricted MAGE-A3 Antigen. Molecular Therapy 2013; 21(suppl): S24.

[68] Robbins PF, Morgan RA, Feldman SA, Yang JC, Sherry RM, Dudley ME, *et al.* Tumor regression in patients with metastatic synovial cell sarcoma and melanoma using genetically engineered lymphocytes reactive with NY-ESO-1. J Clin Oncol 2011; 29(7): 917-24.

[69] Lamers CH, Sleijfer S, van SS, van EP, van KB, Groot C, *et al.* Treatment of metastatic renal cell carcinoma with CAIX CAR-engineered T cells: clinical evaluation and management of on-target toxicity. Mol Ther 2013; 21(4): 904-12.

[70] Park JR, Digiusto DL, Slovak M, Wright C, Naranjo A, Wagner J, *et al.* Adoptive transfer of chimeric antigen receptor re-directed cytolytic T lymphocyte clones in patients with neuroblastoma. Mol Ther 2007; 15(4): 825-33.

[71] Pule MA, Savoldo B, Myers GD, Rossig C, Russell HV, Dotti G, *et al.* Virus-specific T cells engineered to coexpress tumor-specific receptors: persistence and antitumor activity in individuals with neuroblastoma. Nat Med 2008; 14(11): 1264-70.

[72] Louis CU, Savoldo B, Dotti G, Pule M, Yvon E, Myers GD, *et al.* Antitumor activity and long-term fate of chimeric antigen receptor-positive T cells in patients with neuroblastoma. Blood 2011; 118(23): 6050-6.

[73] Ahmed N, Brawley V, Diouf O, Anderson P, Hicks MJ, Wang LL, *et al.* T cells redirected against HER2 for the adoptive immunotherapy for HER2-positive osteosarcoma. Cancer Res 2012; 72(8 (Suppl 1)): Abstract.

[74] Morgan RA, Yang JC, Kitano M, Dudley ME, Laurencot CM, Rosenberg SA. Case report of a serious adverse event following the administration of T cells transduced with a chimeric antigen receptor recognizing ERBB2. Mol Ther 2010; 18(4): 843-51.

[75] Maus MV, Haas AR, Beatty GL, Albelda SM, Levine BL, Liu X, *et al.* T cells expressing chimeric antigen receptors can cause anaphylaxis in humans. Cancer Immunol. Res 2013; 1(1): 26-31.

[76] Davis JL, Theoret MR, Zheng Z, Lamers CH, Rosenberg SA, Morgan RA. Development of human anti-murine T-cell receptor antibodies in both responding and nonresponding patients enrolled in TCR gene therapy trials. Clin Cancer Res 2010; 16(23): 5852-61.
[77] Cohen CJ, Li YF, El-Gamil M, Robbins PF, Rosenberg SA, Morgan RA. Enhanced antitumor activity of T cells engineered to express T-cell receptors with a second disulfide bond. Cancer Res 2007; 67(8): 3898-903.
[78] Linnemann C, Schumacher TN, Bendle GM. T-cell receptor gene therapy: critical parameters for clinical success. J Invest Dermatol 2011; 131(9): 1806-16.
[79] Jorritsma A, Schotte R, Coccoris M, de Witte MA, Schumacher TN. Prospects and limitations of T cell receptor gene therapy. Curr Gene Ther 2011; 11(4): 276-87.
[80] Ochi T, Fujiwara H, Okamoto S, An J, Nagai K, Shirakata T, *et al.* Novel adoptive T-cell immunotherapy using a WT1-specific TCR vector encoding silencers for endogenous TCRs shows marked antileukemia reactivity and safety. Blood 2011; 118(6): 1495-503.
[81] Provasi E, Genovese P, Lombardo A, Magnani Z, Liu PQ, Reik A, *et al.* Editing T cell specificity towards leukemia by zinc finger nucleases and lentiviral gene transfer. Nat Med 2012; 18(5): 807-15.
[82] Torikai H, Reik A, Liu PQ, Zhou Y, Zhang L, Maiti S, *et al.* A foundation for universal T-cell based immunotherapy: T cells engineered to express a CD19-specific chimeric-antigen-receptor and eliminate expression of endogenous TCR. Blood 2012; 119(24): 5697-705.
[83] Hiasa A, Nishikawa H, Hirayama M, Kitano S, Okamoto S, Chono H, *et al.* Rapid alphabeta TCR-mediated responses in gammadelta T cells transduced with cancer-specific TCR genes. Gene Ther 2009; 16(5): 620-8.
[84] Curran KJ, Pegram HJ, Brentjens RJ. Chimeric antigen receptors for T cell immunotherapy: current understanding and future directions. J Gene Med 2012 Jun; 14(6): 405-15.
[85] Maher J. Immunotherapy of malignant disease using chimeric antigen receptor engrafted T cells. ISRN Oncol 2012; 2012: 278093.
[86] Ramos CA, Dotti G. Chimeric antigen receptor (CAR)-engineered lymphocytes for cancer therapy. Expert Opin Biol Ther 2011; 11(7): 855-73.
[87] Yaghoubi SS, Jensen MC, Satyamurthy N, Budhiraja S, Paik D, Czernin J, *et al.* Noninvasive detection of therapeutic cytolytic T cells with 18F-FHBG PET in a patient with glioma. Nat Clin Pract Oncol 2009; 6(1): 53-8.
[88] Mitsuyasu RT, Anton PA, Deeks SG, Scadden DT, Connick E, Downs MT, *et al.* Prolonged survival and tissue trafficking following adoptive transfer of CD4zeta gene-modified autologous CD4(+) and CD8(+) T cells in human immunodeficiency virus-infected subjects. Blood 2000 Aug 1; 96(3): 785-93.
[89] Walker RE, Bechtel CM, Natarajan V, Baseler M, Hege KM, Metcalf JA, *et al.* Long-term *in vivo* survival of receptor-modified syngeneic T cells in patients with human immunodeficiency virus infection. Blood 2000; 96(2): 467-74.
[90] Carpenito C, Milone MC, Hassan R, Simonet JC, Lakhal M, Suhoski MM, *et al.* Control of large, established tumor xenografts with genetically retargeted human T cells containing CD28 and CD137 domains. Proc Natl Acad Sci U S A 2009; 106(9): 3360-5.
[91] Maher J, Brentjens RJ, Gunset G, Riviere I, Sadelain M. Human T-lymphocyte cytotoxicity and proliferation directed by a single chimeric TCRzeta/CD28 receptor. Nat Biotechnol 2002; 20(1): 70-5.
[92] Vera JF, Hoyos V, Savoldo B, Quintarelli C, Giordano Attianese GM, Leen AM, *et al.* Genetic manipulation of tumor-specific cytotoxic T lymphocytes to restore responsiveness to IL-7. Mol Ther 2009; 17(5): 880-8.
[93] Lanitis E, Poussin M, Klattenhoff AW, Song D, Sandaltzopoulos R, June CH, *et al.* Chimeric antigen receptor T Cells with dissociated signaling domains exhibit focused antitumor activity with reduced potential for toxicity *in vivo*. Cancer Immunol Res 2013; 1(1): 43-53.
[94] Wilkie S, van Schalkwyk MC, Hobbs S, Davies DM, van der Stegen SJ, Pereira AC, *et al.* Dual targeting of ErbB2 and MUC1 in breast cancer using chimeric antigen receptors engineered to provide complementary signaling. J Clin Immunol 2012; 32(5): 1059-70.

[95] Kershaw MH, Wang G, Westwood JA, Pachynski RK, Tiffany HL, Marincola FM, *et al.* Redirecting migration of T cells to chemokine secreted from tumors by genetic modification with CXCR2. Hum Gene Ther 2002; 13(16): 1971-80.

[96] Craddock JA, Lu A, Bear A, Pule M, Brenner MK, Rooney CM, *et al.* Enhanced Tumor Trafficking of GD2 Chimeric Antigen Receptor T Cells by Expression of the Chemokine Receptor CCR2b. J Immunother. 2010.

[97] Di Stasi A, De Angelis B, Rooney CM, Zhang L, Mahendravada A, Foster AE, *et al.* T lymphocytes coexpressing CCR4 and a chimeric antigen receptor targeting CD30 have improved homing and antitumor activity in a Hodgkin tumor model. Blood 2009; 113(25): 6392-402.

[98] Dotti G, Savoldo B, Pule M, Straathof KC, Biagi E, Yvon E, *et al.* Human cytotoxic T lymphocytes with reduced sensitivity to Fas-induced apoptosis. Blood 2005; 105(12): 4677-84.

[99] Foster AE, Dotti G, Lu A, Khalil M, Brenner MK, Heslop HE, *et al.* Antitumor activity of EBV-specific T lymphocytes transduced with a dominant negative TGF-beta receptor. J Immunother 2008; 31(5): 500-5.

[100] Wagner HJ, Bollard CM, Vigouroux S, Huls MH, Anderson R, Prentice HG, *et al.* A strategy for treatment of Epstein-Barr virus-positive Hodgkin's disease by targeting interleukin 12 to the tumor environment using tumor antigen-specific T cells. Cancer Gene Ther 2004; 11(2): 81-91.

[101] Pegram HJ, Lee JC, Hayman EG, Imperato GH, Tedder TF, Sadelain M, *et al.* Tumor-targeted T cells modified to secrete IL-12 eradicate systemic tumors without need for prior conditioning. Blood 2012; 119(18): 4133-41.

[102] Chinnasamy D, Yu Z, Kerkar SP, Zhang L, Morgan RA, Restifo NP, *et al.* Local delivery of interleukin-12 using T cells targeting VEGF receptor-2 eradicates multiple vascularized tumors in mice. Clin Cancer Res 2012; 18(6): 1672-83.

[103] Hoyos V, Savoldo B, Quintarelli C, Mahendravada A, Zhang M, Vera J, *et al.* Engineering CD19-specific T lymphocytes with interleukin-15 and a suicide gene to enhance their anti-lymphoma/leukemia effects and safety. Leukemia 2010; 24(6): 1160-70.

[104] Wilkie S, Burbridge SE, Chiapero-Stanke L, Pereira AC, Cleary S, van der Stegen SJ, *et al.* Selective expansion of chimeric antigen receptor-targeted T-cells with potent effector function using interleukin-4. J Biol Chem 2010; 285(33): 25538-44.

[105] Hsu C, Hughes MS, Zheng Z, Bray RB, Rosenberg SA, Morgan RA. Primary human T lymphocytes engineered with a codon-optimized IL-15 gene resist cytokine withdrawal-induced apoptosis and persist long-term in the absence of exogenous cytokine. J Immunol 2005; 175(11): 7226-34.

[106] Quintarelli C, Vera JF, Savoldo B, Giordano Attianese GM, Pule M, Foster AE, *et al.* Co-expression of cytokine and suicide genes to enhance the activity and safety of tumor-specific cytotoxic T lymphocytes. Blood 2007; 110(8): 2793-802.

[107] Kalbasi A, Shrimali RK, Chinnasamy D, Rosenberg SA. Prevention of interleukin-2 withdrawal-induced apoptosis in lymphocytes retrovirally cotransduced with genes encoding an antitumor T-cell receptor and an antiapoptotic protein. J Immunother 2010; 33(7): 672-83.

[108] Bondanza A, Valtolina V, Magnani Z, Ponzoni M, Fleischhauer K, Bonyhadi M, *et al.* Suicide gene therapy of graft-*versus*-host disease induced by central memory human T lymphocytes. Blood 2006; 107(5): 1828-36.

[109] Traversari C, Marktel S, Magnani Z, Mangia P, Russo V, Ciceri F, *et al.* The potential immunogenicity of the TK suicide gene does not prevent full clinical benefit associated with the use of TK-transduced donor lymphocytes in HSCT for hematologic malignancies. Blood 2007; 109(11): 4708-15.

[110] Di Stasi A, Tey SK, Dotti G, Fujita Y, Kennedy-Nasser A, Martinez C, *et al.* Inducible apoptosis as a safety switch for adoptive cell therapy. N Engl J Med 2011; 365(18): 1673-83.

[111] Straathof KC, Pule MA, Yotnda P, Dotti G, Vanin EF, Brenner MK, *et al.* An inducible caspase 9 safety switch for T-cell therapy. Blood 2005; 105(11): 4247-54.

[112] Serafini M, Manganini M, Borleri G, Bonamino M, Imberti L, Biondi A, *et al.* Characterization of CD20-transduced T lymphocytes as an alternative suicide gene therapy approach for the treatment of graft-*versus*-host disease. Hum Gene Ther 2004; 15(1): 63-76.

[113] Bollard CM, Rossig C, Calonge MJ, Huls MH, Wagner HJ, Massague J, *et al.* Adapting a transforming growth factor beta-related tumor protection strategy to enhance antitumor immunity. Blood 2002; 99(9): 3179-87.

[114] Bollard CM, Dotti G, Gottschalk S, Mims MP, Liu H, Gee AP, *et al.* Administration of TGF-beta resistant tumor-specific CTL to patienst with EBV-associated HL and NHL. Molecular Therapy 2012; 20(Supplement 1): S22.

[115] Stephan MT, Ponomarev V, Brentjens RJ, Chang AH, Dobrenkov KV, Heller G, *et al.* T cell-encoded CD80 and 4-1BBL induce auto- and transcostimulation, resulting in potent tumor rejection. Nat Med 2007; 13(12): 1440-9.

[116] Hsu C, Jones SA, Cohen CJ, Zheng Z, Kerstann K, Zhou J, *et al.* Cytokine-independent growth and clonal expansion of a primary human CD8+ T-cell clone following retroviral transduction with the IL-15 gene. Blood 2007; 109(12): 5168-77.

[117] Vanneman M, Dranoff G. Combining immunotherapy and targeted therapies in cancer treatment. Nat Rev Cancer 2012; 12(4): 237-51.

[118] Donia M, Fagone P, Nicoletti F, Andersen RS, Hogdall E, Straten PT, *et al.* BRAF inhibition improves tumor recognition by the immune system: Potential implications for combinatorial therapies against melanoma involving adoptive T-cell transfer. Oncoimmunology 2012; 1(9): 1476-83.

[119] Liu C, Peng W, Xu C, Lou Y, Zhang M, Wargo JA, *et al.* BRAF inhibition increases tumor infiltration by T cells and enhances the antitumor activity of adoptive immunotherapy in mice. Clin Cancer Res 2013; 19(2): 393-403.

[120] Chou J, Voong LN, Mortales CL, Towlerton AM, Pollack SM, Chen X, *et al.* Epigenetic modulation to enable antigen-specific T-cell therapy of colorectal cancer. J Immunother 2012; 35(2): 131-41.

[121] Cruz CR, Gerdemann U, Leen AM, Shafer JA, Ku S, Tzou B, *et al.* Improving T-cell therapy for relapsed EBV-negative Hodgkin lymphoma by targeting upregulated MAGE-A4. Clin Cancer Res 2011; 17(22): 7058-66.

[122] Tivol EA, Borriello F, Schweitzer AN, Lynch WP, Bluestone JA, Sharpe AH. Loss of CTLA-4 leads to massive lymphoproliferation and fatal multiorgan tissue destruction, revealing a critical negative regulatory role of CTLA-4. Immunity 1995; 3(5): 541-7.

[123] Waterhouse P, Penninger JM, Timms E, Wakeham A, Shahinian A, Lee KP, *et al.* Lymphoproliferative disorders with early lethality in mice deficient in Ctla-4. Science 1995; 270(5238): 985-8.

[124] Leach DR, Krummel MF, Allison JP. Enhancement of antitumor immunity by CTLA-4 blockade. Science 1996; 271: 1734-6.

[125] Hodi FS, O'Day SJ, McDermott DF, Weber RW, Sosman JA, Haanen JB, *et al.* Improved survival with ipilimumab in patients with metastatic melanoma. N Engl J Med 2010; 363(8): 711-23.

[126] Ahmadzadeh M, Johnson LA, Heemskerk B, Wunderlich JR, Dudley ME, White DE, *et al.* Tumor antigen-specific CD8 T cells infiltrating the tumor express high levels of PD-1 and are functionally impaired. Blood 2009; 114(8): 1537-44.

[127] Nishimura H, Okazaki T, Tanaka Y, Nakatani K, Hara M, Matsumori A, *et al.* Autoimmune dilated cardiomyopathy in PD-1 receptor-deficient mice. Science 2001; 291(5502): 319-22.

[128] Nishimura H, Nose M, Hiai H, Minato N, Honjo T. Development of lupus-like autoimmune diseases by disruption of the PD-1 gene encoding an ITIM motif-carrying immunoreceptor. Immunity 1999; 11(2): 141-51.

[129] Keir ME, Butte MJ, Freeman GJ, Sharpe AH. PD-1 and its ligands in tolerance and immunity. Annu Rev Immunol 2008; 26: 677-704.

[130] Brahmer JR, Tykodi SS, Chow LQ, Hwu WJ, Topalian SL, Hwu P, *et al.* Safety and activity of anti-PD-L1 antibody in patients with advanced cancer. N Engl J Med 2012; 366(26): 2455-65.

[131] Peggs KS, Quezada SA, Allison JP. Cancer immunotherapy: co-stimulatory agonists and co-inhibitory antagonists. Clin Exp Immunol 2009; 157(1): 9-19.

[132] Overwijk WW, Theoret MR, Finkelstein SE, Surman DR, de Jong LA, Vyth-Dreese FA, *et al.* Tumor regression and autoimmunity after reversal of a functionally tolerant state of self-reactive CD8+ T cells. J Exp Med 2003; 198(4): 569-80.

[133] Lou Y, Wang G, Lizee G, Kim GJ, Finkelstein SE, Feng C, *et al.* Dendritic cells strongly boost the antitumor activity of adoptively transferred T cells *in vivo*. Cancer Res 2004; 64(18): 6783-90.

[134] Song XT, Turnis M, Zhou X, Zhu W, Hong B, Rolins L, *et al.* A Th1-inducing adenoviral vaccine for boosting adoptively transferred T cells. Molecular Therapy 2010; 19(1): 211-7.

[135] Leen AM, Rooney CM, Foster AE. Improving T cell therapy for cancer. Annu Rev Immunol 2007; 25: 243-65.

[136] Ohta A, Gorelik E, Prasad SJ, Ronchese F, Lukashev D, Wong MK, *et al.* A2A adenosine receptor protects tumors from antitumor T cells. Proc Natl Acad Sci U S A 2006; 103(35): 13132-7.

[137] Sitkovsky MV, Kjaergaard J, Lukashev D, Ohta A. Hypoxia-adenosinergic immunosuppression: tumor protection by T regulatory cells and cancerous tissue hypoxia. Clin Cancer Res 2008; 14(19): 5947-52.

[138] Cirri P, Chiarugi P. Cancer associated fibroblasts: the dark side of the coin. Am J Cancer Res 2011; 1(4): 482-97.

[139] Kakarla S, Song XT, Gottschalk S. Cancer-associated fibroblasts as targets for immunotherapy. Immunotherapy 2012; 4(11): 1129-38.

[140] Kakarla S, Chow KK, Mata M, Shaffer DR, Song XT, Wu MF, *et al.* Antitumor effects of chimeric receptor engineered human T cells directed to tumor stroma. Mol Ther 2013; 21(8): 1611-20.

## CHAPTER 3

# NK Cell-Based Immunotherapy

**Adam W. Mailloux and Pearlie K. Epling-Burnette***

*H. Lee Moffitt Cancer Center, SRB 23033, Tampa, FL 33612, USA*

**Abstract:** The debate has been raging for many years about the immune system's ability to identify and destroy emerging tumor cells, and to thereby act as a barrier to cancer development. Investigators have now used both murine models and human studies to offer convincing evidence in support of this concept. Accumulating information about the particular effector molecules and immune cell types involved in this process has formed the basis for rational design of immunotherapies. Both T lymphocytes and Natural killer (NK) cells participate in cancer immune surveillance. Intricate effector mechanisms are involved in providing protection against both malignant and virally infected cells. Our vision of NK cells as therapeutic agents has evolved from the seminal discovery of inhibitory and activating NK receptors. NK cells can recognize tumor cells while preserving normal self, and the understanding of the mechanisms allowing for this preferential recognition pattern has greatly impacted the success of stem cell therapy and immunotherapy. Two main strategies are used by NK cells to recognize tumor targets. A number of tumor cells down-regulate major histocompatibility complex (MHC) class I molecules, protecting against T-cell recognition but releasing the inhibitory breaks in NK cells. The balance of activating and inhibitory NK receptor signals determines whether nascent tumor cells will be recognized and destroyed. In this chapter, the concepts of immune surveillance, immunoediting and NK immunotherapy are discussed. Effective NK immunotherapy may become a reality for many types of cancers in the near future.

**Keywords:** Activation-dependent cellular cytotoxicity, adaptor molecules, adoptive cell therapy, apoptosis, cancer, cytokines, cytotoxicity, immune surveillance, immunoediting, immunotherapy, interferon, interleukin, lymphocyte, killer immunoglobulin-like receptor, major histocompatibility complex, natural killer cell, natural killer cell receptor, signaling, stem cell transplantation, tumor necrosis factor.

## IMMUNE SURVEILLANCE AND THE RATIONALE FOR IMMUNOTHERAPY

### General Principle of Immune Surveillance

The idea that transformed cells are continuously generated, but largely destroyed

***Corresponding author Pearlie K. Epling-Burnette:** H. Lee Moffitt Cancer Center, SRB 23033, Tampa, FL 33612, USA; Tel: 813-745-6177; E-mail: Pearlie.Burnette@moffitt.org

**Jianxun Song (Ed)**

by the immune system through a process of surveillance, was conceived as far back as 1909 [1]. While the role of the immune system in cancer immune surveillance has evolved to a new understanding, there are still difficult concepts to be addressed because tumors, by derivation, represent self. Therefore, these tissues should be non-immunogenic. It is this simplistic logic that prevented meaningful research on tumor immunity for some time. The scientific community challenged the idea of cancer immune surveillance due to the dogma of self-immune privilege. The first evidence supporting the theory of immune surveillance was founded nearly fifty years later when experiments in tumor transplant models suggested that immune reactions against cancer could indeed take place [2]. Identification of immunogenic tumor antigens soon followed [3, 4], but immune surveillance as a theory remained controversial. In the 1990s, when cancer was studied in animal models lacking specific immune components, the concept of tumor immune surveillance became fully appreciated.

One of the earliest approaches used to study the role of the immune system in tumor rejection was carried out with neonatal thymectomy. However, studies of tumor growth in athymic mice produced inconclusive evidence in support of the immune surveillance theory. These early models tested both chemically induced [5, 6] and spontaneous types of cancer [7, 8]. Later, the advent of athymic nude mice, with genetic elimination of key immunologic components, broadened these studies. Again, murine experiments failed to definitively support the concept of cancer immune surveillance. There was no difference in cancer incidence or tumor growth in these immunodeficient mice compared to wild-type mice [9-11], which perpetuated further doubt in the immune surveillance theory.

Athymic mouse models were then shown to retain a significant population of T-cells with functional αβ T-cell receptors [12, 13]. Together with the discovery that γδ T-cells may be thymus-independent [14], the immune deficient status of athymic mouse models came into question. Additionally, it became apparent that the athymic mouse models studied were abnormally sensitive to the particular chemical carcinogen used. In mice, methylcholanthrene is not carcinogenic in its native form. Instead, it becomes carcinogenic through the action of the enzyme aryl hydrocarbon hydroxylase system [15]. It was finally concluded later that the CBA/H mouse strain used in these early studies produces an aryl hydrocarbon hydroxylase isoform with unusually high activity. These mice were so beset with carcinogenesis that immune surveillance potential was overwhelmed [16].

Another immunodeficient animal model, CB-17, was then examined for immune surveillance. CB-17 is a mouse strain with severe-combined immune deficiency

(SCID) and chemically-induced tumors were found to occur significantly more frequently in these mice as compared to wild type controls (BALBc) [17]. Hence, studies in this model yielded different results from the athymic mouse models and were among the first to support the theory of immune surveillance. However, just like its athymic counterparts, the SCID mouse model contained a non-immunological variable which could affect tumor growth. SCID mice have no the active subunit of the DNA-dependant protein kinase enzyme preventing the proper rearrangement of various antigen receptors in lymphocytes [18]. The end result is dysfunctional adaptive immunity, but this same genetic defect also prevents the repair of double-stranded DNA breaks in normal stroma [19], which could ultimately lead to higher incidence of spontaneous cell transformation in SCID mice. This observation cast doubt on the interpretation of the SCID mouse model data.

Ultimately, the immune surveillance model was definitively proven in an animal model in 2001. Mice missing recombination activating gene 1 (RAG-1) and RAG-2 lack all functional natural killer cells (NK), natural killer T-cells (NKT), B, and T lymphocytes while retaining the function of DNA repair mechanisms in non-lymphoid cells [20]. Chemically-induced tumor growth in these mice occurred more rapidly and frequently than in wild type controls, and for the first time, provided irrefutable proof of immune surveillance in an animal model [21]. To date, no evidence exists that these mice have any non-immunological reasons for increased tumor occurrence.

Immune surveillance is now considered as the initial step in the larger process of immunoediting in which transformed cells may be cleared by the immune system. If immune surveillance should fail, an extended period of equilibrium may then ensue, in which selective pressure from the immune system balances oncogenic drift and clonal evolution. Eventually, the neoplasm may escape immune detection all together [22, 23]. This last step also coincides with the onset of active tumor-induced immune suppressive mechanisms, which has been well reviewed [24]. While the canonical effector cells of immunoediting have traditionally been T-cells, it is now well appreciated that innate immunity plays a large role in immune surveillance and clonal evolution [25].

## Role of T-Cells in Immune Surveillance

Additional evidence of immune surveillance comes from the selective depletion of specific subsets of immune cells while leaving the rest of the immune system relatively intact. These types of studies reveal the individual contributions of each respective cell type toward the overall effect of immune surveillance. Furthermore, these studies highlight cell populations with potential benefit when used in cell-based immune therapies against cancer in humans.

The quintessential effector cells for adaptive immunity are T-cells, and indeed these cells commonly infiltrate solid tumors and make up large percentages of the total tumor-infiltrating lymphocytes (TIL). Their presence is a positive prognostic factor for melanoma [26-28], breast cancer [29], bladder cancer [30], colorectal cancer [31-33], prostatic carcinomas [34], adenocarcinomas [35], and glioblastomas/gilomas [36]. Depletion of all T-cells by injecting anti-Thy1 antibody into a mouse results in increased tumor occurrence and growth in a chemically-induced mouse model of cancer, indicating that adaptive effector immunity is involved in immune surveillance [37]. More specifically, depletion of either $CD4^+$ or $CD8^+$ cells inhibited the rejection of transplanted tumors in wild-type mice [22], meaning that both $CD4^+$ helper T-cells ($T_H$) and $CD8^+$ cytotoxic T cells ($T_C$) play important roles in immune surveillance. Furthermore, specific subsets of T-cells were tested by developing transgenic mice lacking the TCRβ gene or the TCRγ gene. Both types of mice displayed increased tumor incidence and growth in fibrosarcoma and spindle cell carcinoma models. However, only the $TCR\gamma^{-/-}$ mice displayed increased tumor incidence and growth in a chemically-induced skin carcinogenesis model [38]. This means that while both αβ and γδ T-cells can play a role in immune surveillance, the contribution of either may vary between cancer types.

## Evidence of NK Cell Involvement in Immune Surveillance

The contributions of specific components of innate immunity toward immune surveillance have also been investigated. Injection of anti-NK1.1 antibody in mice systemically depletes both NK and NKT cells [39]. Mice injected with this antibody generated between two and three times as many chemically-induced tumors as injected controls. Injection of anti-asialo-GM-1 antibody was used to deplete NK cells without affecting NKT cells. Mice injected with this antibody produced identical results to those injected with the anti-NK1.1 antibody, suggesting that NK cells can play the larger role in innate immune surveillance [39]. However, another study utilizing $J\alpha281^{-/-}$ mice, which only lack NKT cells, showed that these mice displayed higher levels of the same chemically-induced tumors as compared to normal controls [37]. Hence, the extent to which NKT cells contribute to immune surveillance is somewhat unclear. Recent work in liver cancer indicates that both NK and NKT play significant roles in immunosurveillance against *de novo* hepatocarcinogenesis [40]. Both NK and NKT cells display heightened constitutive activity compared to their peripheral counterparts, priming them for anti-tumor activity [40-43]. Importantly, the activity of NKT cells in this setting appears to be the production of pro-inflammatory cytokines such as IFN-γ, IL-4, IL-5, IL-13, and TNF-α [40, 41]. This cascade of cytokine production plays a supportive role in downstream NK anti-hepatocellular carcinoma cytotoxicity [44]. It is possible, then, that the increased tumor growth observed in $J\alpha281^{-/-}$ mice may result from the depletion of an NK-supporting cell population, as opposed to the loss of a directly cytotoxic population.

In contrast to NKT cells, NK cells have a profound effect on tumor occurrence. The accelerated tumor growth in mice lacking NK cells seen in these studies [37, 39] appears to be greater than the accelerated tumor growth in mice that lack all or specific types of T-cells [22, 37, 38]. This may indicate that innate effector immunity contributes more toward cancer surveillance than adaptive immunity, although the relative importance may vary between tumor models.

## Effector Mechanisms

Effector cells kill tumor cells through a variety of mechanisms as shown in Fig. **1**.

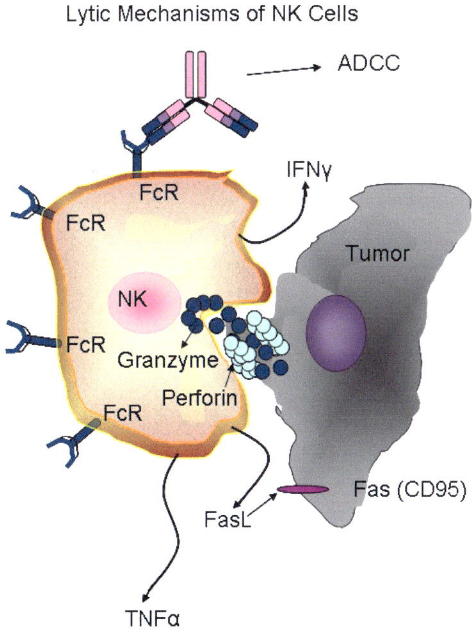


**Figure 1: Lytic Mechanisms.** Mechanisms of tumor killing include antibody dependent cellular cytotoxicity (ADCC), interferon γ and TNFα release, production of FasL and mobilization of lytic granules including granzyme and perforin.

### *IFNγ*

The first experiments to manipulate effector mechanisms of immunity were those that targeted various cytokines associated with tumor immunity. Interferon-gamma (IFN-γ) is secreted by activated antigen-specific T-cells and by activated NK cells. Initiation of this cytokine-mediated cascade of inflammatory events is necessary for beneficial immune response against cancer [45]. In this manner, IFN-γ represents a vital first step in both adaptive and innate immune effector responses. In 1994, antibody-mediated neutralization of endogenous IFN-γ significantly increased the growth of transplanted tumors, while the overexpression of a dominant negative mutation of the IFN-γ receptor α subunit ablated the protective effect of endogenous IFN-γ in both chemically-induced and spontaneous murine tumor models [46]. Similar results were later observed for chemically-induced tumors in mice genetically lacking functional STAT-1, which is required for IFN-γ signal transduction [47]. Finally, IFN-$\gamma^{-/-}$ mice developed a higher incidence of spontaneous lymphomas compared to normal controls [48]. Together, these studies implicate the IFN-γ signaling axis in immune surveillance.

### *IL-12*

Another cytokine involved in beneficial anti-tumor immune response is interleukin-12 (IL-12). IL-12 is secreted by activated effector cells including $T_H$, $T_C$, and NK cells, and is vital for initiating and maintaining a beneficial type-1 immune response and avoiding a suppressive type-2 immune response [49-51]. In chemically induced tumor models, IL-$12^{-/-}$ mice were more susceptible to tumor growth and incidence as compared to wild-type controls [37]. Conversely, wild-type mice that were given exogenous IL-12 at high doses had lower incidence of chemically-induced tumor formation, and exhibited slower growth after onset compared to normal controls [52]. Because IL-12 plays such a crucial role in orchestrating effector populations, these data suggest that an organized and active immune response is required for immune surveillance, as opposed to the mere presence of lymphocytes.

### *Cytotoxic Granules*

While not a cytokine, the secreted protein perforin is essential to cell-mediated cytotoxicity in the context of NK and $T_C$ effector response. Upon recognition of target cells, both $T_C$ and NK cells release lytic granules into the immune synapse [53]. Among other proteins, perforin acts to lyse the target cell by inserting itself into the lipid bilayer and polymerizing in an ever-growing pore. This pore contributes toward cell lysis and allows other lytic proteins to enter the target cell.

Perforin$^{-/-}$ mice displayed higher incidence of chemically-induced tumor formation and growth as compared to wild-type controls [37, 54, 55]. These mice also displayed higher rates of spontaneous lymphomas [56] and lung adenocarcinomas [48] as compared to wild-type controls. Other key components of this granule exocytosis pathway are granzymes A and B, which serve to release pro-inflammatory cytokines [57] and initiate the target cell's intrinsic apoptosis pathways, respectively [58-60]. Effector lymphocyte killing is greatly impaired in cells lacking granzyme B [61, 62]. However, mice lacking either granzyme A or B have yet to display increased incidence of carcinogenesis or tumor growth [48, 63-67], possibly due to a level of redundancy between existing granzymes.

### *Apoptotic Death Pathway*

Molecules involved in the lytic capabilities of effector cells include members of the Tumor necrosis factor (TNF) superfamily including TNFα and the TNF-related apoptosis-inducing ligand (TRAIL). Expression of these molecules is induced on monocytes, NK cells, and dendritic cells during activation [68], and upon ligation with its receptor on target cells, TRAIL induces rapid extrinsic apoptosis. Mice that genetically lack TRAIL generate fibrosarcomas at higher rates than do wild-type control mice [69]. Similar results were obtained when mice were injected with a neutralizing antibody to TRAIL [70]. Another TNF-family protein, CD95/Fas, can also induce extrinsic apoptosis upon ligation to Fas ligand (FasL), and is a major route of cellular cytotoxicity in NK cells [71]. In general, TRAIL and Fas-mediated apoptosis are dependent on the expression of adhesion molecules and on the expression of death receptors, but are independent of inhibitory NK cell receptor expression [72]. In the context of cancer, it is clear that NK cells use both perforin and FasL to kill target cancer cells, but in the case of murine renal cancer, perforin-mediated cytotoxicity prevails [73].

Collectively, these data indicate that immune surveillance depends on lytic function mediated by the apoptotic death pathway, death receptors, and cytokines in both innate and adaptive immune effector cells. A tabulated summary of the evidence supporting immune surveillance in mice can be found in Table **1**.

**Table 1:** Evidence for immune surveillance in mice

| Model | Effect | Cancer Type(s) | Reference(s) |
|---|---|---|---|
| RAG 2 -/- | Lacks T, B, and NKT cells | MCA induced sarcoma | [21] |
| | | Spontaneous intestinal neoplasia | |
| RAG 1-/- | Lacks T, B, and NKT cells | MCA induced sarcoma | [39] |
| | | Spontaneous intestinal neoplasia | |

***Table 1: 1 cont….***

| | | | |
|---|---|---|---|
| RAG 2-/-; STAT1-/- | Lacks T, B, and NKT cells | MCA induced sarcoma | [21] |
| | Lacks IFN α,β,γ signaling | Spontaneous intestinal neoplasia | |
| | | Spontaneous mammary neoplasia | |
| SCID | Lacks T, B, and NKT cells | MCA induced sarcoma | [39] |
| Perforin -/- | Lacks Perforin | MCA induced sarcoma | [37, 48, 54-56] |
| | | Spontaneous lymphoma | |
| TCR Jα281 -/- | Lacks NKT cells | MCA induced sarcoma | [37, 39, 54] |
| α asialo GM1 ab | Lacks NK cells | MCA induced sarcoma | [39] |
| α NK1.1 ab | Lacks NK, NKT cells | MCA induced sarcoma | [37, 39] |
| α Thy1 ab | Lacks T cells | MCA induced sarcoma | [37] |
| αβ T cell -/- | Lacks αβ T cells | MCA induced sarcoma | [38] |
| γδ T cell -/- | Lacks γδ T cells | MCA induced sarcoma | [38] |
| STAT -/- | Lacks IFN α,β,γ signaling | MCA induced sarcoma | [21, 47] |
| STAT1-/-; p53-/- | Lacks IFN α,β,γ signaling | Many transplant models | [47] |
| | | Lacks apoptosis | |
| IFNγR1 receptor -/- | Lacks IFN α,β,γ signaling | MCA induced sarcoma | [21, 47] |
| | | Many transplant models | |
| IFN γ-/- | Lacks IFN γ | MCA induced sarcoma | [48, 54] |
| | | Spontaneous lymphoma | |
| | | Spontaneous lung adenocarcinoma | |
| Perforin-/-; IFNγ-/- | Lacks Perforin, IFN γ | MCA induced sarcoma | [48, 54] |
| | | Spontaneous lymphoma | |
| IL-12-/- | Lacks IL 12 | MCA induced sarcoma | [37] |
| IL-12 | Exogenous IL 12 | MCA induced sarcoma | [52] |
| LMP2 -/- | Lacks LMP2 subunit | Spontaneous uterine neoplasm | [74] |
| GM-CSF-/-; IFNγ-/- | Lacks GM CSF, IFN γ | Spontaneous lymphoma | [75] |
| | | Many transplant models | |
| TRAIL-/- | Lacks TRAIL | MCA induced sarcoma | [69] |
| α TRAIL ab | Lacks TRAIL signaling | MCA induced sarcoma | [70] |
| | | Spontaneous lymphoma | |
| | | Spontaneous sarcoma | |
| α GalCer | Lacks NKT cell activation | MCA induced sarcoma | [76] |

Abbreviations not defined in text: antibody (ab); granulocyte-macrophage colony stimulating factor (GM CSF); methylcholanthrene (MCA).

If immune surveillance exists in mice, then it is easy to predict that immune surveillance also exists in humans, although there is an obvious difficulty in proving this hypothesis. However, unfortunate situations exist where humans enter an immune-deficient state and studies indicate that these patients are more susceptible to cancer. Allogeneic stem cell transplant recipients given immunosuppressive drug regimens are at significantly higher risk of carcinogenesis [77]. The same is true of patients with primary immunodeficiencies such as acquired immune deficiency syndrome (AIDS) [78]. As early immune-deficient mouse models proved difficult to interpret, these human studies have also been plagued with difficulties including independent variables that explain higher cancer rates. The vast majority of cancers occur in the setting of a viral etiology. The fact that immune-suppressed individuals are at greater risk of viral infection sheds doubt on the argument of immune surveillance [79-81]. Additionally, immune clearance of cancer cells with viral etiologies post-carcinogenesis could be attributed to immune reactions against viral antigens, and not to the existence of immune surveillance. In response to these questions, studies were conducted in cancers with non-viral etiology, and immune-deficient patients were confirmed to be at greater risk for the *de novo* genesis of melanoma [82, 83] and for non-Kaposi's sarcomas [84]. These studies provide strong evidence that immune surveillance exists in humans.

## A CASE FOR INNATE IMMUNITY FOR THEREPEUTIC INTERVENTION

The idea of a tumor vaccine has great appeal, and if successful, the immunological memory resulting from such efforts could protect from future neoplasms. However, there are both pros and cons to pursuing adaptive immunotherapy that must be considered. First, adaptive immunotherapy requires detailed knowledge of tumor antigen expression and presentation. To achieve an effective T-cell response, an adequately immunogenic antigen must be identified that is ubiquitously expressed on tumor cells, but that is also absent or significantly reduced in healthy tissue to avoid destructive autoimmunity. The identification of such antigens has been proceeding over the last few decades, and when found, these antigens often display great variability in expression from patient to patient. Another difficulty facing adaptive immunotherapies is the requirement for adequate major histocompatibility complex (MHC) expression, which is required for tumor antigen presentation. The loss of MHC expression is one of the most widely described mechanisms for tumor immune escape [85-87]. This is not to completely discount peptide-based vaccine attempts, as some successes have been obtained. In particular, vaccines targeting the melanoma antigens have shown therapeutic potential [88]. Unfortunately, the vast majority of peptide-based vaccination attempts against established tumors have been unsuccessful. Lastly, clonal evolution or antigen shedding can lead to immunotherapy-resistant variants. To be curative, antigen-specific approaches must eliminate all cancer cells in a single adaptive immune response to avoid the resurgence of antigen negative clones.

In contrast to T-cells, NK cells do not require specific antigen presentation to elicit cytoxicity, but instead rely on a delicate balance of activating and inhibitory signals given by NK-cell receptors bearing immunoreceptor tyrosine-based activation motifs (ITAMs) or immunoreceptor tyrosine-based inhibitory motifs (ITIMs), respectively. In the setting of the tumor microenvironment, the cognate ligands for these receptors can be found not only on tumor cells, but also on surrounding stroma and bystander immune infiltrate. Importantly, MHC class I (MHC-I; HLA class I, or HLA-1 in humans) serves as a major ligand for a large number of the inhibitory killer cell immunoglobulin-like receptor (KIR) family of NK cell receptors. The aforementioned loss of MHC-I on tumor cells that circumvents adaptive immunity actually sensitizes tumor cells to NK cell-mediated cytotoxicity by virtue of lost inhibitory KIR signaling [89, 90], thereby tipping the positive/negative signaling balance toward cytotoxic response (Fig. **2**). The expression of KIRs is inherited by a stochastic process due to extensive polymorphism among KIR haplotypes reflecting not only differing nucleotide sequences, but also gene content [91]. Individuals with little to no activating KIR genes (A haplotype) have a low probability of expressing activating KIRs on any given NK cell, while individuals with multiple activating KIR genes (B haplotype) have a higher probability of expressing activating KIRs on any given NK cell. This results in great variability from person to person regarding NK cell responsiveness to specific HLA-1 types. In a process similar to T-cells, NK cells undergo a selection process during maturation that ensures the presence of at least one inhibitory KIR specific for self HLA-1 [92]. The overall responsiveness of NK is largely determined by the presence and strength of KIR/HLA interaction. Cells with low or mismatched HLA display greater susceptibility to NK cytotoxicity in the presence of activating NK signals. This aspect of basic NK cell biology raises the intriguing possibility of utilizing NK cells from slightly mismatched donors to artificially introduce a KIR/HLA mismatch in cancer patients. This can be done without the need for an exhaustive search for tumor-specific antigens. In the setting of matched KIR/HLA, NK cells with high levels of inhibitory KIR expression are poised to respond in the event of reduced inhibitory signaling or elevated activating signaling. These cells are said to be "licensed" or "armed" [93, 94] displaying a greater potential for cytotoxic response despite the greater level of inhibitory KIR safeguards. In contrast, NK cells expressing low inhibitory KIR expression develop a hyporesponsive state [93], presumably to avoid autoimmune cytotoxicity. The process of dampening the responsiveness of NK cells lacking cognate inhibitory KIRs has been termed "NK cell education" [95] and is somewhat analogous to the selection T-cells undergo during maturation in the thymus, using self-HLA recognition in place of self-antigen presentation. Importantly, these hyporesponsive NK cells can become responsive under enforced activation with high dose IL-2 [93, 96] creating an easy opportunity to overcome NK tolerance *ex vivo* during any adoptive cell transfer (ACT) based therapy.

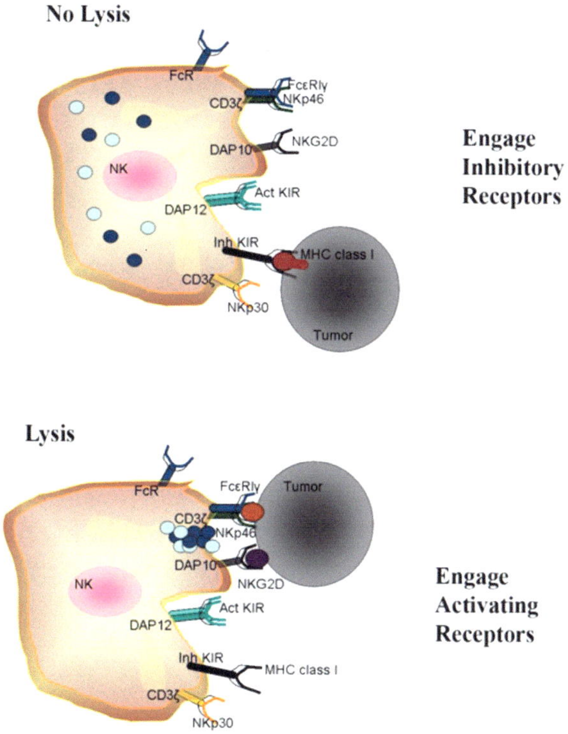


**Figure 2: Control of NK receptor cytolytic activity.** (No Lysis) There is a critical relationship between the interaction and signaling events which lead to lysis or protection of tumor cells. NK cells with unpolarized cytotoxic granules can be found when there is engagement of inhibitory KIR or NKG2 family receptors with MHC class I on the tumor cells. This activated SHP1, which blocks propagation of intracellular signals. (Lysis) Cytolytic activity is induced in the absence of inhibitory signals when activating receptors are engaged. This leads to a signaling cascade mediated by activating adaptor molecules and polarized granule mobilization.

MHC-class I-binding receptors in the murine genome consist of the Ly49 molecules. Like KIR, Ly49 exist in both inhibitory and activating variants.

Ly49A-function was severely reduced in mice with a SHP-1 deficiency [97] and ITIMs of the inhibitory Ly49 receptors bind SHP-1 in similar fashion to inhibitory KIR molecules in humans.

Activating forms of KIR possess a truncated cytoplasmic region, lack ITIM domains [98], and have intracellular ITAMs that comprise two copies of the Yxx(I/L) motif that is precisely spaced six or seven residues apart [99, 100]. Activating KIRs, and other NK activating receptors, associate with a unique adaptor molecule known as DAP12 [101], as shown in Fig. **2**. DAP12 phosphorylation leads to a downstream signaling cascade mediated by ZAP-70 and Syk protein tyrosine kinases and MAPK [102]. In addition to activating KIR and FcR, there is another family of C-lectin-like receptors known as the NKG2-family [103, 104]. This family consists of inhibitory receptors NKG2A, B, E and F, which form a heterodimer with CD94 to recognize the non-classical HLA-E molecule [105], and activating receptors NKG2D and C. The best-characterized of all NK receptor ligands are the stress-inducible MHC class I-restricted chain A (MICA), MICB, and UL16-binding proteins (ULBPs) in humans and Rae-1 in mouse that bind NKG2D [106-110]. NKG2D ligands show stress-related induction by viruses and tumor cells [111, 112]. Cytotoxicity by NKG2D is coupled to the transmembrane adaptor DAP10 for intracellular signaling which delivers cytotoxicity to the tumor. The most potent NK activating molecules include the natural cytotoxicity receptor (NCR) family including NKp46, NKp30, and an inducible receptor NKp44 [113-115]. These receptors trigger tumor cell lysis of many targets by associating with ITAM-containing adaptors, including CD3ζ/FcγR heterodimers, CD3ζ homodimers, and DAP12, as shown in Fig. **2**. These receptors also present cooperation to widen the target range of cytotoxic killing, but specific ligands recognized by these receptors are largely unidentified.

## ADOPTIVE NK CELL TRANSFER AND HEMATOPOETIC STEM CELL TRANSPLANT

Compared to T-cells, NK cells are more easily expanded and activated *ex vivo*. In addition, their shorter lifespan of approximately one month [116] eliminates the fear of prolonged autoimmune induction as an unwanted side effect of NK cell-based therapy. These facts, coupled with the non-antigen specific nature of NK cell cytotoxicity, make the direct application of NK cells an attractive therapeutic strategy for cancer. Autologous NK cells, or NK cells from a HLA matched (or slightly mismatched) donor, can either be delivered directly through adoptive cell transfer (ACT), or reconstituted following hematopoietic stem cell transplant (HSCT), a treatment already native to the standard of care for numerous hematopoietic malignancies. In the case of HSCT, the primary goal is to replace the failing or neoplastic marrow with healthy marrow. Upon reconstitution, the transplanted immune cells may recognize residual tumor and mount an anti-tumor response. This secondary graft-*versus*-tumor (GVT) effect, while beneficial, must be balanced against the possibility of graft-*versus*-host disease (GVHD) in which the graft immune cells attack the healthy normal tissue of the recipient. Often, donor marrow is depleted of T-cells *ex vivo* prior to transplant to help safeguard against GVHD. Unfortunately this also significantly reduces any GVT effect of the HSCT [117]. NK cells are among the first lymphocytes to reconstitute following HSCT, but contribute much less to GVHD than donor T-cells [118]. As such, efforts can be made to utilize donor NK cells to augment the GVT effect of the HSCT. In a retrospective study in which acute myeloid leukemia (AML) patients received HLA-matched HSCT, a greater incidence of tumor relapse was observed in cases where the donor KIR haplotype did not match with the recipient's [119], presumably due to inability of the KIRs on donor NK cells to bind recipient HLA. This data directed investigators to carefully study KIR/KIR matching in the setting of HSCT for AML. Here, it was found that recipient patients with heterozygous HLA-Cw genes (and therefore providing greater opportunity for HLA recognition by KIRs) have significantly worse survival and higher relapse rates compared to homozygous patients [120].

These observations in AML paved the way for studies utilizing direct allogeneic NK adoptive cell therapy. Successful expansion of haploidentical NK cells was first demonstrated in 2005 in a group of patients with metastatic melanoma, renal cell carcinoma, refractory Hodgkin's disease, and refractory AML. The expansion of donor NK cells required high-dose cyclophosphamide and fludarabine regimes to be administered to the recipient prior to adoptive cell therapy. This established the need for lymphodepletion in order to create an available niche for transferred NK cells, and to reduce the competition for homeostatic resources. While only 10% of all patients displayed substantial donor NK cell expansion, that 10% experienced significant anti-tumor effects. This included 30% of AML patients with poor prognosis, who achieved a complete remission. These responding patients displayed higher numbers of circulating donor NK cells compared to non-responding patients suggesting the expansion and persistence of transferred NK cells is required for sustained anti-tumor immunity [121]. Surprisingly, donor/recipient KIR mismatch did not correlate with response to NK adoptive cell therapy in this study. This is perhaps due to the spike in IL-15 observed after lymphodepletion. IL-15 is rudimentary to NK cell homeostatic reconstitution [122], and may have the ability to temporarily alter the expression ratios of KIRs on proliferating NK cells [123]. Despite the inconsistent findings regarding donor/recipient KIR mismatch between HSCT and adoptive cell therapy in this study, future NK infusion studies will likely continue to develop intentional KIR/KIR mismatch as a potential mechanism to enhance anti-tumor activity. Early indications are encouraging, despite the need for continual co-administration of IL-2 [124]. The success of NK-based cellular therapies will depend upon the optimization of donor NK expansion and persistence. It has been suggested that clonal NK cell lines such as NK-92 can be used in lieu of primary NK cells. NK-92 cells lack KIR expression [125], which allows for cytotoxicity against a wide range of malignancies. This approach has the advantage of an inexhaustible source of infusible cells, and less tolerizable NK activity. Irradiated NK-92 adoptive cell therapy has demonstrated safety and some efficacy in a small number of patients [126]. The obvious drawback to this approach is the inherent danger of infusing a patient with a transformed cell line. Further development of this approach may require safeguards to be genetically introduced into NK-92 cells such as the conditional expression of diphtheria toxin receptor to safe guard against this potential risk. In addition, NK-92 cells are dependent on IL-2, making any hypothetical sustained infusion of NK-92 cells dependent on repeated IL-2 injection, which raises toxicity concerns. Variants of the NK-92 cell line displaying independence from IL-2 could be considered for future efforts [127].

## AUGMENTING THE ENDOGENOUS NK CELL RESPONSE

As an alternative to administering new or additional NK cell populations to the patient, many therapies aim to augment endogenous NK populations. NK cell activation and cytotoxicity is highly influenced by contextual cytokines, particularly IL-2, IL-15, IL-12, IL-18, and type I interferon (IFN), and exogenous administration of these cytokines can increase NK activity. Of these, IL-15 is critical for NK development, homeostasis, and survival as IL-15$^{-/-}$ mice lack measureable levels of NK populations and are unable to sustain adoptively transferred wild-type NK cells [128]. The IL-2 receptor shares common $\beta$ and $\gamma$ chains with the IL-15 receptor $\alpha$ chain, which is upregulated during NK cell activation. IL-2 signaling is essential for the induction of lymphokine-activated killer (LAK) activity, and a sustained anti-tumor response relies on continual IL-2 bioavailability [129]. Treatment of cancer patients with IL-2 has demonstrated promising results and is FDA approved for renal cell carcinoma and melanoma. Responding patients demonstrate increased circulating NK numbers, increased NK cytotoxicity, and increased overall survival [130]. However, the toxicity of repeated IL-2 administration is problematic, and thus limits the duration of beneficial increased NK activity to a single IL-2 dose [131]. Administration of IL-15 may provide an alternative to the toxicity seen with repeated doses of IL-2, where it may elicit effective NK activity without the IL-2-associated induction of regulatory T-cells (Tregs) [132]. Clinical trials are currently underway to test the safety and efficacy of intravenous IL-15 administration. The best result may occur through combinations of cytokines. Specifically, IL-12, IL-15, and IL-18 combination was able to provide superior tumoricidal activity in an established murine tumor model of T-cell lymphoma after a single injection. The NK response appeared somewhat sustained, although the effect was dependent on the co-administration of radiation therapy [133].

In addition to direct tumor cytotoxicity, NK cells also serve as a final effector population for antibody-dependent cell-mediated cytotoxicity (ADCC), which constitutes another facet of immunotherapeutic efforts aimed at increasing NK activity to combat cancer. CD16, otherwise known as FcγRIIIa, is transmembrane receptor with high affinity for the FC region of antibodies that is highly expressed on NK cells. Through CD16, NK calls can bind and recognize opsonized cells targeted for cytotoxic destruction [134]. Monoclonal antibodies (mAb) that target tumor-specific antigens can be used to induce ADCC. Successful examples include antibodies targeting CD20 (rituximab), Her2/neu (herceptin), epithelial growth factor receptor (cetuximab), and disialoganglioside (GD2) [135-139]. While not all of the anti-tumor effects of these antibodies can be attributed to ADCC, it is clear that at least a significant portion of the beneficial effects are NK cell dependent. Efforts to enhance the ADCC inducing capability of mAb treatments have been studied in the pre-clinical setting including the co-administration of toll-like rector (TLR) agonists, or functional cross-linking antibodies directed against activating NK cell receptors. CpG, a TLR9 agonist, has been shown to increase NK activity when administered with rituximab in mice with $CD20^+$ orthotropic malignancy [140], and agonistic mAb directed against 4-1BB, an activating NK cell receptor, increases the efficacy of rituximab in murine B-cell lymphoma [141].

## SUMMARY

With many exciting advances in support of the hypothesis of cancer immune surveillance, it is only natural that studies will identify new approaches to harvest the power of the immune system to fight against cancer. Effective cancer immunotherapy may become a reality for many types of tumors. Using new advances in immunotherapy, survival advantage may be recognized in tumors that are currently unresponsive to chemotherapy and radiation.

## ACKNOWLEDGEMENT

Declared None.

## CONFLICT OF INTEREST

The authors confirm that this chapter contents have no conflict of interest.

## REFERENCES

[1] Ehrlich P. Ueber den jetzigen stand der karzinomforschung. Ned Tijdschr Geneeskd 1909; 5(5): 73-290.

[2] Burnet M. Cancer; a biological approach. I. The processes of control. Br Med J 1957; 1(5022): 779-86.

[3] Klein G. Tumor antigens. Annu Rev Microbiol 1966; 20: 223-52.

[4] Old LJ, Boyse EA. Immunology of Experimental Tumors. Annu Rev Med 1964; 15: 167-86.

[5] Grant GA, Miller JF. Effect of neonatal thymectomy on the induction of sarcomata in C57 BL mice. Nature 1965; 205(976): 1124-5.

[6] Trainin N, Linker-Israeli M, Small M, Boiato-Chen L. Enhancement of lung adenoma formation by neonatal thymectomy in mice treated with 7,12-dimethylbenz(a)anthracene or urethan. Int J Cancer 1967; 2(4): 326-36.

[7] Burstein NA, Law LW. Neonatal thymectomy and non-viral mammary tumours in mice. Nature 1971; 231(5303): 450-2.

[8] Sanford BH, Kohn HI, Daly JJ, Soo SF. Long-term spontaneous tumor incidence in neonatally thymectomized mice. J Immunol 1973; 110(5): 1437-9.

[9] Rygaard J, Povlsen CO. The mouse mutant nude does not develop spontaneous tumours. An argument against immunological surveillance. Acta Pathol Microbiol Scand [B] Microbiol Immunol 1974; 82(1): 99-106.

[10] Rygaard J, Povlsen CO. Is immunological surveillance not a cell-mediated immune function? Transplantation 1974; 17(1): 135-6.

[11] Stutman O. Tumor development after 3-methylcholanthrene in immunologically deficient athymic-nude mice. Science 1974; 183(124): 534-6.

[12] Ikehara S, Pahwa RN, Fernandes G, Hansen CT, Good RA. Functional T cells in athymic nude mice. Proc Natl Acad Sci U S A 1984; 81(3): 886-8.

[13] Maleckar JR, Sherman LA. The composition of the T cell receptor repertoire in nude mice. J Immunol 1987; 138(11): 3873-6.

[14] Hayday AC. [gamma][delta] cells: a right time and a right place for a conserved third way of protection. Annu Rev Immunol 2000; 18: 975-1026.

[15] Hornsby PJ, Aldern KA, Harris SE. Methylcholanthrene: a possible pseudosubstrate for adrenocortical 17 alpha-hydroxylase and aryl hydrocarbon hydroxylase. Biochemical pharmacology 1986; 35(19): 3209-19.

[16] Heidelberger C. Chemical carcinogenesis. Annu Rev Biochem 1975; 44: 79-121.

[17] Engel AM, Svane IM, Rygaard J, Werdelin O. MCA sarcomas induced in scid mice are more immunogenic than MCA sarcomas induced in congenic, immunocompetent mice. Scand J Immunol 1997; 45(5): 463-70.

[18] Schuler W, Weiler IJ, Schuler A, *et al.* Rearrangement of antigen receptor genes is defective in mice with severe combined immune deficiency. Cell 1986; 46(7): 963-72.

[19] Featherstone C, Jackson SP. DNA double-strand break repair. Curr Biol 1999; 9(20): R759-61.

[20] Shinkai Y, Rathbun G, Lam KP, *et al.* RAG-2-deficient mice lack mature lymphocytes owing to inability to initiate V(D)J rearrangement. Cell 1992; 68(5): 855-67.

[21] Shankaran V, Ikeda H, Bruce AT, *et al.* IFNgamma and lymphocytes prevent primary tumour development and shape tumour immunogenicity. Nature 2001; 410(6832): 1107-11.

[22] Dunn GP, Old LJ, Schreiber RD. The three Es of cancer immunoediting. Annu Rev Immunol 2004; 22: 329-60.

[23] Dunn GP, Bruce AT, Ikeda H, Old LJ, Schreiber RD. Cancer immunoediting: from immunosurveillance to tumor escape. Nat Immunol 2002; 3(11): 991-8.

[24] Whiteside TL. The tumor microenvironment and its role in promoting tumor growth. Oncogene 2008; 27(45): 5904-12.

[25] O'Sullivan T, Saddawi-Konefka R, Vermi W, *et al.* Cancer immunoediting by the innate immune system in the absence of adaptive immunity. J Exp Med 2012; 209(10): 1869-82.

[26] Clark WH, Jr., Elder DE, Guerry Dt, *et al.* Model predicting survival in stage I melanoma based on tumor progression. J Natl Cancer Inst 1989; 81(24): 1893-904.

[27] Clemente CG, Mihm MC, Jr., Bufalino R, Zurrida S, Collini P, Cascinelli N. Prognostic value of tumor infiltrating lymphocytes in the vertical growth phase of primary cutaneous melanoma. Cancer 1996; 77(7): 1303-10.

[28] Mihm MC, Jr., Clemente CG, Cascinelli N. Tumor infiltrating lymphocytes in lymph node melanoma metastases: a histopathologic prognostic indicator and an expression of local immune response. Lab Invest 1996; 74(1): 43-7.

[29] Rilke F, Colnaghi MI, Cascinelli N, *et al.* Prognostic significance of HER-2/neu expression in breast cancer and its relationship to other prognostic factors. Int J Cancer 1991; 49(1): 44-9.

[30] Lipponen PK, Eskelinen MJ, Jauhiainen K, Harju E, Terho R. Tumour infiltrating lymphocytes as an independent prognostic factor in transitional cell bladder cancer. Eur J Cancer 1992; 29A(1): 69-75.

[31] Nacopoulou L, Azaris P, Papacharalampous N, Davaris P. Prognostic significance of histologic host response in cancer of the large bowel. Cancer 1981; 47(5): 930-6.

[32] Naito Y, Saito K, Shiiba K, *et al.* CD8+ T cells infiltrated within cancer cell nests as a prognostic factor in human colorectal cancer. Cancer Res 1998; 58(16): 3491-4.

[33] Jass JR. Lymphocytic infiltration and survival in rectal cancer. J Clin Pathol 1986; 39(6): 585-9.

[34] Epstein NA, Fatti LP. Prostatic carcinoma: some morphological features affecting prognosis. Cancer 1976; 37(5): 2455-65.

[35] Deligdisch L, Jacobs AJ, Cohen CJ. Histologic correlates of virulence in ovarian adenocarcinoma. II. Morphologic correlates of host response. Am J Obstet Gynecol 1982; 144(8): 885-9.

[36] Palma L, Di Lorenzo N, Guidetti B. Lymphocytic infiltrates in primary glioblastomas and recidivous gliomas. Incidence, fate, and relevance to prognosis in 228 operated cases. J Neurosurg 1978; 49(6): 854-61.

[37] Smyth MJ, Thia KY, Street SE, *et al.* Differential tumor surveillance by natural killer (NK) and NKT cells. J Exp Med 2000; 191(4): 661-8.

[38] Girardi M, Oppenheim DE, Steele CR, *et al.* Regulation of cutaneous malignancy by gammadelta T cells. Science 2001; 294(5542): 605-9.

[39] Smyth MJ, Crowe NY, Godfrey DI. NK cells and NKT cells collaborate in host protection from methylcholanthrene-induced fibrosarcoma. Int Immunol 2001; 13(4): 459-63.

[40] Gao B, Radaeva S, Park O. Liver natural killer and natural killer T cells: immunobiology and emerging roles in liver diseases. J Leukoc Biol 2009; 86(3): 513-28.

[41] de Lalla C, Galli G, Aldrighetti L, *et al.* Production of profibrotic cytokines by invariant NKT cells characterizes cirrhosis progression in chronic viral hepatitis. J Immunol 2004; 173(2): 1417-25.

[42] Ishiyama K, Ohdan H, Ohira M, Mitsuta H, Arihiro K, Asahara T. Difference in cytotoxicity against hepatocellular carcinoma between liver and periphery natural killer cells in humans. Hepatology 2006; 43(2): 362-72.

[43] Ochi M, Ohdan H, Mitsuta H, *et al.* Liver NK cells expressing TRAIL are toxic against self hepatocytes in mice. Hepatology 2004; 39(5): 1321-31.

[44] Miyagi T, Takehara T, Tatsumi T, *et al.* CD1d-mediated stimulation of natural killer T cells selectively activates hepatic natural killer cells to eliminate experimentally disseminated hepatoma cells in murine liver. Int J Cancer 2003; 106(1): 81-9.

[45] Zaidi MR, Merlino G. The two faces of interferon-gamma in cancer. Clinical cancer research: an official journal of the American Association for Cancer Research 2011; 17(19): 6118-24.

[46] Dighe AS, Richards E, Old LJ, Schreiber RD. Enhanced *in vivo* growth and resistance to rejection of tumor cells expressing dominant negative IFN gamma receptors. Immunity 1994; 1(6): 447-56.

[47] Kaplan DH, Shankaran V, Dighe AS, *et al.* Demonstration of an interferon gamma-dependent tumor surveillance system in immunocompetent mice. Proc Natl Acad Sci U S A 1998; 95(13): 7556-61.

[48] Street SE, Trapani JA, MacGregor D, Smyth MJ. Suppression of lymphoma and epithelial malignancies effected by interferon gamma. J Exp Med 2002; 196(1): 129-34.

[49] Hsieh CS, Macatonia SE, Tripp CS, Wolf SF, O'Garra A, Murphy KM. Development of TH1 CD4+ T cells through IL-12 produced by Listeria-induced macrophages. Science 1993; 260(5107): 547-9.

[50] Kobayashi M, Fitz L, Ryan M, *et al.* Identification and purification of natural killer cell stimulatory factor (NKSF), a cytokine with multiple biologic effects on human lymphocytes. J Exp Med 1989; 170(3): 827-45.

[51] Manetti R, Parronchi P, Giudizi MG, *et al.* Natural killer cell stimulatory factor (interleukin 12 [IL-12]) induces T helper type 1 (Th1)-specific immune responses and inhibits the development of IL-4-producing Th cells. J Exp Med 1993; 177(4): 1199-204.

[52] Noguchi Y, Jungbluth A, Richards EC, Old LJ. Effect of interleukin 12 on tumor induction by 3-methylcholanthrene. Proc Natl Acad Sci U S A 1996; 93(21): 11798-801.

[53] Rothstein TL, Mage M, Jones G, McHugh LL. Cytotoxic T lymphocyte sequential killing of immobilized allogeneic tumor target cells measured by time-lapse microcinematography. J Immunol 1978; 121(5): 1652-6.

[54] Street SE, Cretney E, Smyth MJ. Perforin and interferon-gamma activities independently control tumor initiation, growth, and metastasis. Blood 2001; 97(1): 192-7.

[55] van den Broek ME, Kagi D, Ossendorp F, *et al.* Decreased tumor surveillance in perforin-deficient mice. J Exp Med 1996; 184(5): 1781-90.

[56] Smyth MJ, Thia KY, Street SE, MacGregor D, Godfrey DI, Trapani JA. Perforin-mediated cytotoxicity is critical for surveillance of spontaneous lymphoma. J Exp Med 2000; 192(5): 755-60.

[57] Metkar SS, Menaa C, Pardo J, *et al.* Human and mouse granzyme A induce a proinflammatory cytokine response. Immunity 2008; 29(5): 720-33.

[58] Adrain C, Murphy BM, Martin SJ. Molecular ordering of the caspase activation cascade initiated by the cytotoxic T lymphocyte/natural killer (CTL/NK) protease granzyme B. J Biol Chem 2005; 280(6): 4663-73.

[59] Cullen SP, Adrain C, Luthi AU, Duriez PJ, Martin SJ. Human and murine granzyme B exhibit divergent substrate preferences. J Cell Biol 2007; 176(4): 435-44.

[60] Martin SJ, Amarante-Mendes GP, Shi L, *et al.* The cytotoxic cell protease granzyme B initiates apoptosis in a cell-free system by proteolytic processing and activation of the ICE/CED-3 family protease, CPP32, *via* a novel two-step mechanism. The EMBO journal 1996; 15(10): 2407-16.

[61] Pardo J, Bosque A, Brehm R, *et al.* Apoptotic pathways are selectively activated by granzyme A and/or granzyme B in CTL-mediated target cell lysis. J Cell Biol 2004; 167(3): 457-68.

[62] Heusel JW, Wesselschmidt RL, Shresta S, Russell JH, Ley TJ. Cytotoxic lymphocytes require granzyme B for the rapid induction of DNA fragmentation and apoptosis in allogeneic target cells. Cell 1994; 76(6): 977-87.

[63] Davis JE, Smyth MJ, Trapani JA. Granzyme A and B-deficient killer lymphocytes are defective in eliciting DNA fragmentation but retain potent *in vivo* anti-tumor capacity. Euro J Immunol 2001; 31(1): 39-47.

[64] Mullbacher A, Waring P, Tha Hla R, *et al.* Granzymes are the essential downstream effector molecules for the control of primary virus infections by cytolytic leukocytes. Proc Natl Acad Sci U S A 1999; 96(24): 13950-5.
[65] Muller U, Sobek V, Balkow S, *et al.* Concerted action of perforin and granzymes is critical for the elimination of Trypanosoma cruzi from mouse tissues, but prevention of early host death is in addition dependent on the FasL/Fas pathway. Euro J Immunol 2003; 33(1): 70-8.
[66] Riera L, Gariglio M, Valente G, *et al.* Murine cytomegalovirus replication in salivary glands is controlled by both perforin and granzymes during acute infection. Euro J Immunol 2000; 30(5): 1350-5.
[67] Smyth MJ, Street SE, Trapani JA. Cutting edge: granzymes A and B are not essential for perforin-mediated tumor rejection. J Immunol 2003; 171(2): 515-8.
[68] Smyth MJ, Takeda K, Hayakawa Y, Peschon JJ, van den Brink MR, Yagita H. Nature's TRAIL--on a path to cancer immunotherapy. Immunity 2003; 18(1): 1-6.
[69] Cretney E, Takeda K, Yagita H, Glaccum M, Peschon JJ, Smyth MJ. Increased susceptibility to tumor initiation and metastasis in TNF-related apoptosis-inducing ligand-deficient mice. J Immunol 2002; 168(3): 1356-61.
[70] Takeda K, Smyth MJ, Cretney E, *et al.* Critical role for tumor necrosis factor-related apoptosis-inducing ligand in immune surveillance against tumor development. J Exp Med 2002; 195(2): 161-9.
[71] Medvedev AE, Johnsen AC, Haux J, *et al.* Regulation of Fas and Fas-ligand expression in NK cells by cytokines and the involvement of Fas-ligand in NK/LAK cell-mediated cytotoxicity. Cytokine 1997; 9(6): 394-404.
[72] Smyth MJ, Swann J, Kelly JM, *et al.* NKG2D recognition and perforin effector function mediate effective cytokine immunotherapy of cancer. J Exp Med 2004; 200(10): 1325-35.
[73] Seki N, Brooks AD, Carter CR, *et al.* Tumor-specific CTL kill murine renal cancer cells using both perforin and Fas ligand-mediated lysis *in vitro*, but cause tumor regression *in vivo* in the absence of perforin. J Immunol 2002; 168(7): 3484-92.
[74] Hayashi T, Faustman DL. Development of spontaneous uterine tumors in low molecular mass polypeptide-2 knockout mice. Cancer Res 2002; 62(1): 24-7.
[75] Enzler T, Gillessen S, Manis JP, *et al.* Deficiencies of GM-CSF and interferon gamma link inflammation and cancer. J Exp Med 2003; 197(9): 1213-9.
[76] Hayakawa Y, Rovero S, Forni G, Smyth MJ. Alpha-galactosylceramide (KRN7000) suppression of chemical- and oncogene-dependent carcinogenesis. Proc Natl Acad Sci U S A 2003; 100(16): 9464-9.
[77] Penn I, Halgrimson CG, Starzl TE. *De novo* malignant tumors in organ transplant recipients. Transplant Proc 1971; 3(1): 773-8.
[78] Gatti RA, Good RA. Occurrence of malignancy in immunodeficiency diseases. A literature review. Cancer 1971; 28(1): 89-98.
[79] Birkeland SA, Storm HH, Lamm LU, *et al.* Cancer risk after renal transplantation in the Nordic countries, 1964-1986. Int J Cancer 1995; 60(2): 183-9.
[80] Boshoff C, Weiss R. AIDS-related malignancies. Nat Rev Cancer 2002; 2(5): 373-82.
[81] Penn I. Posttransplant malignancies. Transplant Proc 1999; 31(1-2): 1260-2.
[82] Penn I. Malignant melanoma in organ allograft recipients. Transplantation 1996; 61(2): 274-8.
[83] Sheil AG. Cancer after transplantation. World J Surg 1986; 10(3): 389-96.
[84] Penn I. Sarcomas in organ allograft recipients. Transplantation 1995; 60(12): 1485-91.
[85] Ferris RL, Whiteside TL, Ferrone S. Immune escape associated with functional defects in antigen-processing machinery in head and neck cancer. Clin Can Res 2006; 12(13): 3890-5.
[86] Lopez-Albaitero A, Nayak JV, Ogino T, *et al.* Role of antigen-processing machinery in the *in vitro* resistance of squamous cell carcinoma of the head and neck cells to recognition by CTL. J Immunol 2006; 176(6): 3402-9.
[87] Chang CC, Ferrone S. Immune selective pressure and HLA class I antigen defects in malignant lesions. Can Immunol Immunother: CII 2007; 56(2): 227-36.

[88] Raaijmakers MI, Rozati S, Goldinger SM, Widmer DS, Dummer R, Levesque MP. Melanoma immunotherapy: historical precedents, recent successes and future prospects. Immunotherapy 2013; 5(2): 169-82.
[89] Storkus WJ, Alexander J, Payne JA, Dawson JR, Cresswell P. Reversal of natural killing susceptibility in target cells expressing transfected class I HLA genes. Proc Natl Acad Sci U S A 1989; 86(7): 2361-4.
[90] Storkus WJ, Howell DN, Salter RD, Dawson JR, Cresswell P. NK susceptibility varies inversely with target cell class I HLA antigen expression. J Immunol 1987; 138(6): 1657-9.
[91] Parham P. MHC class I molecules and KIRs in human history, health and survival. Nat Rev Immunol 2005; 5(3): 201-14.
[92] Valiante NM, Uhrberg M, Shilling HG, *et al.* Functionally and structurally distinct NK cell receptor repertoires in the peripheral blood of two human donors. Immunity 1997; 7(6): 739-51.
[93] Kim S, Poursine-Laurent J, Truscott SM, *et al.* Licensing of natural killer cells by host major histocompatibility complex class I molecules. Nature 2005; 436(7051): 709-13.
[94] Raulet DH, Vance RE. Self-tolerance of natural killer cells. Nat Rev Immunol 2006; 6(7): 520-31.
[95] Orr MT, Lanier LL. Natural killer cell education and tolerance. Cell 2010; 142(6): 847-56.
[96] Fernandez NC, Treiner E, Vance RE, Jamieson AM, Lemieux S, Raulet DH. A subset of natural killer cells achieves self-tolerance without expressing inhibitory receptors specific for self-MHC molecules. Blood 2005; 105(11): 4416-23.
[97] Nakamura MC, Niemi EC, Fisher MJ, Shultz LD, Seaman WE, Ryan JC. Mouse Ly-49A interrupts early signaling events in natural killer cell cytotoxicity and functionally associates with the SHP-1 tyrosine phosphatase. J Exp Med 1997; 185(4): 673-84.
[98] Uhrberg M, Valiante NM, Shum BP, *et al.* Human diversity in killer cell inhibitory receptor genes. Immunity 1997; 7(6): 753-63.
[99] Lanier LL. NK cell receptors. Annu Rev Immunol 1998; 16: 359-93.
[100] Moretta L, Biassoni R, Bottino C, Mingari MC, Moretta A. Human NK-cell receptors. Immunol Today 2000; 21(9): 420-2.
[101] Lanier LL, Corliss BC, Wu J, Leong C, Phillips JH. Immunoreceptor DAP12 bearing a tyrosine-based activation motif is involved in activating NK cells. Nature 1998; 391(6668): 703-7.
[102] McVicar DW, Taylor LS, Gosselin P, *et al.* DAP12-mediated signal transduction in natural killer cells. A dominant role for the Syk protein-tyrosine kinase. The Journal of biological chemistry 1998; 273(49): 32934-42.
[103] Yabe T, McSherry C, Bach FH, Houchins JP. A cDNA clone expressed in natural killer and T cells that likely encodes a secreted protein. J Exp Med 1990; 172(4): 1159-63.
[104] Houchins JP, Yabe T, McSherry C, Miyokawa N, Bach FH. Isolation and characterization of NK cell or NK/T cell-specific cDNA clones. J Mol Cell Immunol: JMCI 1990; 4(6): 295-304; discussion 5-6.
[105] Braud V, Jones EY, McMichael A. The human major histocompatibility complex class Ib molecule HLA-E binds signal sequence-derived peptides with primary anchor residues at positions 2 and 9. European journal of immunology 1997; 27(5): 1164-9.
[106] Arase H, Lanier LL. Virus-driven evolution of natural killer cell receptors. Microbes and infection/Institut Pasteur 2002; 4(15): 1505-12.
[107] Cosman D, Mullberg J, Sutherland CL, *et al.* ULBPs, novel MHC class I-related molecules, bind to CMV glycoprotein UL16 and stimulate NK cytotoxicity through the NKG2D receptor. Immunity 2001; 14(2): 123-33.
[108] Leong CC, Chapman TL, Bjorkman PJ, *et al.* Modulation of natural killer cell cytotoxicity in human cytomegalovirus infection: the role of endogenous class I major histocompatibility complex and a viral class I homolog. J Exp Med 1998; 187(10): 1681-7.
[109] Sutherland CL, Chalupny NJ, Cosman D. The UL16-binding proteins, a novel family of MHC class I-related ligands for NKG2D, activate natural killer cell functions. Immunol Rev 2001; 181: 185-92.

[110] Sutherland CL, Chalupny NJ, Schooley K, VandenBos T, Kubin M, Cosman D. UL16-binding proteins, novel MHC class I-related proteins, bind to NKG2D and activate multiple signaling pathways in primary NK cells. J Immunol 2002; 168(2): 671-9.

[111] Wu J, Song Y, Bakker AB, *et al.* An activating immunoreceptor complex formed by NKG2D and DAP10. Science 1999; 285(5428): 730-2.

[112] Bauer S, Groh V, Wu J, *et al.* Activation of NK cells and T cells by NKG2D, a receptor for stress-inducible MICA. Science 1999; 285(5428): 727-9.

[113] Sivori S, Pende D, Bottino C, *et al.* NKp46 is the major triggering receptor involved in the natural cytotoxicity of fresh or cultured human NK cells. Correlation between surface density of NKp46 and natural cytotoxicity against autologous, allogeneic or xenogeneic target cells. European journal of immunology 1999; 29(5): 1656-66.

[114] Pende D, Sivori S, Accame L, *et al.* HLA-G recognition by human natural killer cells. Involvement of CD94 both as inhibitory and as activating receptor complex. Euro J Immunol 1997; 27(8): 1875-80.

[115] Vitale M, Bottino C, Sivori S, *et al.* NKp44, a novel triggering surface molecule specifically expressed by activated natural killer cells, is involved in non-major histocompatibility complex-restricted tumor cell lysis. J Exp Med 1998; 187(12): 2065-72.

[116] Ames E, Murphy WJ. Advantages and clinical applications of natural killer cells in cancer immunotherapy. Cancer immunology, immunotherapy 2014; vol. 63, no. 1, pp. 21–28.

[117] Welniak LA, Blazar BR, Murphy WJ. Immunobiology of allogeneic hematopoietic stem cell transplantation. Annu Rev Immunol 2007; 25: 139-70.

[118] Barao I, Murphy WJ. The immunobiology of natural killer cells and bone marrow allograft rejection. Biol Blood Marrow Transplant: journal of the American Society for Blood and Marrow Transplantation 2003; 9(12): 727-41.

[119] Ruggeri L, Capanni M, Urbani E, *et al.* Effectiveness of donor natural killer cell alloreactivity in mismatched hematopoietic transplants. Science 2002; 295(5562): 2097-100.

[120] Sobecks RM, Ball EJ, Maciejewski JP, *et al.* Survival of AML patients receiving HLA-matched sibling donor allogeneic bone marrow transplantation correlates with HLA-Cw ligand groups for killer immunoglobulin-like receptors. Bone Marrow Transplant 2007; 39(7): 417-24.

[121] Miller JS, Soignier Y, Panoskaltsis-Mortari A, *et al.* Successful adoptive transfer and *in vivo* expansion of human haploidentical NK cells in patients with cancer. Blood 2005; 105(8): 3051-7.

[122] Prlic M, Blazar BR, Farrar MA, Jameson SC. *In vivo* survival and homeostatic proliferation of natural killer cells. J Exp Med 2003; 197(8): 967-76.

[123] de Rham C, Ferrari-Lacraz S, Jendly S, Schneiter G, Dayer JM, Villard J. The proinflammatory cytokines IL-2, IL-15 and IL-21 modulate the repertoire of mature human natural killer cell receptors. Arthritis Res Therapy 2007; 9(6): R125.

[124] Curti A, Ruggeri L, D'Addio A, *et al.* Successful transfer of alloreactive haploidentical KIR ligand-mismatched natural killer cells after infusion in elderly high risk acute myeloid leukemia patients. Blood 2011; 118(12): 3273-9.

[125] Maki G, Klingemann HG, Martinson JA, Tam YK. Factors regulating the cytotoxic activity of the human natural killer cell line, NK-92. J Hematother Stem Cell Res 2001; 10(3): 369-83.

[126] Arai S, Meagher R, Swearingen M, *et al.* Infusion of the allogeneic cell line NK-92 in patients with advanced renal cell cancer or melanoma: a phase I trial. Cytotherapy 2008; 10(6): 625-32.

[127] Tam YK, Maki G, Miyagawa B, Hennemann B, Tonn T, Klingemann HG. Characterization of genetically altered, interleukin 2-independent natural killer cell lines suitable for adoptive cellular immunotherapy. Human Gene Therapy 1999; 10(8): 1359-73.

[128] Cooper MA, Bush JE, Fehniger TA, *et al.* *In vivo* evidence for a dependence on interleukin 15 for survival of natural killer cells. Blood 2002; 100(10): 3633-8.

[129] Egilmez NK, Jong YS, Iwanuma Y, *et al.* Cytokine immunotherapy of cancer with controlled release biodegradable microspheres in a human tumor xenograft/SCID mouse model. Cancer Immunol Immunother: CII 1998; 46(1): 21-4.

[130] Sutlu T, Alici E. Natural killer cell-based immunotherapy in cancer: current insights and future prospects. Journal of internal medicine 2009; 266(2): 154-81.

[131] Rosenstein M, Ettinghausen SE, Rosenberg SA. Extravasation of intravascular fluid mediated by the systemic administration of recombinant interleukin 2. J Immunol 1986; 137(5): 1735-42.

[132] Jakobisiak M, Golab J, Lasek W. Interleukin 15 as a promising candidate for tumor immunotherapy. Cytokine & growth factor reviews 2011; 22(2): 99-108.

[133] Ni J, Miller M, Stojanovic A, Garbi N, Cerwenka A. Sustained effector function of IL-12/15/18-preactivated NK cells against established tumors. J Exp Med 2012; 209(13): 2351-65.

[134] Ravetch JV, Bolland S. IgG Fc receptors. Annu Rev Immunol 2001; 19: 275-90.

[135] Navid F, Santana VM, Barfield RC. Anti-GD2 antibody therapy for GD2-expressing tumors. Curr Can Drug Targets 2010; 10(2): 200-9.

[136] Garnock-Jones KP, Keating GM, Scott LJ. Trastuzumab: A review of its use as adjuvant treatment in human epidermal growth factor receptor 2 (HER2)-positive early breast cancer. Drugs 2010; 70(2): 215-39.

[137] Garcia-Foncillas J, Diaz-Rubio E. Progress in metastatic colorectal cancer: growing role of cetuximab to optimize clinical outcome. Clin Transl Oncol: official publication of the Federation of Spanish Oncology Societies and of the National Cancer Institute of Mexico 2010; 12(8): 533-42.

[138] Winter MC, Hancock BW. Ten years of rituximab in NHL. Expert Opinion on Drug Safety 2009; 8(2): 223-35.

[139] Albertini MR, Hank JA, Sondel PM. Native and genetically engineered anti-disialoganglioside monoclonal antibody treatment of melanoma. Cancer Chem Biol Res Modif 2005; 22: 789-97.

[140] Betting DJ, Yamada RE, Kafi K, Said J, van Rooijen N, Timmerman JM. Intratumoral but not systemic delivery of CpG oligodeoxynucleotide augments the efficacy of anti-CD20 monoclonal antibody therapy against B cell lymphoma. J Immunother 2009; 32(6): 622-31.

[141] Kohrt HE, Houot R, Goldstein MJ, *et al.* CD137 stimulation enhances the antilymphoma activity of anti-CD20 antibodies. Blood 2011; 117(8): 2423-32.

**CHAPTER 4**

# The Basics of Cancer Immunity Dc-Based Immunotherapy: Gliomas as a Paradigm Disease?

**Steven De Vleeschouwer***

*Experimental Neurosurgery and Neuroanatomy, Department of Neurosciences, KU Leuven, Belgium*

**Abstract:** Dendritic cell-based vaccines are considered the most advanced examples of active specific immunotherapy against cancer. Dendritic cells, being pivotal for the induction of immunity or tolerance, are not a single cell-type but comprise a large group of cells with differing phenotypes, all with crucial implications for the resulting immune response. To date, cancer vaccines are even being developed for cancers that have traditionally not been regarded as immunogenic, like brain cancer, which might even display underexplored opportunities rather than only hurdles. The major actual challenge is the full integration of the vaccines into the complex interface of the patient as host of the tumor, the tumor micro-environment and the conventional and other therapies applied.

**Keywords:** Brain cancer, combinatorial therapies, dendritic cell, glioma, immune modulation, immune profiles, micro-environment, tumor antigens, tumor vaccine.

## DENDRITIC CELL VACCINATION: PROMISE OR FAILURE?

Using the immune system to tackle cancer has been an appealing concept since more than 100 years with Coley's bacterial toxins being one of the first immunotherapeutic approaches to cancer [1]. Only the last two decades, major improvements in our understanding of the complex interplay of all the cells and systems of our immunity boosted this intention towards clinically applicable approaches [2]. Nevertheless, we're still facing many unsolved problems, leaving us with different degrees of uncertainty about the best tailored approach for the different types of cancer that might be eligible for immunotherapy. In an era, however, of growing interest in 'targeted therapies' and 'personalized medicine', the immune system continues to be the most attractive physiological system to combine cytotoxic actions with specificity. In its most advanced way, 4 decades after the first discovery of the dendritic cell [DC] by Ralph Steinman [3], the

***Corresponding author Steven De Vleeschouwer:** Experimental Neurosurgery and Neuroanatomy, Department of Neurosciences, KU Leuven, Belgium; Tel: +32 16 34 42 90; Fax: +32 16 34 42 41;
E-mail: steven.devleeschouwer@uzleuven.be

**Jianxun Song (Ed)**

induction of an active specific immune response using autologous dendritic cells loaded with different types of relevant tumor antigens has shown to be safe, to be able to mount cellular anti-tumor immune responses and modest to promising clinical results [4]. Interestingly, the existence of several larger Good Medical Practice – [GMP] approved cell therapy facilities may pave the way to test the full potential of these DC-based approaches in well-designed clinical trials to rapidly move forward and establish the correct current and future position of this type of immunotherapy for different cancers [5]. Following this track, immunotherapy based on autologous DC might have the huge advantage to be tested in large, randomized trials which is an inherent problem or limitation for other forms of personalized medicine approaches in which extensive sub-grouping could jeopardize statistical power.

Gliomas and in particular malignant gliomas have never been considered a good paradigm tumor for immunotherapy because of many reasons [6]. Considered poorly immunogenic as compared to malignant melanoma or renal cell carcinoma and residing in a relatively immune-privileged site in the brain, it was believed that a rejective or protective immune response was highly unlikely in HGG patients. Many of the different, perceived objections for the use of immunotherapy in HGG continue to be true and relevant [7]: highly infiltrative beyond the margins of a broken blood brain barrier [BBB], a highly heterogenous phenotype with a lack of commonly expressed, vital tumor antigens, lack of major histocompatibility [MHC] class II molecules, down-regulation of MHC class I molecules, protection against NK activity, notoriously immunosuppressive capacities both locally and systemically, rapidly progressing, need for anti-oedema therapy with steroids are all very well described hurdles. In spite of all these, a rapidly growing number of papers report on feasibility and safety, but also on promising clinical results. In uncontrolled trials, this promise often concerns an important subgroup of patients with a remarkably long survival for this invariantly fatal disease. In controlled trials [several are underway], slight evidence might emerge on its added value to standard of care therapies, although current data still suffer from the shortcomings of low level of evidence or weak experimental or clinical study design.

Dendritic cells, being discovered in the 70's as a curiosum subset of white blood cells [3], consistently gained the status of preferred [cellular] adjuvants of modern immunotherapeutic approaches against cancer. This is mainly due to their remarkably strong antigen presenting capacity in the afferent arm of immunity and their pivotal role of linking innate to adaptive immunity [8, 9]. It is however increasingly being recognized that the source, the subtype, the differentiation, maturation, activation, polarization and antigen loading of these dendritic cells are of utmost importance for the actual performance of these key players of immunity [10-17]. A full spectrum of activities varying from tolerance induction to target tumor rejection can be displayed based on phenotype and engineered functions. Apart from this physiological diversity of these dendritic cells, dendritic cell function can be altered by the tumor and its host's environment [18, 19].

With the progressive unraveling of the many levels involved in an adequate and appropriate immune response, it is being understood that one should not restrict the focus on the immunity as a single-arm, linear cascade of several rigidly determined reactions but rather acknowledge the complex mutual and dynamic interplays of host, tumor, micro-environment, concomitant therapies, different immune cells, cytokines and chemokines to be responsible for the ultimate outcome. This recognition implies that immune monitoring of single- arm immune events [20] will not be able to provide an adequate prediction of the full picture. An integrative, multimodal immune-, host- and tumor-profiling will be needed to reveal underlying mechanisms and predict therapy response, outcome and prognosis. This 'interactome' of host, tumor and immunity might be highly relevant to take the next step to a more comprehensive understanding of the true value of immunotherapy and beyond, including conventional cancer therapies like radiation and chemotherapeutics.

## THE HOST: WHO IS ELIGIBLE FOR DENDRITIC CELL VACCINATION?

To date, 27 papers have reported on the use of DC-based therapy in more than 530 high grade glioma [HGG] patients in almost all varying contexts [21-47], being part of an even larger exploration of all cellular immunotherapy strategies in brain tumors [48]. Many reports are dealing with vaccination therapy in a postoperative setting, some [focusing on diffuse pontine gliomas, DIPG] report on vaccines administered after only a biopsy. Many trials included only relapsed or multi-relapsed HGG patients after standard of care with at least one and often more session[s] of surgery, radiotherapy and chemotherapy and others focus on the setting of newly diagnosed malignant brain tumors. In some reports only World Health Organisation [WHO] grade IV tumors are included whereas in others both WHO grade III and IV tumor patients are being treated. Dendritic cells from different source [13] with different phenotype and maturation status, and generated with different differentiation cocktails, loaded with different types of tumor antigens are used in different dose, frequency and route of administration [15, 17, 49-51]. Most trials require[d] the patients to be fully weaned from steroids for several reasons of documented immune deficiency of patients under corticosteroids [52, 53], but in some other trials, the use of [a low dose of] steroids was allowed. It is clear that such an heterogeneity of the cellular products used, impedes any useful meta-analysis. A universal common finding however seems to be the safety and feasibility of the approach [54]. Moreover, almost regardless the approach and monitoring tools and assays used, some indication of immunological activity is found in about 50% of patients, whereas objective clinical responses are overall being reported in about 15% of cases. It should be noticed however that, apart from the patient's immune profile, basic clinical parameters can [and should] be used to stratify patients in different risk groups [55, 56], highly influencing overall prognosis of the target population of patients, eligible for immunotherapy and enabling an indirect comparison with other types of treatment in a comparable patient population. Probably the strongest independent predictor of outcome remains a pretreatment variable, namely the age of the patient, which is not surprising at all both from the oncological and the immunological point of view [28]. Mounting evidence is emerging that the major benefit of [added] immunotherapy can be found in well-performing, younger patients with a low [residual] tumor burden before the start of the immunotherapy. As such, it can't be recommended anymore to apply immunotherapy in end-stage cancer patients, apart from first-in-humans small phase I trials testing a complete new, unexplored immune strategy. Moreover, the opposite trend, *i.e.,* applying [prophylactic] tumor vaccination strategies in pre-cancerous lesions seems to gain interest [57].

Disturbances in the BBB are notorious for malignant gliomas. Mounting evidence is being gathered that also in several other pathologies, even small defects in the BBB can modify the interaction of astrocytes, neurons and endothelial cells thereby possibly triggering the pathogenic processes in different neuropsychiatric disorders. A disrupted BBB in HGG can be seen as an opportunity to get medicinal products or [cytotoxic] immune cells in the tumor [58]. It remains to be seen however, to what extent, a disrupted BBB in malignant glioma could be a hurdle for therapy rather than a blessing. Anyhow, it is an important hallmark for tumor progression by shaping and conditioning all relevant cells in the tumor micro-environment. After all, its contrast-enhancing appearance on computer tomography [CT] and magnetic resonance imaging [MRI] scans, depending on a regional BBB breakthrough, is the most striking radiological difference with LGG, that generally behave much more indolent in terms of tumor progression.

One of the possible interactions of the tumor with the micro-environment could be lying in the metabolic connections between supporting glia-cells such as astrocytes and glioma tumor cells. No other cancer has such an infiltrative character in its surrounding host tissues as [malignant] gliomas. This alone already indirectly suggests the need for collaboration of the host tissue in the spreading of the disease throughout the brain, with cells like microglia probably playing a pivotal role [59, 60]. Michael Lisanti's group extensively published on the importance of the tumor micro-environment providing 'food' for the tumor by ketogenic metabolism to fuel the tumor's oxidative metabolism associated with tumor growth [61, 62]. Interfering with this mechanism might be crucial to re-edit the tumor micro-environment to change it from a tumor-friendly to a therapy-friendly setting. This environmental reshaping is especially important for the immune system as we know that lactate might influence myeloid derived cells and NK cells in the tumor environment [63]. Modifying this environment could theoretically be done in several ways, often not internally consequent: whether ketogenic diets, shown to reduce glycolytic activity in tumor cells, or substances like NAC [N-acetyl-cystein] inhibiting glycolysis in supportive stromal cells are to be advocated, is still a matter of controversy [64]. It becomes increasingly clear however, that efforts will have to be made to elucidate this important issue to establish the best possible local circumstances to give systemic [and local] therapies a fair chance to control the tumor that has been safely engrafted in its preferred environment. Recent reports even show that the local environment of the brain tumor could educate aspects of systemic immunity [65]. All the above mentioned elements strongly support the need for a more intense 'cross-talk' between the cancer biologist and immunologist [66].

## THE TUMOR: COMPREHENSIVE OR TARGETED IMMUNOTHERAPY?

Anti-tumor immunotherapy historically has been focusing on inherently immunogenic tumors like melanoma, renal cell carcinoma, prostate carcinoma and several hematologic malignancies [4]. At first glance this makes sense, given the rather good accessibility of the targets, the extensive libraries of specific defined tumor rejective antigens and the apparently straight forward immune monitoring opportunities that could support this approach. Often however, the results obtained in surrogate endpoints are more impressive than those in the clinical field [67]. Several explanations can be hypothesized for this phenomenon. First of all, the last decade, many reports made it increasingly clear that the main hurdles to an efficacious immunotherapy against cancer are the tumor-induced immune suppression and immune escape [68]. Many tumors, especially in end-stage disease states, tilt the immune balance, both locally and systemically, towards an immune suppressive modus. The mechanisms for that have extensively being studied and comprise the positive selection of [sometimes more aggressive] antigen-loss variants, the down-regulation of MHC class I molecules on the targeted tumor cells, the production of immunosuppressive cytokines and substances like IL-10, TGF-beta2, Galectin 1 and 3 or the expression of PDL1, Fas and Fas-ligand [69-74]. The influence of the tumor micro-environment on the balances of immune cells, both lymphocytic [regulatory T cells, γδ T cells, CTLA4 expression, zeta-chain down-regulation in T and NK cells,…] or myeloid [IDO expression, MDSC, pro-tumor M2 macrophages attraction and/or priming] is an additional point of concern [75-82]. Many of these mechanisms might gain more impact at more established stages of tumor progression because of the many interactive, positive feedback mechanisms. For all those reasons, it might be more attractive to think about cancer types that are considered to be 'less immunogenic' and as such haven't been extensively sculptured or edited by the immune system. One such tumor type could be malignant gliomas that have been hidden for immunity in the relatively immune privileged brain. Proper exposure of these types of cancer to effective immunological strategies in a minimal residual disease status and maximally reset micro-environment might yield interesting results, as can be seen in the [still moderate numbers of] long-term survivors after such approaches [55].

In an era where molecular markers start to guide personalized therapies in cancer, one should pay attention to indications of predictive [and prognostic] markers, increasingly being identified today. Murat *et al.* [83] already identified a set of genes of immunological importance or with importance for tumor-host interaction, being prognostically important in the outcome of glioblastoma [GBM] treated with radio-and chemotherapy. Prins *et al.* identified the mesenchymal tumor type of GBM [38] as more prone to the effects of immunotherapy, based on gene profiles in tumor samples of vaccinated patients. This goes in line with the recent finding that tumor infiltrating lymphocytes [TIL] in GBM were enriched in the mesenchymal subclass and depleted in the classical subclass and in EGFR-amplified and PTEN-deleted tumors [84]. Although the relevance of a genetic

[85] and epigenetic [86] glioblastoma signature in treatment selection is widely being acknowledged, one should realize the enormous heterogeneity of many cancers and especially GBM as nicely shown in the paper of Barajas *et al.* [87] demonstrating that even the morphological characteristic of the GBM is heavily depending on the specific location of the tumor where the sample is being taken by the neurosurgeon. This should withhold us from exclusively appointing a tumor to a certain cluster based on limited sampling of the complete lesion. Furthermore, the pathological entity of malignant glioma might indeed represent two quite distinct diseases in the pediatric and adult population [88].

An immediate consequence of the variability described in the paragraph above, is the inherent limited value of single-target approaches, often advocated previously in 'targeted therapies' or single-peptide based immune strategies. Prins *et al.* demonstrated that using autologous tumor lysate-loaded DC in glioma patients yields a wider patient eligibility compared to the use of glioma-associated antigen-loaded DC [89]. Although much harder to monitor, it is reasonable to believe that the more comprehensive approaches are going to have more impact on the global lesion. Ultimately, active specific immunotherapy approaches targeting the whole autologous tumor antigen repertoire are about the closest one can get to fully personalized medicine in theory, even more than the personalized peptide vaccines [90]. Both theoretically [91] and in experimental designs [92] or clinical trials [83], the use of glioma stem cells [GSC] as a source of most relevant tumor antigens can be advocated. A problem remaining for the concept of cancer stem cells [93, 94] however, is the still undecided essential phenotypic characteristic a glioma stem cell should display [95, 96]: GSC can be isolated using culturing techniques and selected on morphological criteria like neurosphere-forming units, by membrane molecules expression [CD133, nestin,SOX2,...] or as a negative selection in side-population experiments. To what extent these different prerequisites of GSC are overlapping remains unclear. It can be predicted that the larger trials implementing autologous DC vaccination will yield such an enormous mass of possibly relevant data that computational analysis might become a prerequisite to really capture the larger picture.

## THE IMMUNE SYSTEM: CHECKS AND BALANCES?

In the majority of reports dealing with DC-based immunotherapy against cancer, one is [exclusively] focusing on the well-described paradigm of a single-arm lymphocytic rejective activity of the immune system [97]. Even if regulatory T cells [Treg] are considered to play a very important role [98, 99], with reports suggesting a useful monitoring opportunity of CTLA4 expressing T cells before and after vaccination [100], one should not ignore the importance of a more multifaceted immunity with γδ T cells [101], natural killer [NK] cells [102, 103], NK T cells, macrophages [104, 105] and myeloid derived suppressor cells [MDSC] [106] all playing an important, maybe a major, role in [GBM] tumor immunity. Both pre-clinical and clinical data coming available now, point to the sometimes massive invasion of these cells in the tumor both spontaneously or after treatment [107]. The complex interplay of chemokines, cytokines and cellular invasion still is to be elucidated [108]. The resulting number and types of immune cells infiltrating in the tumor micro-environment can be influenced by conventional, non-immune therapies as such resetting the local balance in favor of or hazardous for a subsequent immunotherapy. Therefore, it might be more relevant to try to define relevant immune profiles of cells in the blood and/or the tumor [if available] that coincide with a preferred response to therapy rather than exclusively monitoring single-arm immune response after vaccination [23]. As for the latter, only a very limited number of reports find a correlation of immune monitoring findings and clinical responses in DC-based vaccination for patients with malignant gliomas [43]. This could make sense, as most of these monitoring tools are applied to the blood compartment of which we know that the correlation with the local representation of immune cells in the brain [-tumor] is very poor, sometimes even negative [own, unpublished data]. The recognition of the involvement of many arms of immunity in building a durable rejective or protective immunity against cancer [-relapse], implies that immune approaches should target either key hubs of innate and adaptive immunity, either combine different complementary strategies to really shift the balance from tolerance to immunity.

## THE MICRO-ENVIRONMENT: RESISTANCE OR COLLABORATION?

As mentioned before, the importance of the tumor micro-environment is increasingly being recognized as pivotal in tumor progression and [immune] therapy response [18]. One most relevant element seems to be hypoxia in tumor areas [109]. Not only is hypoxia a driving force of oxidative stress and might it as such directly drive the metabolic connection between the stromal and the tumor cells, but it also triggers neo-angiogenesis. This neo-angiogenesis is not only supplying substrates for tumor growth, it might also be a key-element in vascular shunting of the tumor thereby impeding a good penetration of anti-tumor products [and cells] rather than facilitating it. Recent observations revealed a remarkable correlation between the vascular endothelial growth factor [VEGF], as pro-angiogenic factor and galectin-1 [Gal-1] as immunosuppressive factor in malignant glioma cells [74]. This opens the question whether hypoxia, oxidative stress and local immune suppression are interrelated phenomena in tumor progression. Moreover, preliminary observations suggest the importance of hypoxia markers to be involved in the recruitment of macrophages into the tumor in already very early stage of hypoxia [unpublished data]. Several efforts have been done to combat GBM with anti-angiogenic agents like bevacizumab and cilengitide. No unequivocal advantage of these substances could be demonstrated in the clinic in spite of the multiple theoretically beneficial interactions they should orchestrate [110]. Vessel recruitment, with tumor cells invading towards and around major existing feeding vessels, in case anti-angiogenics are being used to block the neo-angiogenesis, could be a partial explanation of the modest effects of these agents in glioma-therapy. Combining these angiogenesis-inhibitors with immune approaches seems to be rational, both in terms of preventing the tumor shunt effect and exploiting the correlation between the expression of VEGF and immunosuppressive substances like Gal-1. In that regard, it is interesting to note that the mesenchymal subtype of GBM seems to respond better than the other subtypes [neural, proneural, classical] to immunotherapy [38] whereas it is associated with a resistance to anti-VEGF therapy [111]. It is only a small step from tumor vascular supply through neo-angiogenesis towards the underestimated importance of tumor endothelial cells. In GBM, endothelial proliferation is a traditional pathological hallmark of these tumors, but the pathophysiological meaning remains unclear. Endothelial cells are a major element of the micro-environment and play a role in the local homeostasis over the [disrupted] BBB and in the homing and recruitment of immune cells from the blood compartment [112]. Considering the quite pathognomonic pathological findings of necrosis, endothelial proliferation and pseudopalissading tumor cells around the necrotic areas in GBM, one should really wonder how all these constituents act together and what exactly is their pathophysiological meaning. Therefore, we should plea for an integrative vision on the micro-environment as a complex, and regionally variable contribution of the different players involved: proliferating tumor cells, invading tumor cells, glioma stem cells, necrotic tumor cells, endothelial cells, normal stromal and glia cells and microglia cells in the invaded periphery, all the locally produced cytokines and chemokines and the immune cells of different origin like cytotoxic T cells, regulatory T cells, γδ T cells, NK cells, NK T cells, anti-tumor [M1] or pro-tumor [M2] polarized macrophages and MDSC.

Experimental data using monocyte galactose/N-acetylgalactosamine-specific C-type lectin stimulated immunotherapy in B57BL/6 mice demonstrated regional specificity of the phenotype of monocyte derived cells of the brain [113]. To fully integrate all these factors, we will need multi-layer analyses, preferentially with computational immunohistochemistry [IHC]. Not only the type of cell, but also its preferential appearance and location in or around the necrotic areas, in the proliferative bulk of tumor cells, in the invaded periphery or the perivascular spaces of the tumor might all be equally important.

Even then, we should realize that we know far more about these parts of the tumor that usually get resected neurosurgically, whereas the residing and remaining enemy are the [non-resected] peripheral tumor parts, often showing low density infiltration of tumor cells, beyond the intraoperative detection threshold even if intraoperative fluorescence guided techniques are being used routinely at the moment. These tumor cells probably behave different from those being currently investigated after harvesting during the operation. Establishing such a ‘cellular interactome’ as a key signature of the tumor seems to be mandatory to understand its capacity to progress so rapidly.

Whether or not, useful and easy accessible [blood] biomarkers will be found for malignant glioma to guide therapy and prognosis, is still a matter of debate [114]. More and more biomarkers are coming from glioma tissue analysis and examples as $O^6$-methylguanine-DNA- methyltransferase [MGMT] promotor hypermethylation in the elderly GBM or 1p19q co-deletions in anaplastic astrocytomas [115], isocitrate dehydrogenase-1 [IDH1] mutations [116] found their way to daily life, clinical decision making. Particularly relevant to immune therapy strategies, might be the PTEN loss in gliomas: this can increase PDL1 expression in the tumor installing an additional immune suppressive pathway protecting against conventional T cell attacks. The search for useful serum markers, possibly able to monitor [new forms] of therapy for malignant gliomas is difficult. Nevertheless, modest steps are being set with investigating the meaning of elevated serum markers like Galectin-1 [117], a galactoside binding protein that already showed its prognostic meaning in pathology samples of gliomas [118]. The latter would be very interesting as it might be related not only to chemotherapy resistance and angiogenesis, but also to immunosuppression by the tumor. As such, attempts to modify its expression and secretion in order to influence the tumor micro-environment could be followed during treatment and eventually prove useful in glioma immunotherapy too.

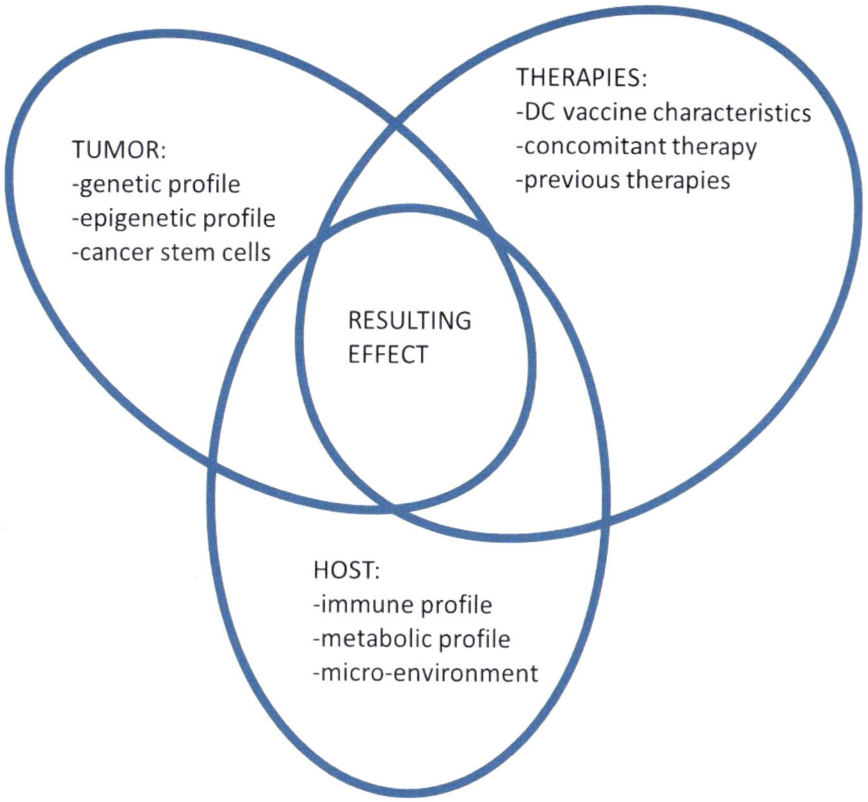


**Visual presentation** of the 'interactome' concept in which the final resulting effect of any intervention will depend on a complex interplay of therapy characteristics, the targeted tumor and the patient, 'hosting' the tumor.

## THE DENDRITIC CELL: AN ABSOLUTE SUPERIOR ADJUVANT OR PLASTIC REGULATOR?

To date, no real doubt exists about the superiority of dendritic cells as an adjuvant for active specific immunotherapy in terms of its ability to raise a protective or rejective immune response [119]. Many items of the DC biology itself however remain a matter of debate. Most trials of DC-based immunotherapy are using monocyte-derived dendritic cells, although several other sources are possible too. Mature DC seem to be preferred over immature DC [120] because of the latter's ability to lead to tolerance induction and its inferior migration capacities [121]. Especially in terms of migration, the use of prostaglandin E2 [PGE2] remains controversial: is it necessary to up-regulate CCR7 on the DC or is it to be avoided because of the stimulation of CCL22 production and Treg attraction [122]? Maturation of DC can be expressed as up-regulated co-stimulatory molecules like

CD80 [51] and CD86 [50] and up-regulated MHC class II molecules both important for a proper presentation and co-stimulation in the interaction process with the T cell [16]. A marker often referred to however, is CD83 to measure maturity: probably it represents a capacity of the DC to enhance T cell proliferation and inhibit T cell apoptosis enabling a continued expansion of the primed T cells beyond 6 weeks *i.e.,* lead to more durable T cell responses [123]. The differentiation cocktails used to treat the precursor cell population with can be quite different [124], as are maturation cocktails: comparison analysis has demonstrated the crucial involvement of especially TNFα in the cocktail to correlate with favorable clinical responses [125]. For additional activation of the injected DC, several Toll-like receptor [TLR] agonists have been tested clinically of which imiquimod/resiquimod [TLR 7 agonist], poly I:C [TLR 3 agonist] and clinical grade LPS [TLR4 agonist] are the most common. The polarization of the DC inducing Th0, Th1, Th2 or Th17 responses, is an ongoing issue, although the majority of data point towards a classical Th1 polarisation with substantial IL12 production as the most desirable phenotype [126]. Th17 polarisation seems to gain some interest in the field, but data are less established [127]. According to some recent data on the use of oncolytic viral strains against cancer [128], the development of especially anti-tumor antibodies [humoral immunity] after an oncolytic viral therapy might even correlate to a worse outcome, suggesting Th2 type of responses could be less preferred.

The classical interaction with the lymphocytes is currently being seen as a 4-steps process [129]: TCR engagement leading to specificity by avidity, co-stimulation binding leading to T cell expansion, polarization of the immunity towards a Th1 type immunity [with IFN-γ production] through DC interaction with the lymphocyte and finally regulation of the T cell homing properties resulting in homing of the primed T cells in the target organ. Especially the latter aspect is not well understood yet, but of utmost importance to make sure the primed lymphocytes are able to track, find and control the remaining tumor cells. Although this is the ruling paradigm, we should not forget that more complex interaction with regulatory T cells and MDSC are parts of the actual biological process, influencing the end result to a high extent. Thereby, once more, we cannot ignore the impact of the [progressing] tumor on the DC: tumor-altered DC are the reality and one should refrain from [too] easy extrapolations of data from healthy volunteers' DC to cancer patients' DC [19]. This might be particularly relevant given the fact that especially the nature of the DC-derived signal 2 [co-stimulation *versus* co-inhibition] in this 4-steps model, determines the resulting T cell responses and promotes as such, either immunity or tolerance [130]. In the future, newer approaches directly targeting *in vivo* DC like *e.g.*, the increasingly used nanoparticles to load DC *in vivo* and raise an anti-tumor immune response might be the start of a complete new form of active specific immunity and cancer vaccines [131]. Getting even closer to the real, comprehensive phenotype of the tumor cell [and its environmental cells], to design future strategies of vaccination could be an opportunity, especially for those tumors arising in relatively immune privileged sites like the brain. In that regard, the concept of split immunity in which vital tumor cells from tumors of immune privileged sites, are injected in an immune accessible environment, could indeed be another future approach to get more powerful vaccines for these patients [132].

## THE SOURCE OF ANTIGENS: KEY TARGETING OR GENERAL BOMBING?

The capacity of the DC to induce a robust, tumor-specific and clinically meaningful immune response is not solely depending on its basic phenotype. Equally important are the tumor antigens used to load the DC with. These can be very different and comprise peptides, proteins, apoptotic or necrotic bodies, whole tumor cell lysates, RNA. The most relevant and still exclusive capacity of the DC to cross-present peptides derived from exogenous antigens on MHC class I molecules renders the DC the most professional APC to date, although the full understanding of this process has not been reached yet [133]. More and more however, the importance of immunogenic types of cell death and apoptosis is being recognized as the preferred way to generate the right source of tumor antigens: several danger-associated molecular patterns [DAMP's] like calreticulin, ATP, HSP 70 or 90, HMGB1 have been identified to play a role in the appropriate activation and polarization of the DC [134]. The single-peptide approach from the beginning, ideal to perform easy to interpret, straight-forward immune monitoring, is being replaced by either a rational combination of multiple peptides [polypeptide-approach] or whole tumor cell preparations, which by definition are resembling most to the target but are notoriously difficult to monitor. As proof of the principle, the former are preferred, but as most rational approach for durable clinical benefit, the latter appear to be superior. Whether highly engineered DC preparations [135] are being preferred over the more 'dirty' vaccines, rather is a matter of taste than of scientific estimation at the moment. Especially if we succeed in feeding the DC with more appropriate sources of tumor antigens, displayed in a context of immunogenic apoptosis with DAMP's [or engineered pathogen-associated molecular patterns, PAMP's], there might be no real need to molecularly tailor the differentiation, maturation and activation process of the DC

[136]. Anyhow, after it has been shown by Prins *et al.* [38] that DC vaccination strategies do not exhibit a classical dose-response effect, recent data even suggest that reducing the number of DC injected pro injection site [to 5x10e6 or less cells pro injection site] might even improve the migration to the draining lymph nodes instead of the opposite [137].

## COMBINATORIAL THERAPIES: SYNERGY OR OPPOSITION?

Considering all the above mentioned elements of DC vaccination, it is becoming increasingly clear that the phenotypic engineering of the DC will have some, but albeit modest advantages in terms of clinical results. Far more important will be the intelligent modulation of the local [and systemic] micro-environment of the cancer patient's tumor, probably in a broader field than what has been done before [138]. Combinatorial strategies aimed to overcome one of the major hurdles to effective immunotherapy *i.e.* immune-editing and antigen loss in tumor cells may be essential to produce robust anti-tumor responses [139]. A remarkable parallel can be seen between the immunity characteristics in case of a chronic inflammatory disease and cancer [140]. Also for this next step, glioblastoma can be a paradigm tumor. Already for more than a decade, the opportunities of correctly combining chemotherapy with immunotherapy become obvious [141, 142]. Several explanations can be found for this synergy in both directions going from immunogenic apoptosis induction by chemotherapy, clearing of chemo-resistant tumor sub-clones by immunotherapy [143], exploiting thymic-independent homeostatic T cell proliferation in the reconstitution phase after chemo to yield a higher percentages of specifically primed anti-tumor T cells by the vaccine [141], to deleting regulatory T cell pools by *e.g.* cyclophosphamide [144] or deleting MDSC-pools by gemcitabine [145]. Exploring these rational combinations will be one of the major challenges to move the field forward in the coming decade. To that end, we should start thinking about less conventional routes to the brain, like the transnasal route which has been underexplored for a long period [146]. Correctly balancing all useful insights in this matter, will not be easy. In that regard, the importance of autophagy, a major cytotoxic mechanism induced in the glioblastoma cell by *e.g.,* temozolomide, the most commonly used chemotherapeutic against GBM at the moment, is just one example of the controversy. Although combined postoperative treatment with radiotherapy and temozolomide is the golden standard today, one should realize that autophagy is a multifaceted phenomenon proving useful to combat early stages of cancer but maybe rather harmful in later stages of the disease. In that regards, already in 2006 Sotelo *et al.* [147] conducted an interesting trial with the autophagy inhibitor, chloroquine [CQ] in GBM, actually resulting in a better outcome for the study group. Very recently, an intriguing link between blocking autophagy by chloroquine and the tumor micro-environment has been described by Maes *et al.* [148]: tumors were less hypoxic and necrotic and displayed less invasiveness and metastasis after CQ treatment. A full integration of DC-based vaccination in the standard-of-care postoperative radio-chemotherapy for patients with GBM, is feasible and possibly beneficial [23] but it might even be more rational to exploit the combination with the autophagy-inhibitor included in the schedule.

Another major role is to be suspected for rationally combining immune-relevant targeted therapies with tumor vaccination [149]. Several fully humanized monoclonal antibodies [mAb] are currently being used [and tested] in several cancer therapies, many of them acting through a modified immune responses. Anti-PD1, anti-PDL1, daclizumab [anti-CD25] or anti-CTLA4 mAb [ipilimumab] are all examples of targeted therapies that should be tested in combination with DC vaccination. Especially the latter combination might prove useful in GBM immunotherapy, given the quite impressive results of ipilimumab in malignant melanomas [in combination with a gp100 vaccine] [150] AND the finding that changes in CTLA4 expression on Treg cells after tumor vaccination seemed to correlate with clinical outcome in a small cohort of vaccinated GBM patients [100]. In addition to the aforementioned commonly described molecules, new relevant substances like galectins [1, 3] are gaining interest and might be key-hub molecules in more than one biological pathway involved in cancer progression [151]. It is reasonable to state that we just reached the end of the beginning, rather than the beginning of the end of immunotherapy for [brain] cancer.

## ACKNOWLEDGEMENTS

Declared None.

## CONFLICT OF INTEREST

The authors confirm that this chapter contents have no conflict of interest.

### REFERENCES

[1] Brunschwig A. THE Efficacy of "Coley's Toxin" in the treatment of sarcoma: an experimental study. Ann Surg 1939; 109(1): 109-113.

[2] Nestle FO, Banchereau J, Hart D. Dendritic cells: On the move from bench to bedside. Nat Med 2001; 7(7): 761-5.

[3] Steinman RM, Cohn ZA. Identification of a novel cell type in peripheral lymphoid organs of mice. I. Morphology, quantitation, tissue distribution. J Exp Med 1973; 137(5): 1142-1162.

[4] Ridgway D. The first 1000 dendritic cell vaccinees. Cancer Invest 2003; 21: 873-886.

[5] Schuler G, Schuler-Thurner B, Steinman RM. The use of dendritic cells in cancer immunotherapy. Curr Opin Immunol 2003; 15(2): 138-47.

[6] Weller RO, Engelhardt B, Phillips MJ. Lymphocyte targeting of the central nervous system: a review of afferent and efferent CNS-immune pathways. Brain Pathol 1996; 6(3): 275-288.

[7] Dix AR, Brooks WH, Roszman TL, Morford LA. Immune defects observed in patients with primary malignant brain tumors. J Neuroimmunol 1999; 100(1-2): 216-32.

[8] Banchereau J, Briere F, Caux C, Davoust J, Lebecque S, Liu YJ *et al.* Immunobiology of dendritic cells. Annu Rev. Immunol 2000; 18: 767-811.

[9] Steinman RM. The dendritic cell system and its role in immunogenicity. Annu Rev Immunol 1991; 9: 271-296.

[10] Ashley DM, Faiola B, Nair S, Hale LP, Bigner DD, Gilboa E. Bone marrow-generated dendritic cells pulsed with tumor extracts or tumor RNA induce antitumor immunity against central nervous system tumors. J Exp Med 1997; 186: 1177-1182.

[11] Björck P. Development of dendritic cells and their use in tumor therapy. Clin Immunol 1999; 92: 119-127.

[12] Caux C, Massacrier C, Vanbervliet B, Dubois B, Durand I, Cella M *et al.* CD34+ hematopoietic progenitors from human cord blood differentiate along two independent dendritic cell pathways in response to granulocyte-macrophage colony-stimulating factor plus tumor necrosis factor alpha: II. Functional analysis. Blood 1997; 90: 1458-1470.

[13] Caux C. Developmental pathways of human dendritic cells. Hematol Cell Therapy 1998; 40: 82-86.

[14] Dubsky P, Ueno H, Piqueras B, Connolly J, Banchereau J, Palucka AK. Human dendritic cell subsets for vaccination J Clin Immunol 2005; 25(6): 551-572.

[15] Fong L, Brockstedt D, Benike C, Wu L, Engleman EG. Dendritic cells injected *via* different routes induce immunity in cancer patients. J Immunol 2001; 166: 4254-4259.

[16] Liu YJ. Dendritic cell subsets and lineages, and their functions in innate and adaptive immunity. Cell 2001; 106(3): 259-62.

[17] Okada N, Tsujino M, Hagiwara Y, Tada A, Tamura Y, Mori K *et al.* Administration route-dependent vaccine efficiency of murine dendritic cells pulsed with antigens. Br J Cancer 2001; 84(11): 1564-70.

[18] Fricke I, Gabrilovich DI. Dendritic cells and tumor microenvironment: a dangerous liaison. Immunol Invest 2006; 35(3-4): 459-483.

[19] Hargadon KM. Tumor-altered dendritic cell function: implications for anti-tumor immunity. Front Immunol 2013; 4: 192.

[20] Nagorsen D, Scheibenbogen C, Thiel E, Keilholz U. Immunological monitoring of cancer vaccine therapy. Expert Opin Biol Ther 2004; 4(10): 1677-1684.

[21] Ardon H, Van Gool S, Lopes IS, Maes W, Sciot R, Wilms G *et al.* Integration of autologous dendritic cell-based immunotherapy in the primary treatment for patients with newly diagnosed glioblastoma multiforme: a pilot study. J Neurooncol 2010; 99(2): 261-72.

[22] Ardon H, De Vleeschouwer S, Van Calenbergh F, Claes L, Kramm CM, Rutkowski S *et al.* Adjuvant dendritic cell-based tumour vaccination for children with malignant brain tumours. Pediatr Blood Cancer 2010; 54(4): 519-525.

[23] Ardon H, Van Gool SW, Verschuere T, Maes W, Fieuws S, Sciot R *et al.* Integration of autologous dendritic cell-based immunotherapy in the standard of care treatment for patients with newly diagnosed glioblastoma: results of the HGG-2006 phase I/II trial. Cancer Immunol Immunother 2012; 61(11): 2033-2044.

[24] Caruso DA, Orme LM, Neale AM, Radcliff FJ, Amor GM, Maixner W *et al.* Results of a phase 1 study utilizing monocyte-derived dendritic cells pulsed with tumor RNA in children and young adults with brain cancer. Neuro Oncol 2004; 6(3): 236-246.

[25] Chang CN, Huang YC, Yang DM, Kikuta K, Wei KJ, Kubota T *et al.* A phase I/II clinical trial investigating the adverse and therapeutic effects of a postoperative autologous dendritic cell tumor vaccine in patients with malignant glioma. J Clin Neurosci 2011; 18(8): 1048-1054.

[26] Cho DY, Yang WK, Lee HC, Hsu DM, Lin HL, Lin SZ *et al.* Adjuvant immunotherapy with whole-cell lysate dendritic cells vaccine for glioblastoma multiforme: a phase II clinical trial. World Neurosurg 2012; 77(5-6): 736-744.

[27] De Vleeschouwer S, Van Calenbergh F, Demaerel P, Flamen P, Rutkowski S, Kaempgen E *et al.* Transient local response and persistent tumor control of recurrent malignant glioma treated with combination therapy including dendritic cell therapy. J Neurosurg [pediatrics] 2004; 100: 492-497.

[28] De Vleeschouwer S, Fieuws S, Rutkowski S, Van Calenbergh F, Van Loon J, Goffin J *et al.* Postoperative adjuvant dendritic cell-based immunotherapy in patients with relapsed glioblastoma multiforme. Clin Cancer Res 2008; 14(10): 3098-3104.

[29] Fadul CE, Fisher JL, Hampton TH, Lallana EC, Li Z, Gui J *et al.* Immune response in patients with newly diagnosed glioblastoma multiforme treated with intranodal autologous tumor lysate-dendritic cell vaccination after radiation chemotherapy. J Immunother 2011; 34(4): 382-389.

[30] Jie X, Hua L, Jiang W, Feng F, Feng G, Hua Z. Clinical application of a dendritic cell vaccine raised against heat-shocked glioblastoma. Cell Biochem Biophys 2012; 62(1): 91-99.

[31] Kikuchi T, Akasaki Y, Irie M, Homma S, Abe T, Ohno T. Results of a phase I clinical trial of vaccination of glioma patients with fusions of dendritic and glioma cells. Cancer Immunol Immunother 2001; 50(7): 337-44.

[32] Kikuchi T, Akasaki Y, Abe T, Fukuda T, Saotome H, Ryan JL *et al.* Vaccination of glioma patients with fusions of dendritic and glioma cells and recombinant human interleukin 12. J Immunother 2004; 27(6): 452-459.

[33] Liau LM, Black KL, Martin NA, Sykes SN, Bronstein JM, Jouben-Steele L *et al.* Treatment of a Glioblastoma patient by vaccination with autologous dendritic cells pulsed with allogeneic Major Histocompatibility Complex Class I-matched tumor peptides: Case report. Neurosurgical Focus 2000; 9: on line.

[34] Liau LM, Prins RM, Kiertscher SM, Odesa SK, Kremen TJ, Giovannone AJ *et al.* Dendritic cell vaccination in glioblastoma patients induces systemic and intracranial T-cell responses modulated by the local central nervous system tumor microenvironment. Clin Cancer Res 2005; 11(15): 5515-5525.

[35] Okada H, Lieberman FS, Walter KA, Lunsford LD, Kondziolka DS, Bejjani GK *et al.* Autologous glioma cell vaccine admixed with interleukin-4 gene transfected fibroblasts in the treatment of patients with malignant gliomas. J Transl Med 2007; 5: 67.

[36] Okada H, Kalinski P, Ueda R, Hoji A, Kohanbash G, Donegan TE *et al.* Induction of CD8+ T-cell responses against novel glioma-associated antigen peptides and clinical activity by vaccinations with {alpha}-type 1 polarized dendritic cells and polyinosinic-polycytidylic acid stabilized by lysine and carboxymethylcellulose in patients with recurrent malignant glioma. J Clin Oncol 2011; 20; 29(3): 330-336.

[37] Phuphanich S, Wheeler CJ, Rudnick JD, Mazer M, Wang H, Nuno MA *et al.* Phase I trial of a multi-epitope-pulsed dendritic cell vaccine for patients with newly diagnosed glioblastoma. Cancer Immunol Immunother 2013; 62(1): 125-135.

[38] Prins RM, Soto H, Konkankit V, Odesa SK, Eskin A, Yong WH *et al.* Gene expression profile correlates with T-cell infiltration and relative survival in glioblastoma patients vaccinated with dendritic cell immunotherapy. Clin Cancer Res 2011; 17(6): 1603-1615.

[39] Rutkowski S, De Vleeschouwer S, Kaempgen E, Wolff JEA, Kuhl J, Demaerel P *et al.* Surgery and adjuvant dendritic cell-based tumour vaccination for patients with relapsed malignant glioma, a feasibility study. Br J Cancer 2004; 91: 1656-1662.

[40] Sampson JH, Archer GE, Mitchell DA, Heimberger AB, Herndon JE, Lally-Goss D *et al.* An epidermal growth factor receptor variant III-targeted vaccine is safe and immunogenic in patients with glioblastoma multiforme. Mol Cancer Ther 2009; 8(10): 2773-2779.

[41] Walker DG, Laherty R, Tomlinson FH, Chuah T, Schmidt C. Results of a phase I dendritic cell vaccine trial for malignant astrocytoma: potential interaction with adjuvant chemotherapy. J Clin Neurosci 2008; 15(2): 114-121.

[42] Wheeler CJ, Black KL, Liu G, Ying H, Yu JS, Zhang W *et al.* Thymic CD8[+] T cell production strongly influences tumor antigen recognition and age-dependent glioma mortality. J Immunol 2003; 171: 4927-4933.

[43] Wheeler CJ, Black KL, Liu G, Mazer M, Zhang XX, Pepkowitz S *et al.* Vaccination elicits correlated immune and clinical responses in glioblastoma multiforme patients. Cancer Res 2008; 68(14): 5955-5964.

[44] Yamanaka R, Abe T, Yajima N, Tsuchiya N, Homma J, Kobayashi T *et al.* Vaccination of recurrent glioma patients with tumour lysate-pulsed dendritic cells elicits immune responses: results of a clinical phase I/II trial. Br J Cancer 2003; 89: 1172-1179.

[45] Yamanaka R, Homma J, Yajima N, Tsuchiya N, Sano M, Kobayashi T *et al.* Clinical evaluation of dendritic cell vaccination for patients with recurrent glioma: results of a clinical phase I/II trial. Clin Cancer Res 2005; 11(11): 4160-4167.

[46] Yu JS, Wheeler CJ, Zeltzer PM, Ying H, Finger DN, Lee PK *et al.* Vaccination of malignant glioma patients with peptide-pulsed dendritic cells elicits systemic cytotoxicity and intracranial T-cell infiltration. Cancer Res 2001; 61: 842-847.

[47] Yu JS, Liu G, Ying H, Yong WH, Black KL, Wheeler CJ. Vaccination with tumor lysate-pulsed dendritic cells elicits antigen-specific, cytotoxic T-cells in patients with malignant glioma. Cancer Res 2004; 64: 4973-4979.

[48] Badhiwala J, Decker WK, Berens ME, Bhardwaj RD. Clinical trials in cellular immunotherapy for brain/CNS tumors. Expert Rev Neurother 2013; 13(4): 405-424.

[49] Breckpot K, Corthals J, Bonehill A, Michiels A, Tuyaerts S, Aerts C *et al.* Dendritic cells differentiated in the presence of IFN-{beta} and IL-3 are potent inducers of an antigen-specific CD8+ T cell response. J Leukoc Biol 2005; 78(4): 898-908.

[50] McLellan AD, Starling GC, Williams LA, Hock BD, Hart DNJ. Activation of human peripheral blood dendritic cells induces the CD86 co-stimulatory molecule. Eur J Immunol 1995; 25: 2064-2068.

[51] Nishio M, Spielman J, Lee RK, Nelson DL, Podack ER. CD80 [B7.1] and CD54 [intracellular adhesion molecule-1] induce target cell susceptibility to promiscuous cytotoxic T cell lysis. J Immunol 1996; 157: 4347-4353.

[52] Fessler BJ, Paliogianni F, Hama N, Balow JE, Boumpas DT. Glucocorticoids modulate CD28 mediated pathways for interleukin 2 production in human T cells - Evidence for posttranscriptional regulation. Transplantation 1996; 62: 1113-1118.

[53] Girndt M, Sester U, Kaul H, Hunger F, Kohler H. Glucocorticoids inhibit activation-dependent expression of costimulatory molecule B7-1 in human monocytes. Transplantation 1998; 66: 370-375.

[54] De Vleeschouwer S, Rapp M, Sorg RV, Steiger HJ, Stummer W, Van Gool S *et al.* Dendritic cell vaccination in patients with malignant gliomas: current status and future directions. Neurosurgery 2006; 59(5): 988-999.

[55] De Vleeschouwer S, Ardon H, Van Calenbergh F, Sciot R, Wilms G, Van Loon J *et al.* Stratification according to HGG-IMMUNO RPA model predicts outcome in a large group of patients with relapsed malignant glioma treated by adjuvant postoperative dendritic cell vaccination. Cancer Immunol Immunother 2012; 61(11): 2105-2112.

[56] Mirimanoff RO, Gorlia T, Mason W, van den Bent MJ, Kortmann RD, Fisher B *et al.* Radiotherapy and temozolomide for newly diagnosed glioblastoma: recursive partitioning analysis of the EORTC 26981/22981-NCIC CE3 phase III randomized trial. J Clin Oncol 2006; 24(16): 2563-2569.

[57] Gray A, Raff AB, Chiriva-Internati M, Chen SY, Kast WM. A paradigm shift in therapeutic vaccination of cancer patients: the need to apply therapeutic vaccination strategies in the preventive setting. Immunol Rev 2008; 222: 316-327.

[58] Bellone M, Mondino A, Corti A. Vascular targeting, chemotherapy and active immunotherapy: teaming up to attack cancer. Trends Immunol 2008; 29(5): 235-241.

[59] Gehrmann J, Matsumoto Y, Kreutzberg GW. Microglia: intrinsic immuneffector cell of the brain. Brain Res Brain Res Rev 1995; 20: 269-287.

[60] Graeber MB, Scheithauer BW, Kreutzberg GW. Microglia in brain tumors. Glia 2002; 40: 252-259.

[61] Bonuccelli G, Tsirigos A, Whitaker-Menezes D, Pavlides S, Pestell RG, Chiavarina B *et al.* Ketones and lactate "fuel" tumor growth and metastasis: Evidence that epithelial cancer cells use oxidative mitochondrial metabolism. Cell Cycle 2010; 9(17): 3506-3514.

[62] Martinez-Outschoorn UE, Lin Z, Trimmer C, Flomenberg N, Wang C, Pavlides S *et al.* Cancer cells metabolically "fertilize" the tumor microenvironment with hydrogen peroxide, driving the Warburg effect: implications for PET imaging of human tumors. Cell Cycle 2011; 10(15): 2504-2520.

[63] Husain Z, Huang Y, Seth P, Sukhatme VP. Tumor-derived lactate modifies antitumor immune response: effect on myeloid-derived suppressor cells and NK cells. J Immunol 2013; 191(3): 1486-1495.

[64] Danial NN, Hartman AL, Stafstrom CE, Thio LL. How does the ketogenic diet work? Four potential mechanisms. J Child Neurol 2013; 28(8): 1027-1033.

[65] Masson F, Calzascia T, Berardino-Besson W, de Tribolet N, Dietrich PY, Walker PR. Brain microenvironment promotes the final functional maturation of tumor-specific effector CD8+ T cells. J Immunol 2007; 179(2): 845-853.

[66] Prendergast GC, Jaffee EM. Cancer immunologists and cancer biologists: why we didn't talk then but need to now. Cancer Res 2007; 67(8): 3500-3504.

[67] Nagorsen D, Scheibenbogen C, Marincola FM, Letsch A, Keilholz U. Natural T cell immunity against cancer. Clin Cancer Res 2003; 9(12): 4296-4303.

[68] Dunn GP, Bruce AT, Ikeda H, Old LJ, Schreiber RD. Cancer immunoediting: from immunosurveillance to tumor escape. Nat Immunol 2002; 3(11): 991-998.

[69] Bergwelt-Baildon MS, Popov A, Saric T, Chemnitz J, Classen S, Stoffel MS *et al.* CD25 and indoleamine 2,3-dioxygenase are up-regulated by prostaglandin E2 and expressed by tumor-associated dendritic cells *in vivo*: additional mechanisms of T-cell inhibition. Blood 2006; 108(1): 228-237.

[70] Garin MI, Chu CC, Golshayan D, Cernuda-Morollon E, Wait R, Lechler RI. Galectin-1: a key effector of regulation mediated by CD4+CD25+ T cells. Blood 2007; 109(5): 2058-2065.

[71] Grauer O, Poschl P, Lohmeier A, Adema GJ, Bogdahn U. Toll-like receptor triggered dendritic cell maturation and IL-12 secretion are necessary to overcome T-cell inhibition by glioma-associated TGF-beta2. J Neurooncol 2007; 82(2): 151-161.

[72] Nagata S. Fas ligand and immune evasion. Nat Med 1996; 2: 1306-1307.

[73] Okazaki T, Honjo T. PD-1 and PD-1 ligands: from discovery to clinical application. Int Immunol 2007; 19(7): 813-824.

[74] Verschuere T, Toelen J, Maes W, Poirier F, Boon L, Tousseyn T *et al.* Glioma-derived galectin-1 regulates innate and adaptive antitumor immunity. Int J Cancer 2013; 134(4): 873-84.

[75] Chambers CA, Kuhns MS, Egen JG, Allison JP. CTLA-4-mediated inhibition in regulation of T cell responses: mechanisms and manipulation in tumor immunotherapy. Annu Rev Immunol 2001; 19: 565-94.

[76] Chung CD, Patel VP, Moran M, Lewis LA, Miceli MC. Galectin-1 induces partial TCR zeta-chain phosphorylation and antagonizes processive TCR signal transduction. J Immunol 2000; 165(7): 3722-3729.

[77] Curiel TJ. Tregs and rethinking cancer immunotherapy. J Clin Invest 2007; 117(5): 1167-1174.

[78] El Andaloussi A, Lesniak MS. An increase in CD4+CD25+FOXP3+ regulatory T cells in tumor-infiltrating lymphocytes of human glioblastoma multiforme. Neuro-oncol 2006; 8(3): 234-243.

[79] Kusmartsev S, Gabrilovich DI. Effect of tumor-derived cytokines and growth factors on differentiation and immune suppressive features of myeloid cells in cancer. Cancer Metastasis Rev 2006; 25(3): 323-331.

[80] Mantovani A, Sozzani S, Locati M, Allavena P, Sica A. Macrophage polarization: tumor-associated macrophages as a paradigm for polarized M2 mononuclear phagocytes. Trends Immunol 2002; 23(11): 549-555.

[81] Sica A, Larghi P, Mancino A, Rubino L, Porta C, Totaro MG *et al.* Macrophage polarization in tumour progression. Semin Cancer Biol 2008; 18(5): 349-355.

[82] Yamaguchi T, Sakaguchi S. Regulatory T cells in immune surveillance and treatment of cancer. Semin Cancer Biol 2006; 16(2): 115-123.

[83] Murat A, Migliavacca E, Gorlia T, Lambiv WL, Shay T, Hamou MF *et al.* Stem cell-related "self-renewal" signature and high epidermal growth factor receptor expression associated with resistance to concomitant chemoradiotherapy in glioblastoma. J Clin Oncol 2008; 26(18): 3015-3024.

[84] Rutledge WC, Kong J, Gao J, Gutman DA, Cooper L, Appin C *et al.* Tumor-infiltrating lymphocytes in glioblastoma are associated with specific genomic alterations and related to transcriptional class. Clin Cancer Res 2013; 19(18): 4951-60

[85] Verhaak RG, Hoadley KA, Purdom E, Wang V, Qi Y, Wilkerson MD *et al.* Integrated genomic analysis identifies clinically relevant subtypes of glioblastoma characterized by abnormalities in PDGFRA, IDH1, EGFR, and NF1. Cancer Cell 2010; 17(1): 98-110.

[86] Sturm D, Witt H, Hovestadt V, Khuong-Quang DA, Jones DT, Konermann C *et al.* Hotspot mutations in H3F3A and IDH1 define distinct epigenetic and biological subgroups of glioblastoma. Cancer Cell 2012; 22(4): 425-437.

[87] Barajas RF, Jr., Phillips JJ, Parvataneni R, Molinaro A, Essock-Burns E, Bourne G *et al.* Regional variation in histopathologic features of tumor specimens from treatment-naive glioblastoma correlates with anatomic and physiologic MR Imaging. Neuro Oncol 2012; 14(7): 942-954.
[88] Jones C, Perryman L, Hargrave D. Paediatric and adult malignant glioma: close relatives or distant cousins? Nat Rev Clin Oncol 2012; 9(7): 400-413.
[89] Prins RM, Wang X, Soto H, Young E, Lisiero DN, Fong B *et al.* Comparison of glioma-associated antigen peptide-loaded *versus* autologous tumor lysate-loaded dendritic cell vaccination in malignant glioma patients. J Immunother 2013; 36(2): 152-157.
[90] Itoh K, Yamada A. Personalized peptide vaccines: a new therapeutic modality for cancer. Cancer Sci 2006; 97(10): 970-976.
[91] Houben R, Wischhusen J, Menaa F, Synwoldt P, Schrama D, Brocker EB *et al.* Melanoma stem cells: targets for successful therapy? J Dtsch Dermatol Ges 2008; 6(7): 541-546.
[92] Pellegatta S, Poliani PL, Corno D, Menghi F, Ghielmetti F, Suarez-Merino B *et al.* Neurospheres enriched in cancer stem-like cells are highly effective in eliciting a dendritic cell-mediated immune response against malignant gliomas. Cancer Res 2006; 66(21): 10247-10252.
[93] Rahman R, Heath R, Grundy R. Cellular immortality in brain tumours: an integration of the cancer stem cell paradigm. Biochim Biophys Acta 2009; 1792(4): 280-288.
[94] Vescovi AL, Galli R, Reynolds BA. Brain tumour stem cells. Nat Rev Cancer 2006; 6(6): 425-436.
[95] Bleau AM, Hambardzumyan D, Ozawa T, Fomchenko EI, Huse JT, Brennan CW *et al.* PTEN/PI3K/Akt pathway regulates the side population phenotype and ABCG2 activity in glioma tumor stem-like cells. Cell Stem Cell 2009; 4(3): 226-235.
[96] Zeppernick F, Ahmadi R, Campos B, Dictus C, Helmke BM, Becker N *et al.* Stem cell marker CD133 affects clinical outcome in glioma patients. Clin Cancer Res 2008; 14(1): 123-129.
[97] Okada H. Brain tumor immunotherapy with type-1 polarizing strategies. Ann N Y Acad Sci 2009; 1174: 18-23.
[98] Grauer OM, Nierkens S, Bennink E, Toonen LW, Boon L, Wesseling P *et al.* CD4+FoxP3+ regulatory T cells gradually accumulate in gliomas during tumor growth and efficiently suppress antiglioma immune responses *in vivo*. Int J Cancer 2007; 121(1): 95-105.
[99] Zhou G, Drake CG, Levitsky HI. Amplification of tumor-specific regulatory T cells following therapeutic cancer vaccines. Blood 2006; 10(2): 628-636.
[100] Fong B, Jin R, Wang X, Safaee M, Lisiero DN, Yang I *et al.* Monitoring of regulatory T cell frequencies and expression of CTLA-4 on T cells, before and after DC vaccination, can predict survival in GBM patients. PLoS ONE 2012; 7(4): e32614.
[101] Peng G, Wang HY, Peng W, Kiniwa Y, Seo KH, Wang RF. Tumor-Infiltrating gammadelta T Cells Suppress T and Dendritic Cell Function *via* Mechanisms Controlled by a Unique Toll-like Receptor Signaling Pathway. Immunity 2007; 27(2): 334-348.
[102] Ferlazzo G, Tsang ML, Moretta L, Melioli G, Steinman RM, Munz C. Human dendritic cells activate resting natural killer [NK] cells and are recognized *via* the NKp30 receptor by activated NK cells. J Exp Med 2002; 195(3): 343-51.
[103] Kalinski P, Mailliard RB, Giermasz A, Zeh HJ, Basse P, Bartlett DL *et al.* Natural killer-dendritic cell cross-talk in cancer immunotherapy. Expert Opin Biol Ther 2005; 5(10): 1303-1315.
[104] Hagemann T, Lawrence T, McNeish I, Charles KA, Kulbe H, Thompson RG *et al.* "Re-educating" tumor-associated macrophages by targeting NF-kappaB. J Exp Med 2008; 205(6): 1261-1268.
[105] Martinez FO, Sica A, Mantovani A, Locati M. Macrophage activation and polarization. Front Biosci 2008; 13: 453-461.
[106] Kusmartsev S, Gabrilovich DI. Role of immature myeloid cells in mechanisms of immune evasion in cancer. Cancer Immunol Immunother 2006; 55(3): 237-245.
[107] Dunn GP, Dunn IF, Curry WT. Focus on TILs: Prognostic significance of tumor infiltrating lymphocytes in human glioma. Cancer Immun 2007; 7: 12.
[108] Birnbaum T, Roider J, Schankin CJ, Padovan CS, Schichor C, Goldbrunner R *et al.* Malignant gliomas actively recruit bone marrow stromal cells by secreting angiogenic cytokines. J Neurooncol 2007; 83(3): 241-247.
[109] Nair S, Boczkowski D, Moeller B, Dewhirst M, Vieweg J, Gilboa E. Synergy between tumor immunotherapy and antiangiogenic therapy. Blood 2003; 102: 964-971.

[110] Rinne ML, Lee EQ, Nayak L, Norden AD, Beroukhim R, Wen PY *et al.* Update on bevacizumab and other angiogenesis inhibitors for brain cancer. Expert Opin Emerg Drugs 2013; 18(2): 137-153.
[111] Piao Y, Liang J, Holmes L, Zurita AJ, Henry V, Heymach JV *et al.* Glioblastoma resistance to anti-VEGF therapy is associated with myeloid cell infiltration, stem cell accumulation, and a mesenchymal phenotype. Neuro Oncol 2012; 14(11): 1379-1392.
[112] Dzenko KA, Song L, Ge S, Kuziel WA, Pachter JS. CCR2 expression by brain microvascular endothelial cells is critical for macrophage transendothelial migration in response to CCL2. Microvasc Res 2005; 70(1-2): 53-64.
[113] Kushchayev SV, Sankar T, Eggink LL, Kushchayeva YS, Wiener PC, Hoober JK *et al.* Monocyte galactose/N-acetylgalactosamine-specific C-type lectin receptor stimulant immunotherapy of an experimental glioma. Part 1: stimulatory effects on blood monocytes and monocyte-derived cells of the brain. Cancer Manag Res 2012; 4: 309-23.
[114] Holdhoff M, Yovino SG, Boadu O, Grossman SA. Blood-based biomarkers for malignant gliomas. J Neurooncol 2013; 113(3): 345-352.
[115] Weller M, Stupp R, Hegi ME, van den BM, Tonn JC, Sanson M *et al.* Personalized care in neuro-oncology coming of age: why we need MGMT and 1p/19q testing for malignant glioma patients in clinical practice. Neuro Oncol 2012; 14 Suppl 4: iv100-8.
[116] Hartmann C, Hentschel B, Wick W, Capper D, Felsberg J, Simon M *et al.* Patients with IDH1 wild type anaplastic astrocytomas exhibit worse prognosis than IDH1-mutated glioblastomas, and IDH1 mutation status accounts for the unfavorable prognostic effect of higher age: implications for classification of gliomas. Acta Neuropathol 2010; 120(6): 707-718.
[117] Verschuere T, Van Woensel M, Fieuws S, Lefranc F, Mathieu V, Kiss R *et al.* Altered galectin-1 serum levels in patients diagnosed with high-grade glioma. J Neurooncol 2013; 115 (1), 9-17.
[118] Le Mercier M, Fortin S, Mathieu V, Kiss R, Lefranc F. Galectins and gliomas. Brain Pathol 2010; 20(1): 17-27.
[119] Gilboa E. DC-based cancer vaccines. J Clin Invest 2007; 117(5): 1195-1203.
[120] Lesterhuis WJ, Aarntzen EH, de V, I, Schuurhuis DH, Figdor CG, Adema GJ *et al.* Dendritic cell vaccines in melanoma: from promise to proof? Crit Rev Oncol Hematol 2008; 66(2): 118-134.
[121] de Vries IJ, Krooshoop DJ, Scharenborg NM, Lesterhuis WJ, Diepstra JH, Van Muijen GN *et al.* Effective migration of antigen-pulsed dendritic cells to lymph nodes in melanoma patients is determined by their maturation state. Cancer Res 2003; 63(1): 12-17.
[122] Muthuswamy R, Urban J, Lee JJ, Reinhart TA, Bartlett D, Kalinski P. Ability of mature dendritic cells to interact with regulatory T cells is imprinted during maturation. Cancer Res 2008; 68(14): 5972-5978.
[123] Hirano N, Butler MO, Xia Z, Ansen S, Bergwelt-Baildon MS, Neuberg D *et al.* Engagement of CD83 ligand induces prolonged expansion of CD8+ T cells and preferential enrichment for antigen specificity. Blood 2006; 107(4): 1528-1536.
[124] Koski GK, Cohen PA, Roses RE, Xu S, Czerniecki BJ. Reengineering dendritic cell-based anti-cancer vaccines. Immunol Rev 2008; 222: 256-76.
[125] McIlroy D, Gregoire M. Optimizing dendritic cell-based anticancer immunotherapy: maturation state does have clinical impact. Cancer Immunol Immunother 2003; 52(10): 583-591.
[126] Carreno BM, Becker-Hapak M, Huang A, Chan M, Alyasiry A, Lie WR *et al.* IL-12p70-producing patient DC vaccine elicits Tc1-polarized immunity. J Clin Invest 2013; 123(8): 3383-3394.
[127] Weaver CT, Harrington LE, Mangan PR, Gavrieli M, Murphy KM. Th17: an effector CD4 T cell lineage with regulatory T cell ties. Immunity 2006; 24(6): 677-688.
[128] Parker JN, Bauer DF, Cody JJ, Markert JM. Oncolytic viral therapy of malignant glioma. Neurotherapeutics 2009; 6(3): 558-569.
[129] Kalinski P, Urban J, Narang R, Berk E, Wieckowski E, Muthuswamy R. Dendritic cell-based therapeutic cancer vaccines: what we have and what we need. Future Oncol 2009; 5(3): 379-390.
[130] Bakdash G, Sittig SP, van Dijk T, Figdor CG, de Vries IJ. The nature of activatory and tolerogenic dendritic cell-derived signal II. Front Immunol 2013; 4: 53.
[131] Serda RE. Particle platforms for cancer immunotherapy. Int J Nanomedicine 2013; 8: 1683-96.
[132] Volovitz I, Marmor Y, Azulay M, Machlenkin A, Goldberger O, Mor F *et al.* Split immunity: immune inhibition of rat gliomas by subcutaneous exposure to unmodified live tumor cells. J Immunol 2011; 187(10): 5452-5462.

[133] Neefjes J, Sadaka C. Into the intracellular logistics of cross-presentation. Front Immunol 2012; 3: 31.
[134] Garg AD, Dudek AM, Agostinis P. Cancer immunogenicity, danger signals, and DAMPs: What, when, and how? Biofactors 2013; 39(4): 355-367.
[135] Bubenik J. Genetically engineered dendritic cell-based cancer vaccines [review]. Int J Oncol 2001; 18(3): 475-8.
[136] van der Most RG, Currie A, Robinson BW, Lake RA. Cranking the immunologic engine with chemotherapy: using context to drive tumor antigen cross-presentation towards useful antitumor immunity. Cancer Res 2006; 66(2): 601-604.
[137] Aarntzen EH, Srinivas M, Bonetto F, Cruz LJ, Verdijk P, Schreibelt G *et al.* Targeting of 111In-labeled dendritic cell human vaccines improved by reducing number of cells. Clin Cancer Res 2013; 19(6): 1525-1533.
[138] Mocellin S, Nitti D. Therapeutics targeting tumor immune escape: towards the development of new generation anticancer vaccines. Med Res Rev 2008; 28(3): 413-444.
[139] Monjazeb AM, Zamora AE, Grossenbacher SK, Mirsoian A, Sckisel GD, Murphy WJ. Immunoediting and antigen loss: overcoming the achilles heel of immunotherapy with antigen non-specific therapies. Front Oncol 2013; 3: 197.
[140] Baniyash M. TCR zeta-chain downregulation: curtailing an excessive inflammatory immune response. Nat Rev Immunol 2004; 4(9): 675-687.
[141] Jameson SC. Maintaining the norm: T-cell homeostasis. Nat Rev Immunol 2002; 2(8): 547-556.
[142] Zitvogel L, Kepp O, Kroemer G. Immune parameters affecting the efficacy of chemotherapeutic regimens. Nat Rev Clin Oncol 2011; 8(3): 151-160.
[143] Liu G, Akasaki Y, Khong HT, Wheeler CJ, Das A, Black KL *et al.* Cytotoxic T cell targeting of TRP-2 sensitizes human malignant glioma to chemotherapy. Oncogene 2005; 24(33): 5226-5234.
[144] Ghiringhelli F, Menard C, Puig PE, Ladoire S, Roux S, Martin F *et al.* Metronomic cyclophosphamide regimen selectively depletes CD4+CD25+ regulatory T cells and restores T and NK effector functions in end stage cancer patients. Cancer Immunol Immunother 2007; 56(5): 641-648.
[145] Nowak AK, Robinson BW, Lake RA. Synergy between chemotherapy and immunotherapy in the treatment of established murine solid tumors. Cancer Res 2003; 63(15): 4490-4496.
[146] van Woensel M, Wauthoz N, Rosière R, Amighi K, Mathieu V, Lefranc F, Van Gool S and De Vleeschouwer S. Formulations for intranasal delivery of pharmacological agents to combat brain disease: a new opportunity to tackle GBM? Cancers 2013; 5: 1020-1048.
[147] Sotelo J, Briceno E, Lopez-Gonzalez MA. Adding chloroquine to conventional treatment for glioblastoma multiforme: a randomized, double-blind, placebo-controlled trial. Ann Intern Med 2006; 144(5): 337-343.
[148] Maes H, Rubio N, Garg AD, Agostinis P. Autophagy: shaping the tumor microenvironment and therapeutic response. Trends Mol Med 2013; 19(7): 428-446.
[149] Begley J, Ribas A. Targeted therapies to improve tumor immunotherapy. Clin Cancer Res 2008; 14(14): 4385-4391.
[150] McDermott D, Haanen J, Chen TT, Lorigan P, O'Day S. Efficacy and safety of ipilimumab in metastatic melanoma patients surviving more than 2 years following treatment in a phase III trial [MDX010-20]. Ann Oncol 2013; 24(10): 2694-8.
[151] Verschuere T, De Vleeschouwer S, Lefranc F, Kiss R, Van Gool SW. Galectin-1 and immunotherapy for brain cancer. Expert Rev Neurother 2011; 11(4): 533-543.

## CHAPTER 5

# Cytokines in Cancer Immunotherapy: The *Yin* and *Yang* Aspects of IL-12 Family of Cytokines

**Zhenzhen Liu[1], Yun Shi[1,2], Ming-Song Li[2] and Xue-Feng Bai[1,*]**

*[1]Department of Pathology and Comprehensive Cancer Center, The Ohio State University, Columbus, OH, USA and [2]Department of Gastroenterology, Nanfang Hospital, Southern Medical University, Guangzhou, China*

**Abstract:** During the past decades, a large body of evidence has revealed that cytokine-based immunotherapy can potently stimulate anti-tumor immune responses and are beneficial for cancer patients. IL-12 is recognized as a prototype cytokine that can induce type 1 (Th1/Tc1) anti-tumor immune responses. However, clinical trials using IL-12 as a single regime, or as a vaccine substance, have demonstrated limited effectiveness in the majority of cases. Recent evidence suggests that IL-12 induces T cell terminal differentiation/exhaustion and thus T cell responses could not be sustained to resulting in tumor rejection. Thus, evaluation of other novel cytokines such as IL-27 that has potent anti-tumor activity yet induces sustained immune responses is highly desired. In this book chapter, we will discuss the *Yin* and *Yang* aspects of IL-12 family of cytokines (*i.e.*, IL-12, IL-23, IL-27 and IL-35) in cancer pathogenesis and immunotherapy.

**Keywords:** Cancer immunotherapy, Cytokine, IL-12, IL-23, IL-27, IL-35, T cells, Th1, Tim-3.

## INTRODUCTION

In the past decades, a number of cytokines have been introduced into cancer clinical trials. To date, IFN-α and IL-2 are the two notable cytokines that have attained FDA approval for the treatments of various cancers to be used as a single agent. IFN-α is suitable for the treatment of stage II/III melanoma, some hematological malignancies, HIV/AIDS-associated Kaposi's sarcoma, and advanced renal cancer [1, 2]. Administration of high-dose IL-2 results in impartial clinical responses around 15-20% of melanoma, and about 25% of renal cell carcinoma patients [3, 4]. Systemic administration of GM-CSF also shows a certain degree of clinical benefits in prostate cancer, lung metastatic cancer and melanoma [5-7].

***Corresponding author Xue-Feng Bai:** Department of Pathology and Comprehensive Cancer Center, The Ohio State University, Columbus, OH, USA; Tel: 0030-2610969332; E-mail: Xue-Feng.Bai@osumc.edu

Jianxun Song (Ed)

IL-12 is recognized as a prototype of cytokines and a master regulator of type 1 (Th1/Tc1) responses [8, 9]. However, unlike its significant anti-cancer activities known in a number of preclinical investigations [10-14], clinical trials using IL-12 as a single agent, or as a vaccine substance, have demonstrated limited effectiveness in the majority of cases [9, 15-17]. IL-12 also exhibits significant toxicity, presumably due to excessive induction of interferon gamma [18, 19]. Recent evidence further suggests that IL-12 up-regulates the expression of Tim-3 on T cells and induces T cell terminal differentiation/exhaustion, and thus, T cell responses could not be sustained to resulting in tumor rejection [20]. On the other hand, recent other studies [21, 22] have revealed that T cells with concomitant memory and terminally differentiated phenotype are more efficient in rejecting tumors than T cells that are extreme in type 1 (Th1/Tc1) differentiation. Thus, novel cytokines that can induce concomitant memory and effector phenotype in T cells with low toxicity should be evaluated as cancer therapeutics. Recent studies from our laboratory [23] and others [22, 24, 25] have revealed that IL-12 family of cytokines such as IL-27 may be an ideal candidate that can induce optimal anti-tumor CTL responses. In this book chapter, we will discuss the *Yin* and *Yang* aspects of novel IL-12 family of cytokines (*i.e.*, IL-23, IL-27 and IL-35) in cancer pathogenesis and immunotherapy.

## CYTOKINE MEMBERS OF IL-12 FAMILY

The cytokines of IL-12 family members are a unique group of heterodimeric cytokines. Currently, there are four main members, which include IL-12, IL-23, IL-27, and IL-35 [26]. One characteristic of this family of cytokines is that they often share the same subunits. IL-12 shares p40 with IL-23; IL-27 shares EBI3 with IL-35, whereas IL-12 shares p35 with IL-35. Another characteristic of IL-12 family members is that cytokine receptors also have common chains. IL-12Rβ1 pairs with either IL-12Rβ2 or IL-23R to form the receptors IL-12 or IL-23; IL-12Rβ2 also binds to gp130 to form IL-35 receptor, whereas gp130 is also a component of the receptor for IL-27. The downstream signaling pathways for IL-12 family of cytokines are mainly mediated by the JAK-STAT proteins (Fig. **1**). Since the JAK/STAT signaling pathways are essential for mediating biological responses induced by a variety of cytokines, the function of a cytokine is dependent on which members of the JAK and STAT families are activated by its binding to the receptor. IL-12 signals mainly *via* p-STAT4 [27]; IL-23 can mediate signaling through p-STAT3 and p-STAT4 [28, 29]; IL-27 can phosphorylate STAT1 and STAT3 [30, 31], and IL-35 mainly activates STAT1 and STAT4 [32]. Thus, cytokine members of IL-12 family have different roles in immune regulation as well as cancer pathogenesis. Both IL-12 and IL-23 are pro-inflammatory cytokines facilitating Th1 and Th17 development [33-35]; IL-27 holds pro-inflammatory as well as anti-inflammatory properties in a context dependent manner [36, 37] while IL-35 has been shown to be produced by Treg cells and displayed potent immune-regulatory effects [38]. Given their essential roles in regulating T cell differentiation, IL-12 family of cytokines has been the focus of attention for having the potential to enhance tumor-specific T cells to eradicate cancer. In the following section, we will review the biological functions of cytokine members of the IL-12 family in tumor immunity and discuss their therapeutic applications in current preclinical and clinical trials.

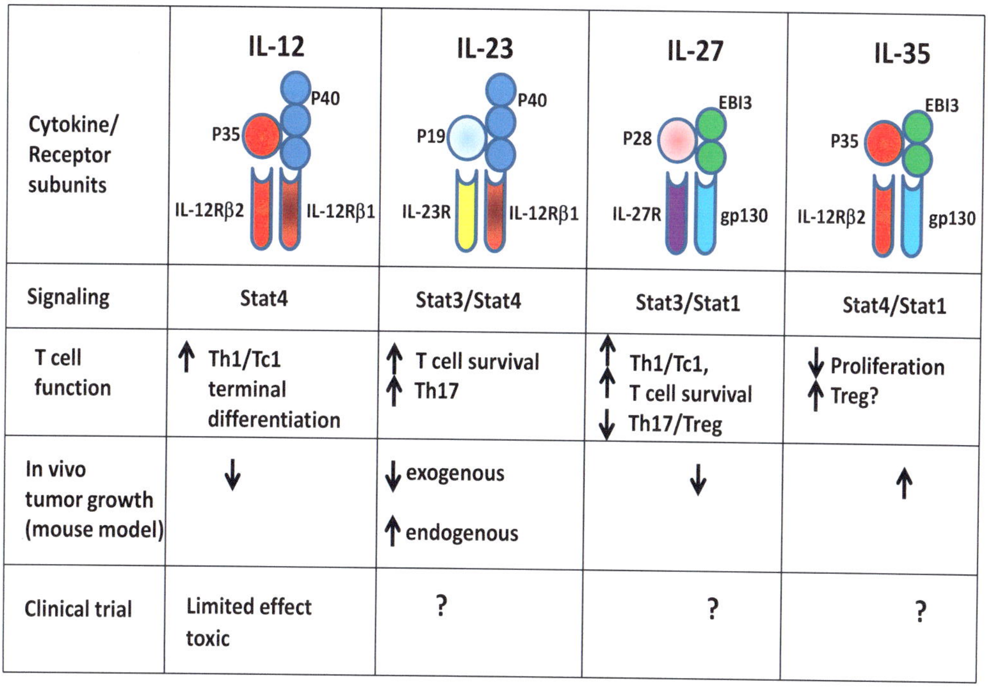


**Figure 1.** The role of IL-12 family of cytokines in cancer pathogenesis and immunotherapy. ↑ =enhance; ↓ =inhibit.

## ROLE OF IL-12 FAMILY MEMBERS IN CANCER PATHOGENESIS AND IMMUNOTHERAPY

### 1. IL-12

IL-12 is a disulfide-linked heterodimeric cytokine, which is composed of a p35 light chain (35kD) and a p40 heavy chain (40kD). IL-12 is mainly produced by antigen presenting cells (APCs) in response to various stimuli [39]. IL-12 is well known to control infectious and malignant diseases by inducing Th1 response [8, 40, 41] and enhancing the cytotoxicity of NK cells and cytotoxic T lymphocytes

[42-44]. Recombinant IL-12 has been verified in many murine tumor models with nearly complete tumor regression and prolonged survival time of animals [45-51]. An IL-12 gene has been genetically over-expressed in various tumor cell lines, including melanoma, colon carcinoma, breast cancer, and ovarian cancer [10, 11, 52], and it has been demonstrated that tumor-derived IL-12 mediates potent antitumor immune responses and leads to tumor rejection. Work from the Surgery Branch in NIH/NCI showed that the local delivery of murine IL-12 by antigen-specific T cells (pmel-1) resulted in significant tumor regression in established B16 melanoma model [53]. The mechanism regarding how IL-12 mediates its potent antitumor activity varies by species, tumor models, doses and schedule of IL-12 administration, delivery method, and the tumor microenvironment. For example, it has been shown that administration of high-dose IL-12 rejected melanoma through NK cells, whereas low-dose IL-12 appeared to activate NKT cells [54].

Recombinant IL-12 has been used in several clinical trials to treat cancer patients, including metastatic melanoma, renal cell cancer, T-cell lymphoma, AIDS-related Kaposi sarcoma, and non-Hodgkins lymphoma [16, 17, 55-57]. The objective response rates in above trials were low. However, many patients who did respond had maintained cytokine levels in the serum, such as IFN-γ, IL-15, and IL-18, indicating that IL-12 has considerable promise for treating cancer patients. It remains unclear why IL-12 trial in cancer patients is not very effective. A recent study suggests that IL-12 can up-regulate the expression of Tim-3 on T cells and induces T cell terminal differentiation/exhaustion, and thus IL-12-induced T cell responses could not be sustained to resulting in tumor rejection [20]. The clinical application of IL-12 was also hindered by dose-limiting toxicities and two treatment deaths in early clinical trials [58, 59]. To control the toxicities and side effects of IL-12, recent studies have dedicated to developing new delivery methods to express IL-12 at tumor sites, including IL-12 administration using a virus-based, gene-modified, or cell-based approach. One study involves the administration of IL-12 through injecting adenoviral vector encoding human IL-12 (Ad.IL-12) intratumorally into patients with advanced cancers, such as pancreatic, colorectal, and primary liver malignancy [60]. In another trial IL-12 plasmid was delivered into metastatic melanoma lesions through electroporation [61]. Kang *et al.* transduced allogeneic or autologous fibroblasts with viral vectors containing the human IL-12 gene and peritumorally injected into patients with disseminated cancer. The side effects of this treatment were comparatively controlled, and tumor burdens were reduced [62]. In July 2011, the NIH approved a phase I clinical trial of new agent NHS-IL12 for the therapy of solid tumors. The

NHS-IL12 comprises two IL-12 heterodimers, in which each fused to one of the H-chains of the NHS76 antibody that has an affinity for both single- and double-stranded DNA. This delivery method would help avoid side effects and enhance the IL-12-mediated antitumor activity. IL-12 has also been used as an adjuvant for vaccination in several clinical trials treating metastatic melanoma and kidney cancer [63-65]. Overall, the IL-12 therapy has shown limited efficacy with significant toxicity in the treatment of cancer.

## 2. IL-23

IL-23 consists of the subunit of IL-12p40, and the IL-23-specific subunit of p19, which is about 40% similar to IL-12p35 in the overall sequence. The co-expression of p40 and p19 has been observed in activated dendritic cells and phagocytic cells. IL-23 not only shares the same subunit of p40 with IL-12 but also has a common receptor unit, IL-12Rβ1. T cells, NK cells, macrophages, and dendritic cells express the IL-23R. As compared to IL-12, IL-23 mainly plays role in naive $CD4^+$ T cells and preferentially in memory $CD4^+$ T cells [66]. Connected with IL-6 and TGF-β1, IL-23 can drive naive $CD4^+$ T cells to differentiate into Th17 cells, and has been shown to be crucial to the pathogenesis of T cell-mediated inflammatory diseases [67, 68].

IL-23 has displayed both anti-tumor and pro-tumor effects in previous studies. Recombinant IL-23 reduces B-ALL cell growth *in vitro* and in preclinical models by inhibiting proliferation and inducing apoptosis of tumor cells [69]. Over-expression of IL-23 in mouse colon carcinoma or B16 melanoma significantly inhibits tumor growth and metastasis [70-72]. Administration of high-dose IL-23 resulted in slower tumor growth and longer survival time of mice bearing fibrosarcoma [73]. In contrast to exogenous IL-23, endogenous IL-23 has been shown to enhance tumor incidence and growth. The deficiency of IL-23 or IL-23R not only decreases tumor incidence but also inhibits tumor growth [74]. IL-23 promotes inflammatory responses, increases angiogenesis, and the infiltration of macrophages, but reduces cytotoxic $CD8^+$ T cell infiltration [74]. Furthermore, IL-23p19 is over-expressed in most human cancers. The differential effects of exogenous and endogenous IL-23 in tumor growth suggest that the dual roles of the immune system in suppressing and promoting cancer formation. Currently, IL-23 or IL-23 targeted therapy has not been introduced into clinical trials of cancer patients.

## 3. IL-27

IL-27 is a heterodimeric cytokine, which is composed of two subunits, including EBI3 and p28 [75]. Similar to IL-12 and IL-23, EBI3 and p28 co-expression in a single cell is required for IL-27 to exert its biological functions [75]. The expression of human IL-27 has been found in monocytes, monocyte-derived DCs, endothelial cells, and trophoblast cells [75, 76], while the expression of murine IL-27 has been verified in activated microglia cells and macrophages [75, 77]. It has been shown that signaling through toll-like receptors (TLR) are crucial inducers of IL-27. Stimulation of macrophages with agonists [poly (I:C)], LPS, R848 for TLR3, TLR4, and TLR7/8 correspondingly resulted in concurrent expression of EBI3 and p28 [78]. The expression of EBI3 in DCs was substantially decreased in the lack of TLR2, TLR4, TLR9, or MyD88, suggesting that TLR stimulation is required for IL-27 expression [79]. In addition, the expression of EBI3 in DCs was induced through the activation of the transcription factors NF-κB and PU-1 [79]. Human IL-27p28 mRNA was specially induced by Toll/IL-1R-containing adaptor inducing IFN-β-coupled TLR ligands, and IRF3 activation is a chief switch for the synthesis of IL-27 [80]. Besides TLR ligands, many host-derived factors, such as CD40L, IL-1β, IFN-α, IFN-β, and IFN-γ, can up-regulate IL-27 expression as well [78, 81]. In contrast, the nucleotide ATP negatively regulates the expression of IL-27 [82].

Researchers from different groups transfected the IL-27 gene into a number of tumor cell lines, evaluated tumorigenesis in mice, and found that tumor-derived IL-27 can trigger potent antitumor immune responses leading to almost complete tumor rejection. For instance, mouse colon carcinoma Colon 26 cells transfected with the IL-27-expressing vector exhibited minimal tumor growth that was mediated mainly by $CD8^+$ T cell expression of IFN-γ and T-bet [24, 25, 83-85]. While in poorly immunogenic tumors (*e.g.*, B16F10 melanoma), IL-27 can give its antitumor effects using different mechanisms, including enhancing NK cell responses [72], inhibiting angiogenesis [86], and directly suppressing tumor cell proliferation [87]. IL-27 also activates NK-mediated antibody-dependent cellular cytotoxicity (ADCC) in the head and neck squamous cell carcinoma [88]. In mice bearing TBJ neuroblastoma tumors, IL-27 mediates overall tumor regression by up-regulating the expression of MHC class I on tumor cells, and enhancing the generation of both tumor-specific immune responsiveness and immunologic memory responses [84]. In lung cancer model, both over-expression of IL-27 and treatment with rIL-27 directly inhibit expression of vimentin, COX-2, and its metabolite (PGE2) in lung cancer cells [89]. Collectively, IL-27-induced immunological and non-immunological effects both contribute to its potent antitumor activities.

It is noteworthy that the induction of CTL response seems to be the most important component of IL-27-mediated antitumor effects. However, the underlying mechanisms of how IL-27 promotes anti-tumor immune responses are not fully understood. IL-27 is likely to induce $CD8^+$ T cells to express T-bet, IL-12Rβ2, and granzyme B. Recently, we proposed [90] several new mechanisms by which IL-27 enhances anti-tumor CTL responses and tumor rejection. First, IL-27 can confer a survival advantage for CTL cells; Second, IL-27 can induce tumor antigen-specific CTL cells to produce a large amount of IL-10, which contributes to CTL-mediated tumor rejection; Third, IL-27 can induce a unique memory phenotype of precursor cell (MPC) in activated $CD8^+$ T cells, characterized by up-regulation of SOCS3, Bcl-6, and Sca-1, and give rise to memory $CD8^+$ T cells. Finally, IL-27 can suppress the development of Treg cells in the tumor microenvironment, which can indirectly enhance antitumor CTL responses [91, 92]. Given the potent antitumor effect of IL-27 in preclinical models, using IL-27 or IL-27-based strategies should provide an effective option for immunotherapy of human cancer. At this stage, IL-27-based cancer immunotherapy has not been translated into clinical settings.

## 4. IL-35

IL-35 is a newly identified cytokine member of IL-12 family. Like other members in the family, IL-35 is a heterodimeric molecule, which is composed of an IL-12α-chain p35 and an IL-27β-chain EBI3 [38, 93, 94]. $Foxp3^+CD4^+CD25^+$ regulatory T cells (Tregs) [38] or a regulatory T cell population induced by IL-35 could secrete IL-35 [32]. IL-35 signals were mediated by a unique heterodimer of receptor chains (*i.e.*, IL-12Rβ2 and gp130), or the homodimers of each chain in target cells [32]. Different from the other members of IL-12 family, IL-35 is a potent immunosuppressive cytokine. It has been shown to suppress the proliferation of T cells by inducing cell-cycle arrest in G1 phase deprived of inducing apoptosis [32, 38, 95]. Loss of IL-35 decreases *in vivo* suppressive ability of Tregs [38]. IL-35-deficient Tregs lost to control the homeostatic expansion of effector T cells as well as cure established colitis, as compared to wild type Tregs. Furthermore, IL-35 has been shown to suppress Th17 development *in vivo* and ameliorate collagen-induced arthritis (CIA) [94]. Several other studies have also reported that IL-35 serves as an immunomodulatory role in many disease conditions [95-99].

Although the expression and function of IL-35 have only been determined in Tregs, gene-expression analysis revealed that IL-35 may have much broader tissue distribution [100]. Reports indicate the upregulation of EBI3 and p35 expressions in placental trophoblasts [101], and EBI3 associates with p35 in the extract of the trophoblastic components of human full-term normal placenta [93]. EBI3 is also detected in Hodgkin lymphoma cells [102], acute myeloid leukemia cells [103], and lung cancer cells [104]. IL-12p35 [102], but not IL-27p28 [105], was detectable in $EBI3^+$ tumor cells; therefore, it is likely that some cancer cells can produce IL-35 but not IL-27. In the tumor microenvironment, $Foxp3^+$ Tregs and other Tregs are accumulated as tumor progresses [106, 107]; they can provide another source of IL-35. In addition, tumor-infiltrating dendritic cells were found to express EBI3 [102, 105], which could be an additional source of IL-35. Taken together, IL-35 could be an important factor in the tumor microenvironment that impacts tumor-specific T cell responses and tumor progression. We have recently reported that IL-35 is abundantly produced in human cancer tissues. Moreover, tumor-derived IL-35 increases $CD11b^+Gr1^+$ myeloid cell accumulation and tumor angiogenesis [108]. Similarly, Wu *et al.* observed that acute myeloid leukemia patients have increased plasma concentrations of IL-35 [109]. In addition, IL-35 is essential for the immunosuppressive ability of human prostate tumor antigen-specific $CD8^+$ Treg cells, indicating that IL-35 is a pro-tumor cytokine by strengthening the tumor immunosuppressive environment [110]. Thus, blocking IL-35 or IL-35 receptor may be a promising therapy to treat cancer patients.

## CONCLUDING REMARKS AND FUTURE DIRECTIONS

Cytokine-based cancer immunotherapy has shown some success in certain cancer patients. However, the limited success of current cytokine-based cancer immunotherapy warrants further evaluation of novel cytokines. Clinical and experimental studies [20-22] have revealed that IL-12 causes T cell terminal differentiation, which is in favor of T cell effector function, but insufficient to cause tumor rejection. These observations warrant novel thinking of using IL-12 family of cytokines as therapeutics for cancer based on their differential functions (Fig. **1**). In this regard, the following characteristics of IL-27 highly support the idea that IL-27 should be evaluated in cancer clinical trial. *First*, IL-27 has a similar ability in inducing type 1 responses to IL-12. However, unlike IL-12, IL-27 has potent survival promoting effect of T lymphocytes [23]. Thus, IL-27 is more likely to stimulate sustained antitumor T cell responses. *Second*, IL-27 can directly inhibit the growth of some type of cancer cells (presumably due to IL-27R expression). *Third*, IL-27 also has potent anti-inflammation effect, it has the potential to suppress cancer associated inflammation or inflammation-associated cancer. Thus, it is anticipated that IL-27 therapy may be particularly beneficial to those cancer types that inflammation is a driven force for cancer progression. Although endogenous IL-23 enhances tumor growth [74], exogenous IL-23 is inhibitory in different tumor models [70-73]. Thus, IL-23 as a therapeutic agent should also be evaluated in cancer patients. In contrast to other IL-12 family members, IL-35 has a potent pro-tumor effect and is likely expressed in the tumor microenvironment of human cancer [108], therefore, IL-35 blockade should be beneficial to cancer patients.

## ACKNOWLEDGEMENTS

Declared None.

## CONFLICT OF INTEREST

The authors confirm that this chapter contents have no conflict of interest.

## REFERENCES

[1] Dranoff G. Cytokines in cancer pathogenesis and cancer therapy. Nat Rev Cancer 2004; 4(1): 11-22.
[2] Rini BI, Halabi S, Rosenberg JE, Stadler WM, Vaena DA, Archer L, *et al.* Phase III trial of bevacizumab plus interferon alfa *versus* interferon alfa monotherapy in patients with metastatic renal cell carcinoma: final results of CALGB 90206. J Clin Oncol 2010; 28(13): 2137-43.
[3] Fyfe G, Fisher RI, Rosenberg SA, Sznol M, Parkinson DR, Louie AC. Results of treatment of 255 patients with metastatic renal cell carcinoma who received high-dose recombinant interleukin-2 therapy. J Clin Oncol 1995; 13(3): 688-96.
[4] Rosenberg SA, Lotze MT, Yang JC, Topalian SL, Chang AE, Schwartzentruber DJ, *et al.* Prospective randomized trial of high-dose interleukin-2 alone or in conjunction with lymphokine-activated killer cells for the treatment of patients with advanced cancer. J Natl Cancer Inst 1993; 85(8): 622-32.
[5] Spitler LE, Grossbard ML, Ernstoff MS, Silver G, Jacobs M, Hayes FA, *et al.* Adjuvant therapy of stage III and IV malignant melanoma using granulocyte-macrophage colony-stimulating factor. J Clin Oncol 2000; 18(8): 1614-21.
[6] Rini BI, Weinberg V, Bok R, Small EJ. Prostate-specific antigen kinetics as a measure of the biologic effect of granulocyte-macrophage colony-stimulating factor in patients with serologic progression of prostate cancer. J Clin Oncol 2003; 21(1): 99-105.
[7] Anderson PM, Markovic SN, Sloan JA, Clawson ML, Wylam M, Arndt CA, *et al.* Aerosol granulocyte macrophage-colony stimulating factor: a low toxicity, lung-specific biological therapy in patients with lung metastases. Clin Cancer Res 1999; 5(9): 2316-23
[8] Colombo MP, Trinchieri G. Interleukin-12 in anti-tumor immunity and immunotherapy. Cytokine Growth Factor Rev 2002; 13(2): 155-68.
[9] Del Vecchio M, Bajetta E, Canova S, Lotze MT, Wesa A, Parmiani G, *et al.* Interleukin-12: biological properties and clinical application. Clin Cancer Res 2007; 13(16): 4677-85.
[10] Coughlin CM, Salhany KE, Wysocka M, Aruga E, Kurzawa H, Chang AE, *et al.* Interleukin-12 and interleukin-18 synergistically induce murine tumor regression which involves inhibition of angiogenesis. J Clin Invest 1998; 101(6): 1441-52.
[11] Kaufman HL, Flanagan K, Lee CS, Perretta DJ, Horig H. Insertion of interleukin-2 (IL-2) and interleukin-12 (IL-12) genes into vaccinia virus results in effective anti-tumor responses without toxicity. Vaccine 2002; 20(13-14): 1862-9.
[12] Li Q, Carr AL, Donald EJ, Skitzki JJ, Okuyama R, Stoolman LM, *et al.* Synergistic effects of IL-12 and IL-18 in skewing tumor-reactive T-cell responses towards a type 1 pattern. Cancer Res 2005; 65(3): 1063-70.
[13] Yoshimoto T, Nagai N, Ohkusu K, Ueda H, Okamura H, Nakanishi K. LPS-stimulated SJL macrophages produce IL-12 and IL-18 that inhibit IgE production *in vitro* by induction of IFN-gamma production from CD3intIL-2R beta+ T cells. J Immunol 1998; 161(3): 1483-92.
[14] Yoshimoto T, Takeda K, Tanaka T, Ohkusu K, Kashiwamura S, Okamura H, *et al.* IL-12 up-regulates IL-18 receptor expression on T cells, Th1 cells, and B cells: synergism with IL-18 for IFN-gamma production. J Immunol 1998; 161(7): 3400-7.

[15] Rosenberg SA, Yang JC, Restifo NP. Cancer immunotherapy: moving beyond current vaccines. Nat Med 2004; 10(9): 909-15.

[16] Atkins MB, Robertson MJ, Gordon M, Lotze MT, DeCoste M, DuBois JS, *et al.* Phase I evaluation of intravenous recombinant human interleukin 12 in patients with advanced malignancies. Clin Cancer Res 1997; 3(3): 409-17.

[17] Younes A, Pro B, Robertson MJ, Flinn IW, Romaguera JE, Hagemeister F, *et al.* Phase II clinical trial of interleukin-12 in patients with relapsed and refractory non-Hodgkin's lymphoma and Hodgkin's disease. Clin Cancer Res 2004; 10(16): 5432-8.

[18] Car BD, Eng VM, Schnyder B, LeHir M, Shakhov AN, Woerly G, *et al.* Role of interferon-gamma in interleukin 12-induced pathology in mice. Am J Pathol 1995; 147(6): 1693-707.

[19] Ryffel B. Interleukin-12: role of interferon-gamma in IL-12 adverse effects. Clin Immunol Immunopathol 1997; 83(1): 18-20.

[20] Yang ZZ, Grote DM, Ziesmer SC, Niki T, Hirashima M, Novak AJ, *et al.* IL-12 upregulates TIM-3 expression and induces T cell exhaustion in patients with follicular B cell non-Hodgkin lymphoma. J Clin Invest 2012; 122(4): 1271-82.

[21] Hirschhorn-Cymerman D, Budhu S, Kitano S, Liu C, Zhao F, Zhong H, *et al.* Induction of tumoricidal function in CD4+ T cells is associated with concomitant memory and terminally differentiated phenotype. J Exp Med 2012; 209(11): 2113-26.

[22] Curran MA, Geiger TL, Montalvo W, Kim M, Reiner SL, Al-Shamkhani A, *et al.* Systemic 4-1BB activation induces a novel T cell phenotype driven by high expression of Eomesodermin. J Exp Med 2013; 210(4): 743-55.

[23] Liu Z, Liu JQ, Talebian F, Wu LC, Li S, Bai XF. IL-27 enhances the survival of tumor antigen-specific CD8(+) T cells and programs them into IL-10-producing, memory precursor-like effector cells. Eur J Immunol 2013; 43(2): 468-79.

[24] Hisada M, Kamiya S, Fujita K, Belladonna ML, Aoki T, Koyanagi Y, *et al.* Potent antitumor activity of interleukin-27. Cancer Res 2004; 64(3): 1152-6.

[25] Salcedo R, Stauffer JK, Lincoln E, Back TC, Hixon JA, Hahn C, *et al.* IL-27 mediates complete regression of orthotopic primary and metastatic murine neuroblastoma tumors: role for CD8+ T cells. J Immunol 2004; 173(12): 7170-82.

[26] Vignali DA, Kuchroo VK. IL-12 family cytokines: immunological playmakers. Nat Immunol 2012; 13(8): 722-8.

[27] Thierfelder WE, van Deursen JM, Yamamoto K, Tripp RA, Sarawar SR, Carson RT, *et al.* Requirement for Stat4 in interleukin-12-mediated responses of natural killer and T cells. Nature 1996; 382(6587): 171-4.

[28] Oppmann B, Lesley R, Blom B, Timans JC, Xu Y, Hunte B, *et al.* Novel p19 protein engages IL-12p40 to form a cytokine, IL-23, with biological activities similar as well as distinct from IL-12. Immunity 2000; 13(5): 715-25.

[29] Parham C, Chirica M, Timans J, Vaisberg E, Travis M, Cheung J, *et al.* A receptor for the heterodimeric cytokine IL-23 is composed of IL-12Rbeta1 and a novel cytokine receptor subunit, IL-23R. J Immunol 2002; 168(11): 5699-708.

[30] Lucas S, Ghilardi N, Li J, de Sauvage FJ. IL-27 regulates IL-12 responsiveness of naive CD4+ T cells through Stat1-dependent and -independent mechanisms. Proc Natl Acad Sci U S A 2003; 100(25): 15047-52.

[31] Hibbert L, Pflanz S, De Waal Malefyt R, Kastelein RA. IL-27 and IFN-alpha signal *via* Stat1 and Stat3 and induce T-Bet and IL-12Rbeta2 in naive T cells. J Interferon Cytokine Res 2003; 23(9): 513-22.

[32] Collison LW, Delgoffe GM, Guy CS, Vignali KM, Chaturvedi V, Fairweather D, *et al.* The composition and signaling of the IL-35 receptor are unconventional. Nat Immunol 2012; 13(3): 290-9.

[33] Cua DJ, Sherlock J, Chen Y, Murphy CA, Joyce B, Seymour B, *et al.* Interleukin-23 rather than interleukin-12 is the critical cytokine for autoimmune inflammation of the brain. Nature 2003; 421(6924): 744-8.

[34] Kastelein RA, Hunter CA, Cua DJ. Discovery and biology of IL-23 and IL-27: related but functionally distinct regulators of inflammation. Annu Rev Immunol 2007; 25: 221-42

[35] Diveu C, McGeachy MJ, Boniface K, Stumhofer JS, Sathe M, Joyce-Shaikh B, *et al.* IL-27 blocks RORc expression to inhibit lineage commitment of Th17 cells. J Immunol 2009; 182(9): 5748-56.

[36] Chen Q, Ghilardi N, Wang H, Baker T, Xie MH, Gurney A, *et al.* Development of Th1-type immune responses requires the type I cytokine receptor TCCR. Nature 2000; 407(6806): 916-20.
[37] Hall AO, Silver JS, Hunter CA. The immunobiology of IL-27. Adv Immunol 2012; 115: 1-44.
[38] Collison LW, Workman CJ, Kuo TT, Boyd K, Wang Y, Vignali KM, *et al.* The inhibitory cytokine IL-35 contributes to regulatory T-cell function. Nature 2007; 450(7169): 566-9.
[39] Trinchieri G. Interleukin-12: a cytokine produced by antigen-presenting cells with immunoregulatory functions in the generation of T-helper cells type 1 and cytotoxic lymphocytes. Blood 1994; 84(12): 4008-27.
[40] Trinchieri G, Scott P. The role of interleukin 12 in the immune response, disease and therapy. Immunol Today 1994; 15(10): 460-3.
[41] Decken K, Kohler G, Palmer-Lehmann K, Wunderlin A, Mattner F, Magram J, *et al.* Interleukin-12 is essential for a protective Th1 response in mice infected with Cryptococcus neoformans. Infection and Immunity 1998; 66(10): 4994-5000.
[42] Perussia B, Chan SH, D'Andrea A, Tsuji K, Santoli D, Pospisil M, *et al.* Natural killer (NK) cell stimulatory factor or IL-12 has differential effects on the proliferation of TCR-alpha beta+, TCR-gamma delta+ T lymphocytes, and NK cells. J Immunol 1992; 149(11): 3495-502.
[43] Chehimi J, Starr SE, Frank I, Rengaraju M, Jackson SJ, Llanes C, *et al.* Natural killer (NK) cell stimulatory factor increases the cytotoxic activity of NK cells from both healthy donors and human immunodeficiency virus-infected patients. J Experimental Medicine 1992; 175(3): 789-96.
[44] Chan SH, Kobayashi M, Santoli D, Perussia B, Trinchieri G. Mechanisms of IFN-gamma induction by natural killer cell stimulatory factor (NKSF/IL-12). Role of transcription and mRNA stability in the synergistic interaction between NKSF and IL-2. J Immunol 1992; 148(1): 92-8.
[45] Brunda MJ, Luistro L, Warrier RR, Wright RB, Hubbard BR, Murphy M, *et al.* Antitumor and antimetastatic activity of interleukin 12 against murine tumors. The J Experimental Medicine 1993; 178(4): 1223-30.
[46] Boggio K, Di Carlo E, Rovero S, Cavallo F, Quaglino E, Lollini PL, *et al.* Ability of systemic interleukin-12 to hamper progressive stages of mammary carcinogenesis in HER2/neu transgenic mice. Cancer Res 2000; 60(2): 359-64.
[47] Nastala CL, Edington HD, McKinney TG, Tahara H, Nalesnik MA, Brunda MJ, *et al.* Recombinant IL-12 administration induces tumor regression in association with IFN-gamma production. J Immunol 1994; 153(4): 1697-706.
[48] Hill HC, Conway TF, Jr., Sabel MS, Jong YS, Mathiowitz E, Bankert RB, *et al.* Cancer immunotherapy with interleukin 12 and granulocyte-macrophage colony-stimulating factor-encapsulated microspheres: coinduction of innate and adaptive antitumor immunity and cure of disseminated disease. Cancer Res 2002; 62(24): 7254-63.
[49] Hess SD, Egilmez NK, Bailey N, Anderson TM, Mathiowitz E, Bernstein SH, *et al.* Human CD4+ T cells present within the microenvironment of human lung tumors are mobilized by the local and sustained release of IL-12 to kill tumors *in situ* by indirect effects of IFN-gamma. J Immunol 2003; 170(1): 400-12.
[50] Nair RE, Jong YS, Jones SA, Sharma A, Mathiowitz E, Egilmez NK. IL-12 + GM-CSF microsphere therapy induces eradication of advanced spontaneous tumors in her-2/neu transgenic mice but fails to achieve long-term cure due to the inability to maintain effector T-cell activity. J Immunother 2006; 29(1): 10-20.
[51] Watkins SK, Li B, Richardson KS, Head K, Egilmez NK, Zeng Q, *et al.* Rapid release of cytoplasmic IL-15 from tumor-associated macrophages is an initial and critical event in IL-12-initiated tumor regression. European journal of immunology 2009; 39(8): 2126-35.
[52] Rao JB, Chamberlain RS, Bronte V, Carroll MW, Irvine KR, Moss B, *et al.* IL-12 is an effective adjuvant to recombinant vaccinia virus-based tumor vaccines: enhancement by simultaneous B7-1 expression. J Immunol 1996; 156(9): 3357-65.
[53] Kerkar SP, Muranski P, Kaiser A, Boni A, Sanchez-Perez L, Yu Z, *et al.* Tumor-specific CD8+ T cells expressing interleukin-12 eradicate established cancers in lymphodepleted hosts. Cancer Res 2010; 70(17): 6725-34.
[54] Kawamura T, Takeda K, Mendiratta SK, Kawamura H, Van Kaer L, Yagita H, *et al.* Critical role of NK1+ T cells in IL-12-induced immune responses *in vivo*. J Immunol 1998; 160(1): 16-9.

[55] Portielje JE, Kruit WH, Schuler M, Beck J, Lamers CH, Stoter G, *et al.* Phase I study of subcutaneously administered recombinant human interleukin 12 in patients with advanced renal cell cancer. Clin Cancer Res 1999; 5(12): 3983-9.
[56] Rook AH, Wood GS, Yoo EK, Elenitsas R, Kao DM, Sherman ML, *et al.* Interleukin-12 therapy of cutaneous T-cell lymphoma induces lesion regression and cytotoxic T-cell responses. Blood 1999; 94(3): 902-8.
[57] Ansell SM, Witzig TE, Kurtin PJ, Sloan JA, Jelinek DF, Howell KG, *et al.* Phase 1 study of interleukin-12 in combination with rituximab in patients with B-cell non-Hodgkin lymphoma. Blood 2002; 99(1): 67-74.
[58] Cohen J. IL-12 deaths: explanation and a puzzle. Science 1995; 270(5238): 908.
[59] Leonard JP, Sherman ML, Fisher GL, Buchanan LJ, Larsen G, Atkins MB, *et al.* Effects of single-dose interleukin-12 exposure on interleukin-12-associated toxicity and interferon-gamma production. Blood 1997; 90(7): 2541-8.
[60] Sangro B, Mazzolini G, Ruiz J, Herraiz M, Quiroga J, Herrero I, *et al.* Phase I trial of intratumoral injection of an adenovirus encoding interleukin-12 for advanced digestive tumors. J Clin Oncol 2004; 22(8): 1389-97.
[61] Daud AI, DeConti RC, Andrews S, Urbas P, Riker AI, Sondak VK, *et al.* Phase I trial of interleukin-12 plasmid electroporation in patients with metastatic melanoma. J Clin Oncol 2008; 26(36): 5896-903.
[62] Kang WK, Park C, Yoon HL, Kim WS, Yoon SS, Lee MH, *et al.* Interleukin 12 gene therapy of cancer by peritumoral injection of transduced autologous fibroblasts: outcome of a phase I study. Human Gene Therapy 2001; 12(6): 671-84.
[63] Peterson AC, Harlin H, Gajewski TF. Immunization with Melan-A peptide-pulsed peripheral blood mononuclear cells plus recombinant human interleukin-12 induces clinical activity and T-cell responses in advanced melanoma. J Clin Oncol 2003; 21(12): 2342-8.
[64] Gollob JA, Veenstra KG, Parker RA, Mier JW, McDermott DF, Clancy D, *et al.* Phase I trial of concurrent twice-weekly recombinant human interleukin-12 plus low-dose IL-2 in patients with melanoma or renal cell carcinoma. J Clin Oncol 2003; 21(13): 2564-73.
[65] Alatrash G, Hutson TE, Molto L, Richmond A, Nemec C, Mekhail T, *et al.* Clinical and immunologic effects of subcutaneously administered interleukin-12 and interferon alfa-2b: phase I trial of patients with metastatic renal cell carcinoma or malignant melanoma. J Clin Oncol 2004; 22(14): 2891-900.
[66] Lankford CS, Frucht DM. A unique role for IL-23 in promoting cellular immunity. J Leukocyte Biol 2003; 73(1): 49-56.
[67] Aggarwal S, Ghilardi N, Xie MH, de Sauvage FJ, Gurney AL. Interleukin-23 promotes a distinct CD4 T cell activation state characterized by the production of interleukin-17. J Biol Chem 2003; 278(3): 1910-4.
[68] Langrish CL, Chen Y, Blumenschein WM, Mattson J, Basham B, Sedgwick JD, *et al.* IL-23 drives a pathogenic T cell population that induces autoimmune inflammation. J Experimental Medicine 2005; 201(2): 233-40.
[69] Cocco C, Canale S, Frasson C, Di Carlo E, Ognio E, Ribatti D, *et al.* Interleukin-23 acts as antitumor agent on childhood B-acute lymphoblastic leukemia cells. Blood 2010; 116(19): 3887-98.
[70] Lo CH, Lee SC, Wu PY, Pan WY, Su J, Cheng CW, *et al.* Antitumor and antimetastatic activity of IL-23. J Immunol 2003; 171(2): 600-7.
[71] Wang YQ, Ugai S, Shimozato O, Yu L, Kawamura K, Yamamoto H, *et al.* Induction of systemic immunity by expression of interleukin-23 in murine colon carcinoma cells. International Journal of Cancer 2003; 105(6): 820-4.
[72] Oniki S, Nagai H, Horikawa T, Furukawa J, Belladonna ML, Yoshimoto T, *et al.* Interleukin-23 and interleukin-27 exert quite different antitumor and vaccine effects on poorly immunogenic melanoma. Cancer Res 2006; 66(12): 6395-404.
[73] Kaiga T, Sato M, Kaneda H, Iwakura Y, Takayama T, Tahara H. Systemic administration of IL-23 induces potent antitumor immunity primarily mediated through Th1-type response in association with the endogenously expressed IL-12. J Immunol 2007; 178(12): 7571-80.
[74] Langowski JL, Zhang X, Wu L, Mattson JD, Chen T, Smith K, *et al.* IL-23 promotes tumour incidence and growth. Nature 2006; 442(7101): 461-5.
[75] Pflanz S, Timans JC, Cheung J, Rosales R, Kanzler H, Gilbert J, *et al.* IL-27, a heterodimeric cytokine composed of EBI3 and p28 protein, induces proliferation of naive CD4(+) T cells. Immunity 2002; 16(6): 779-90.

[76] Larousserie F, Pflanz S, Coulomb-L'Hermine A, Brousse N, Kastelein R, Devergne O. Expression of IL-27 in human Th1-associated granulomatous diseases. J Pathol 2004; 202(2): 164-71.

[77] Sonobe Y, Yawata I, Kawanokuchi J, Takeuchi H, Mizuno T, Suzumura A. Production of IL-27 and other IL-12 family cytokines by microglia and their subpopulations. Brain Res 2005; 1040(1-2): 202-7.

[78] Pirhonen J, Siren J, Julkunen I, Matikainen S. IFN-alpha regulates Toll-like receptor-mediated IL-27 gene expression in human macrophages. J Leukoc Biol 2007; 82(5): 1185-92.

[79] Wirtz S, Becker C, Fantini MC, Nieuwenhuis EE, Tubbe I, Galle PR, *et al.* EBV-induced gene 3 transcription is induced by TLR signaling in primary dendritic cells *via* NF-kappa B activation. J Immunol 2005; 174(5): 2814-24.

[80] Molle C, Nguyen M, Flamand V, Renneson J, Trottein F, De Wit D, *et al.* IL-27 synthesis induced by TLR ligation critically depends on IFN regulatory factor 3. J Immunol 2007; 178(12): 7607-15.

[81] Villarino AV, Huang E, Hunter CA. Understanding the pro- and anti-inflammatory properties of IL-27. J Immunol 2004; 173(2): 715-20.

[82] Schnurr M, Toy T, Shin A, Wagner M, Cebon J, Maraskovsky E. Extracellular nucleotide signaling by P2 receptors inhibits IL-12 and enhances IL-23 expression in human dendritic cells: a novel role for the cAMP pathway. Blood 2005; 105(4): 1582-9.

[83] Chiyo M, Shimozato O, Iizasa T, Fujisawa T, Tagawa M. Antitumor effects produced by transduction of dendritic cells-derived heterodimeric cytokine genes in murine colon carcinoma cells. Anticancer Res 2004; 24(6): 3763-7.

[84] Salcedo R, Hixon JA, Stauffer JK, Jalah R, Brooks AD, Khan T, *et al.* Immunologic and therapeutic synergy of IL-27 and IL-2: enhancement of T cell sensitization, tumor-specific CTL reactivity and complete regression of disseminated neuroblastoma metastases in the liver and bone marrow. J Immunol 2009; 182(7): 4328-38.

[85] Zhu S, Lee DA, Li S. IL-12 and IL-27 sequential gene therapy *via* intramuscular electroporation delivery for eliminating distal aggressive tumors. J Immunol 2010; 184(5): 2348-54.

[86] Shimizu M, Shimamura M, Owaki T, Asakawa M, Fujita K, Kudo M, *et al.* Antiangiogenic and antitumor activities of IL-27. J Immunol 2006; 176(12): 7317-24.

[87] Yoshimoto T, Morishima N, Mizoguchi I, Shimizu M, Nagai H, Oniki S, *et al.* Antiproliferative activity of IL-27 on melanoma. J Immunol 2008; 180(10): 6527-35.

[88] Matsui M, Kishida T, Nakano H, Yoshimoto K, Shin-Ya M, Shimada T, *et al.* Interleukin-27 activates natural killer cells and suppresses NK-resistant head and neck squamous cell carcinoma through inducing antibody-dependent cellular cytotoxicity. Cancer Res 2009; 69(6): 2523-30.

[89] Ho MY, Leu SJ, Sun GH, Tao MH, Tang SJ, Sun KH. IL-27 directly restrains lung tumorigenicity by suppressing cyclooxygenase-2-mediated activities. J Immunol 2009; 183(10): 6217-26.

[90] Liu Z, Yu J, Carson WE, 3rd, Bai XF. The role of IL-27 in the induction of anti-tumor cytotoxic T lymphocyte response. Am J Transl Res 2013; 5(5): 470-80.

[91] Neufert C, Becker C, Wirtz S, Fantini MC, Weigmann B, Galle PR, *et al.* IL-27 controls the development of inducible regulatory T cells and Th17 cells *via* differential effects on STAT1. Eur J Immunol 2007; 37(7): 1809-16.

[92] Huber M, Steinwald V, Guralnik A, Brustle A, Kleemann P, Rosenplanter C, *et al.* IL-27 inhibits the development of regulatory T cells *via* STAT3. Int Immunol 2008; 20(2): 223-34.

[93] Devergne O, Birkenbach M, Kieff E. Epstein-Barr virus-induced gene 3 and the p35 subunit of interleukin 12 form a novel heterodimeric hematopoietin. Proc Natl Acad Sci U S A 1997; 94(22): 12041-6.

[94] Niedbala W, Wei XQ, Cai B, Hueber AJ, Leung BP, McInnes IB, *et al.* IL-35 is a novel cytokine with therapeutic effects against collagen-induced arthritis through the expansion of regulatory T cells and suppression of Th17 cells. Eur J Immunol 2007; 37(11): 3021-9.

[95] Collison LW, Chaturvedi V, Henderson AL, Giacomin PR, Guy C, Bankoti J, *et al.* IL-35-mediated induction of a potent regulatory T cell population. Nat Immunol 2010; 11(12): 1093-101.

[96] Seyerl M, Kirchberger S, Majdic O, Seipelt J, Jindra C, Schrauf C, *et al.* Human rhinoviruses induce IL-35-producing Treg *via* induction of B7-H1 (CD274) and sialoadhesin (CD169) on DC. Eur J Immunol 2010; 40(2): 321-9.

[97] Whitehead GS, Wilson RH, Nakano K, Burch LH, Nakano H, Cook DN. IL-35 production by inducible costimulator (ICOS)-positive regulatory T cells reverses established IL-17-dependent allergic airways disease. J Allergy and Clin Immunol 2012; 129(1): 207-15 e1-5.

[98] Liu F, Tong F, He Y, Liu H. Detectable expression of IL-35 in CD4+ T cells from peripheral blood of chronic hepatitis B patients. Clin Immunol 2011; 139(1): 1-5.

[99] Kochetkova I, Golden S, Holderness K, Callis G, Pascual DW. IL-35 stimulation of CD39+ regulatory T cells confers protection against collagen II-induced arthritis *via* the production of IL-10. J Immunol 2010; 184(12): 7144-53.

[100] Li X, Mai J, Virtue A, Yin Y, Gong R, Sha X, *et al.* IL-35 is a novel responsive anti-inflammatory cytokine--a new system of categorizing anti-inflammatory cytokines. PLoS One 2012; 7(3): e33628.

[101] Devergne O, Coulomb-L'Hermine A, Capel F, Moussa M, Capron F. Expression of Epstein-Barr virus-induced gene 3, an interleukin-12 p40-related molecule, throughout human pregnancy: involvement of syncytiotrophoblasts and extravillous trophoblasts. Am J Pathol 2001; 159(5): 1763-76.

[102] Niedobitek G, Pazolt D, Teichmann M, Devergne O. Frequent expression of the Epstein-Barr virus (EBV)-induced gene, EBI3, an IL-12 p40-related cytokine, in Hodgkin and Reed-Sternberg cells. J Pathol 2002; 198(3): 310-6.

[103] Poleganov MA, Bachmann M, Pfeilschifter J, Muhl H. Genome-wide analysis displays marked induction of EBI3/IL-27B in IL-18-activated AML-derived KG1 cells: critical role of two kappaB binding sites in the human EBI3 promotor. Molecular Immunology 2008; 45(10): 2869-80.

[104] Nishino R, Takano A, Oshita H, Ishikawa N, Akiyama H, Ito H, *et al.* Identification of Epstein-Barr virus-induced gene 3 as a novel serum and tissue biomarker and a therapeutic target for lung cancer. Clin Cancer Res 2011; 17(19): 6272-86.

[105] Larousserie F, Bardel E, Pflanz S, Arnulf B, Lome-Maldonado C, Hermine O, *et al.* Analysis of interleukin-27 (EBI3/p28) expression in Epstein-Barr virus- and human T-cell leukemia virus type 1-associated lymphomas: heterogeneous expression of EBI3 subunit by tumoral cells. Am J Pathol 2005; 166(4): 1217-28.

[106] Liyanage UK, Moore TT, Joo HG, Tanaka Y, Herrmann V, Doherty G, *et al.* Prevalence of regulatory T cells is increased in peripheral blood and tumor microenvironment of patients with pancreas or breast adenocarcinoma. J Immunol 2002; 169(5): 2756-61.

[107] Wolf D, Wolf AM, Rumpold H, Fiegl H, Zeimet AG, Muller-Holzner E, *et al.* The expression of the regulatory T cell-specific forkhead box transcription factor FoxP3 is associated with poor prognosis in ovarian cancer. Clin Cancer Res 2005; 11(23): 8326-31.

[108] Wang Z, Liu JQ, Liu Z, Shen R, Zhang G, Xu J, *et al.* Tumor-Derived IL-35 Promotes Tumor Growth by Enhancing Myeloid Cell Accumulation and Angiogenesis. J Immunol 2013; 190(5): 2415-23.

[109] Wu H, Li P, Shao N, Ma J, Ji M, Sun X, *et al.* Aberrant expression of Treg-associated cytokine IL-35 along with IL-10 and TGF-beta in acute myeloid leukemia. Oncology Letters 2012; 3(5): 1119-23.

[110] Olson BM, Jankowska-Gan E, Becker JT, Vignali DA, Burlingham WJ, McNeel DG. Human prostate tumor antigen-specific CD8+ regulatory T cells are inhibited by CTLA-4 or IL-35 blockade. J Immunol 2012; 189(12): 5590-601.

# CHAPTER 6

# Genetically Engineered T Cell Immunotherapy for Gliomas and Other Solid Tumors

**Richard G. Everson, Colin C. Malone, Kate L. Erickson, Elena I. Fomchenko, Robert M. Prins, Linda M. Liau and Carol A. Kruse***

*Department of Neurosurgery, David Geffen School of Medicine, University of California, Los Angeles, CA 90095, USA*

**Abstract:** Cell-based therapeutics, once very popular, were relegated to background mode because of the seemingly complex and highly technical nature of producing the cells at specialized facilities. However, they once again are emerging as promising biomedicines with the potential to substantially impact cancer. The resurgence in adoptive immunotherapy comes with renewed interest in our ability to endow cells with novel attributes by genetic modification. We now have techniques at our disposal to enable the creation of designer therapeutics since the T cells now are handled beyond simple manipulation with growth factors. For cellular immunotherapies, T cells can be expanded and manipulated *ex vivo* prior to adoptive transfer into the host to achieve a novel immune function and with signaling capability. Also, genetic engineering of T cells has been successfully implemented to redirect the specificity of cytotoxic T lymphocytes towards tumor-associated antigens without MHC restriction. Over 70 Investigative New Drug applications are listed on the Food and Drug Administration maintained website www.clinicaltrials.gov that involve genetically engineered T lymphocytes or T cells endowed with chimeric antigen receptors. While the majority of these trials focus on treatment of hematopoietic diseases generally involving B cells, here, we focus on the description of clinical trials currently testing these modified T cells in patients with solid tumors and even more specifically, for those involving treatment of primary malignant brain tumors.

**Keywords:** Adenocarcinomas, adoptive immunotherapy, adoptive transfer, astrocytomas, cellular therapy, chimeric antigen receptor, CTL, cytotoxic lymphocytes, gliomas, human leukocyte antigens, immunotherapy, immunotherapy, major histocompatibility complex, melanoma, prostate cancer, solid tumors, T cell receptor, tumor associated antigens.

## INTRODUCTION

### T Cell Immunotherapy Historical Perspective

While rare, oncologists occasionally observe spontaneous regression of tumors in

***Corresponding author Carol A. Kruse:** Department of Neurosurgery, David Geffen School of Medicine, University of California, Los Angeles, CA 90095, USA; Tel: (310) 267-2535; E-mail: ckruse@mednet.ucla.edu

Jianxun Song (Ed)

patients who develop infections or other disease complications that are accompanied with immune cell activation [1]. These anecdotal accounts have spurred interest in developing immunotherapies for cancer [2, 3]. In the early 1980s, cellular therapy with *ex vivo* expanded T cells came to the forefront when the recombinant form of Interleukin-2 (IL-2), also known as T cell growth factor, became available. A flurry of clinical trials were conducted that embraced amongst other effector cells, the use of *in vitro* tumor-sensitized cytotoxic T lymphocytes (CTL), *in situ* sensitized, *in vitro* expanded tumor infiltrating lymphocytes (TIL), or short-term cultured, nonspecifically-activated lymphokine activated killer (LAK) cells [4]. A schematic of an adoptive cell transfer approach involving isolation of patient lymphocytes from peripheral blood, their *ex vivo* activation and expansion, followed by transfer of the activated cells back into the tumor bearing host, is shown in Fig. **1**.

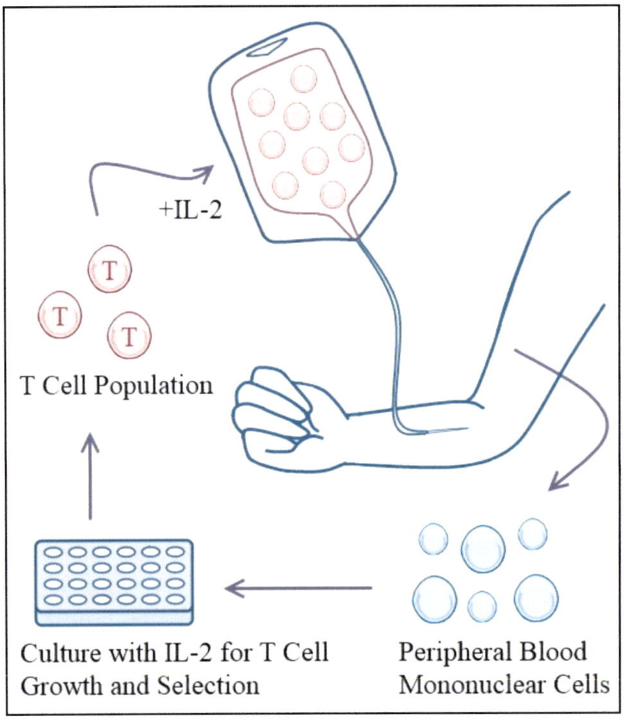


**Figure 1:** Schematic showing one version of an adoptive immunotherapy strategy.

Adoptive cell transfer strategies have sometimes been more successful when 1) appropriate lymphodepleting conditioning regimens are used to neutralize endogenous immunosuppressive cells, such as T regulatory (Treg) or myeloid derived suppressor cells (MDSC), and 2) high-doses of IL-2 are infused for T cell supportive function [5-7]. In studies conducted at the National Institutes of Health (NIH), successful tumor targeting and sustained tumor regressions were obtained with TIL [8]. The protocols commonly employed depletion of immunosuppressive cells with fludarabine and cyclophosphamide prior to infusion with adoptively transferred T cells. Additionally, the adoptive transfer of T cells was accompanied with IL-2, which helps maintain functionality and persistence of the transferred cells. Even with lymphodepletion and IL-2 administration, however, many cancers remain refractory, as peripheral tolerance and tumor immune evasion mechanisms, such as down regulation of MHC antigens and lack of co-stimulatory signals, render the compensatory actions by tumors too overwhelming for immune therapies [5].

T lymphocytes are capable of exquisite specificity. If T cell mediated immunosurveillance functions are working properly, aberrant cells should be recognized and eliminated by our immune system before they become a problem. Thus, when one is diagnosed with cancer, a defect in the person's endogenous immune function should be suspected. Theoretically, corrective measures employing *ex vivo* manipulation with growth factors and patient immune cells should retrain them for enhanced immune function. In the majority of clinical trials, autologous effector T cells derived from the patient were used for therapy, although when placed within the immune semi-privileged sanctuary of the brain, allogeneic cells derived from nonimmunosuppressed donors as sources of effector cells were also tested [9]. One example of the latter is an adoptive cell transfer strategy for recurrent malignant gliomas developed by Kruse and colleagues. Lymphocytes derived from healthy histoincompatible donors were combined with irradiated patient derived lymphocytes [10, 11]. The resultant mixed lymphocyte reaction sensitized the allogeneic donor lymphocytes to patient major histocompatibility complex (MHC) antigens. These alloresponsive T cells were then expanded *ex vivo* with IL-2 and subsequently implanted directly into the brain tumor resection cavity. Preclinical studies indicate the T cells placed into this immune-protected environment are capable of trafficking to and eliminating tumor cells displaying MHC antigens while sparing neuroglia that do not [12]. Patients with recurrent grade III astrocytomas treated with multiple CTL infusates enjoyed long-term survival [13], thus justifying a larger dose-escalation study (clinicaltrials.gov NCT 01144247) to treat recurrent gliomas and meningiomas. The trial is currently underway at UCLA to confirm the safety of this therapeutic modality. Trials such as this offer simplicity in approach and reduced regulatory oversight, compared to those using genetically engineered T cells that require Recombinant Advisory Committee (RAC) approval.

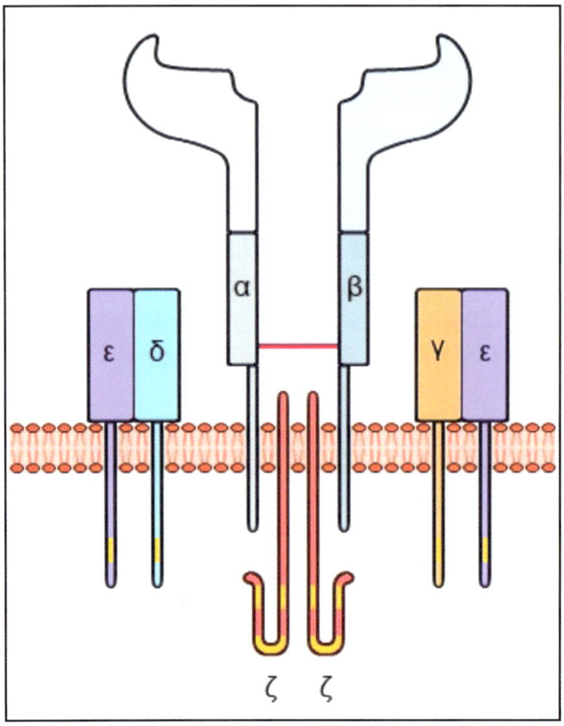


**Figure 2:** The conventional T Cell Receptor. The alpha and beta subunits are responsible for antigen binding, while the accessory CD3 molecules initiate a signaling cascade through ITAM sequences (shown in yellow) upon TCR binding.

## T Cell Receptor Interactions with HLA and Signaling

T cell signaling is mediated by the T cell receptor (TCR). The conventional TCR is a heterodimer composed of alpha and beta protein chains that are translated independently from two separate genes. The alpha and beta chains have variable regions which result in TCR specificity towards an antigen when it is presented in the context of the binding groove of a MHC antigen. Cluster of Differentiation 8 (CD8) positive CTL recognize short amino acid peptide sequences that are displayed by class I MHC molecules. CD4 positive helper-inducer T cells recognize longer peptides bound to MHC class II molecules. In humans, the MHC antigens are termed Human Leukocyte Antigens (HLA), where serotypic class I antigens are termed HLA-A, B, C and class II are HLA-DR, DP, DQ. Each person has 2 alleles, paternal and maternal, that encode HLA. HLA genes are highly polymorphic. Advancements in HLA typing techniques have revealed the vast diversity within HLA serotype families due to genetic polymorphism of the HLA molecule [14, 15]. For example, there are many molecular subtypes within the

HLA-A serotype, distinguishable from each other by only one or a few amino acids, and therefore are better defined by molecular HLA typing techniques using real time polymerase chain reaction (RT-PCR) sequence specific primers (SSP) or by sequence-based typing (SBT).

The TCR is alone unable to induce activation of a lymphocyte. For this, the T cell requires both the TCR as well as six other accessory molecules which make up the CD3 complex (Fig. **2**). The TCR accessory molecules include CD3γ, CD3δ, and two subunits each of CD3ε and CD3ζ. Each CD3 subunit contains an immunoreceptor tyrosine-based activation motif (ITAM), which is a conserved 4-amino acid sequence. These motifs are critical for transducing signal from TCR binding to the antigenic peptide-HLA complex [16]. The tyrosine on these motifs becomes phosphorylated upon TCR binding resulting in T cell activation by induction of downstream signaling cascades [16]. One reason we dwelled specifically on the clinical trial employing alloreactive T cells for therapy, more so than others, is that alloreactivity is the result of T cells encountering a foreign HLA molecule(s) that is sufficiently similar to self to allow TCR-HLA interactions, yet sufficiently different to trigger the activation of a subset of those cells [17].

TCR signaling in mature CD8 lymphocytes leads to cytolysis by the perforin-granzyme pathway, or results in apoptosis of the target cells displaying the antigen to which it is sensitized. Also, an alternative killing mechanism involves that induced by cytokines, the secretion of which is induced by T or other immune cells involved with immune cell supportive function.

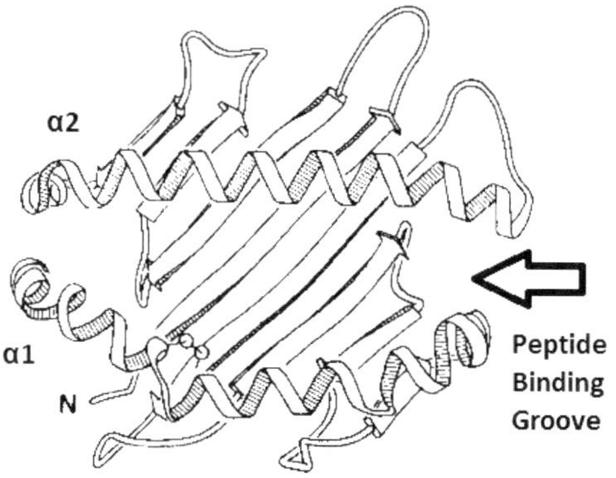


**Figure 3:** Top view of the HLA-A α1 and α2 chains and the peptide binding groove where the amino acid sequence presented would sit at the interface of the TCR with the HLA molecule. Figure adapted from Bjorkman, *et al.* [18].

## Genetic Engineering Techniques

The mechanisms of T cell signaling are now being exploited by genetic engineering techniques to direct T cells to recognize novel antigen(s) that are either overexpressed or expressed exclusively on tumor cells relative to healthy, surrounding tissue cells. Two major methods are being used for T cell genetic engineering. The first is introduction of exogenous alpha and beta T cell receptor genes into T cells to create a cell population with monoclonal specificity towards one TAA. Because this introduced TCR is specific not just to the antigenic peptide sequence but also to the binding groove of the HLA (Fig. **3**) [18], one restriction of this therapy is that it can only target tumors of a particular HLA haplotype (*e.g.* A2). The other technique is the use of an artificial T cell receptor called a Chimeric Antigen Receptor (CAR), which pairs the binding domain of an antibody with the signaling domains of the T cell receptor (Fig. **4**).

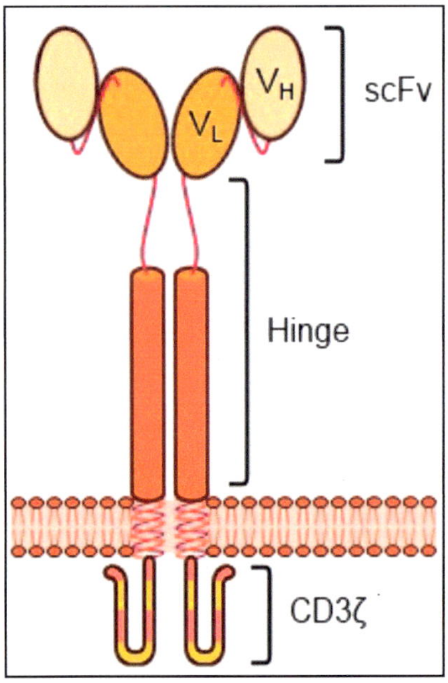


**Figure 4:** A first-generation chimeric antigen receptor. The T cell receptor is shown with antibody variable fragments, hinge, transmembrane, and CD3ζ regions.

Genetically engineering T cells to express CAR allows TAA recognition in an MHC independent fashion [19, 20]. These receptors, in addition to activating the cell killing program upon ligation of the receptor with a TAA, can also provide critical costimulatory signals to drive heightened responses. However, the formidable active immunosuppressive molecules produced by many cancers [5], especially solid tumors, can interfere with the sustained activation of CAR T cells necessary to induce regression of many established tumors.

## GENETICALLY ENGINEERED T CELL RECEPTORS

The first successful utilization of genetically introduced TCR alpha and beta genes, isolated from patient lymphocytes, were directed against the MART-1 melanocyte antigen, which is highly expressed in many melanoma cases but also expressed in normal melanocytes [21]. Later studies with mice expressing transgenic HLA were used to produce new, higher avidity T cell receptors. These studies also demonstrated objective clinical responses but the higher avidity T cell receptors also showed targeted melanocyte destruction in normal tissues [22].

One of the drawbacks of TCR introduction is the mispairing of endogenous TCR alpha and beta proteins with the exogenously introduced TCR alpha beta genes. Advances in modifying T cell receptors have yielded various strategies to circumvent this problem. Modifications include the introduction of cysteine amino acids that allow for new disulfide bonds that support conformational changes allowing exogenous TCR monomers to pair more favorably with each other as opposed to crosspairing with endogenous receptors [23]. Other improvements involve using different T cell subsets, which do not express alpha beta TCR, as well as the use of engineering cytokines into the vectors used so the T cells will respond more robustly to the genetically modified TCR [24].

Many strategies are being developed to enhance the introduction of TCR into the lymphocytes, as they are notoriously difficult to transduce [25], and also are designed to incorporate molecules in them that may react to prodrug so that there is an element of safety in their use for cancer treatment [26, 27]. Objective responses have been observed in clinical trials. Although many tumor types are being used to test their safety/efficacy, here we will focus on their use for solid tumors.

## CHIMERIC ANTIGEN RECEPTORS

The primary advantage of CAR to genetically introduced TCR is the CAR ability to bind tumor antigen through the single-chain variable fragment which does not require HLA interaction. The drawback from the CAR design is its inability to bind tumor antigens expressed intracellularly [28]. The basic design of a CAR involves a domain constructed from $V_H$ and $V_L$ regions of a monoclonal antibody targeted to a TAA (Fig. **4**). The $V_H$ and $V_L$ are linked to hinge sequences and a transmembrane sequence which helps to stabilize the CAR. An intracellular domain, generally containing a CD3 zeta and its corresponding ITAMs, are also included. The single-chain variable region of the CAR can also be replaced by a cytokine signaling domain or other ligands that bind to the targeted antigen. The hinge and transmembrane domain region of the CARs have been substituted by different investigators in different variations of the construct but are often from CD8 alpha sequences or other integral proteins.

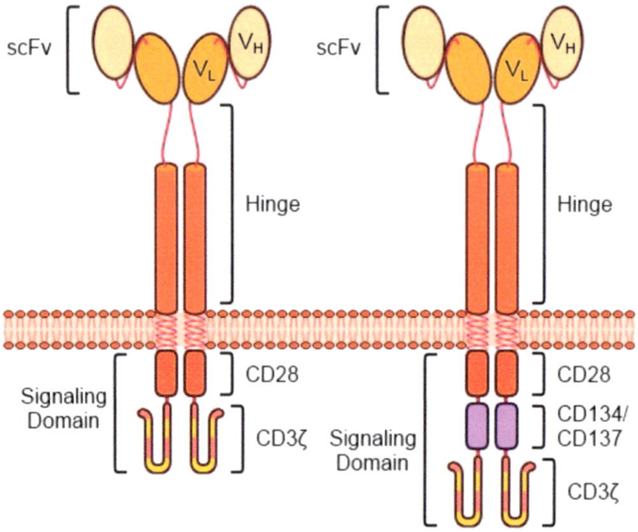


**Figure 5:** Designs of second-generation (left) and third-generation (right) chimeric antigen receptors. While the intracellular signaling domains used will vary from one trial to another, one constant is the CD3 zeta sequence.

From both *in vivo* and *in vitro* studies, CAR-modified T cells have been found to lack stability or persistence relative to CAR T cells that have been modified to include other intracellular signaling domains aside from CD3 zeta. The most commonly included intracellular region is that of CD28 cytoplasmic signaling domain. This allows cells to have greater *in vivo* persistence and improved activation profiles. The inclusion of a CD28 costimulatory sequence in the design of these constructs was an improvement that gave them a designation as second-generation CAR (Fig. **5**). Recent clinical trials of anti-CD19 second generation CARs utilized in B cell lymphomas have shown impressive CAR T cell persistence *in vivo* over long periods after treatment [29, 30]. CAR T cell persistence has correlated with increased survival. Trials are underway for many tumor types using newer second generation CARs as well as third generation CARs. Third generation CARs (Fig. **5**) include additional cytoplasmic stimulatory domains from other key T cell signaling molecules such as CD134 and/or CD137 (also termed 4-1BB) that improve their *in vivo* performance over first and second generation CAR.

## CLINICAL STUDIES – USE OF TCR OR CAR T CELLS FOR SOLID TUMORS

We obtained information at www.clinicaltrials.gov on the clinical studies involving TCR and CAR T cells. We placed in the search terms: T Cell Receptor, Chimeric Antigen Receptor, TCR, CAR, Adoptive T cell therapy, and Cancer. This is a burgeoning field as 437 protocols were listed. The majority are for B cell malignancies, such as refractory non-Hodgkins lymphomas, and relapsed or refractory lymphocytic leukemias in adults and children. They have been used successfully with second generation or third generation CAR T cells targeting CD19 and usually accompanied with costimulation by CD28 or CD137 [30-32]. For this review, we focused on solid tumors. To provide timely information for the eBook readers, which may include both physicians and patients, we considered here only the trials presently recruiting patients and those listing US treatment sites. This information is summarized in Table **1** and lists 18 protocols that are open for patients with solid tumors. A synopsis of these 18 trials follows where we provide information regarding the center and lead investigator, and the NCT identifier on clinicaltrials.gov. We also give the protocol title, the phase of the trial with expected enrollment number, some eligibility criteria and literature references. For purposes of discussion, Table **1** lists the trials offered in order of a specific manufacture site. Since the production of genetically engineered T cells requires specialized laboratories that employ Good Manufacturing Practice/Good Laboratory Practice recommendations, the number of manufacturing facilities is limited but those that do exist often are used for T cell generation for multiple diseases.

**Table 1**: Clinical trials open for patient enrollment that involve TCR and CAR T cell treatment of solid tumors

| Center/Investigator/NCT* | Therapy/Protocol | Phase/Enrollment No. | Eligibility [References] |
|---|---|---|---|
| NIH Clinical Center, Bethesda, MD/<br>Steven A. Rosenberg<br>NCT01218867 | Autologous CTL Expressing a<br>CAR Targeting VEGFR-2<br>(Fludarabine + Cyclophosphamide/IL-2) | I/II - 118 | Recurrent or Non-responder<br>Renal Cancer & Metastatic Melanoma<br>[2, 33] |

*Table 1: contd….*

| | | | |
|---|---|---|---|
| NIH Clinical Center, Bethesda, MD/<br>Steven A. Rosenberg<br>NCT01583686 | Autologous CTL Expressing a CAR Targeting Mesothelin<br>(Fludarabine + Cyclophosphamide/IL-2) | I/II - 136 | Recurrent or Progressive – Mesothelioma & Pancreatic Cancer<br>[2] |
| NIH Clinical Center, Bethesda, MD/<br>Steven A. Rosenberg<br>NCT00670748 | Autologous PBL Expressing a TCR Targeting NY-ESO-1<br>(Fludarabine + Cyclophosphamide/IL-2) | II - 102 | Metastatic Cancer<br>Metastatic Melanoma<br>Metastatic Renal Cancer<br>[2, 34] |
| NIH Clinical Center, Bethesda, MD/<br>Udai S Kammula<br>NCT01495572 | Autologous PBL Expressing<br>anti-MART (p27-35) TCR<br>(Fludarabine + Cyclophosphamide/IL-2) | II - 57 | Metastatic Melanoma<br>[2, 21] |
| NIH Clinical Center (US site),<br>Bethesda, MD/<br>Fiona Thistlethwaite<br>NCT01795976 | Autologous CTL Expressing a TCR Targeting NY-ESO antigen<br>(Cyclophosphamide/IL-2) | I - 28 | Recurrent or Progressive – Esophageal Cancer<br>[34] |
| Memorial Sloan-Kettering Cancer Center, New York City, NY/<br>Susan Slovin<br>NCT01140373 | Autologous CTL Expressing a CAR Targeting Prostate Specific Membrane Antigen (PSMA)<br>(Cyclophosphamide) | I - 18 | Progressive Metastatic Prostate Cancer (Castrate)<br>[35] |
| Roger Williams Medical Institute, Providence, RI/<br>Richard P Junghans<br>NCT00673829 | Autologous PBL Expressing anti-CEA (Carcinoembryonic Antigen) CAR<br>(With or without IL-2) | Ia/Ib - 26 | Metastatic or Advanced Unresectable Breast Cancer<br>[36] |
| Roger Williams Medical Institute, Providence, RI/<br>Richard P Junghans<br>NCT01723306 | Autologous PBL Expressing Second Generation anti-CEA (Carcinoembryonic Antigen) CAR<br>(With or without IL-2) | II - 48 | CEA positive Adenocarcinomas-Gastric, Lung, Colorectal and other Solid Tumors<br>[36] |
| Roger Williams Medical Institute, Providence, RI/<br>Steven C Katz<br>NCT01373047 | Autologous PBL Expressing Second Generation anti-CEA (Carcinoembryonic Antigen) CAR | Phase I - 6 | CEA positive Liver Metastasis [36] |
| Roger Williams Medical Institute, Providence, RI/<br>Richard P Junghans<br>NCT00664196 | Phase Ia/Ib Trial of Anti-PSMA Designer T Cells in Advanced Prostate Cancer After Non-Myeloablative Conditioning<br>(Fludarabine + Cyclophosphamide/IL-2) | Ia/Ib - 18 | Advanced Prostate Cancer<br>[36] |

***Table 1: contd….***

| | | | |
|---|---|---|---|
| UCLA Jonsson Comprehensive Cancer Center, Westwood, CA/ Arun Singh NCT01697527 | Autologous PBMC Expressing anti-NY-ESO-1 (p27-35) TCR (Fludarabine + Cyclophosphamide/IL-2) | II - 22 | Stage IV or locally advanced malignant disease [37, 38] |
| UCLA Jonsson Comprehensive Cancer Center, Westwood, CA/ Antoni Ribas NCT00910650 | Autologous CTL expressing a TCR (F5) targeting MART-1 p126-135 (Fludarabine + Cyclophosphamide/IL-2) | II - 22 | Stage IIIc and IV-Melanoma [37, 38] |
| Washington University, St. Louis, MO/ Univ Pennsylvania, Philadelphia, PA/ Gerald P Linette NCT01350401 | Autologous T cells expressing anti-NY-ESO TCR (C259) | I - 6 | Stage III and IV-Unresectable Metastatic Melanoma [39] |
| Baylor College of Medicine, Houston, TX/ Stephen Gottschalk NCT00889954 | Autologous PBL expressing anti-HER2 CAR and vector expressing a receptor to downregulate TGF-β signaling | I - 18 | Stage III and IV-Breast Cancer, Colon, Esophageal, Gastric, Lung and Prostate Cancers [40-42] |
| Baylor College of Medicine, Houston, TX/ Neil Ahmed NCT00902044 | Autologous T cells expressing anti-HER2 CAR | I - 36 | Progressive or Metastatic Sarcoma or Osteosarcoma [40-42] |
| Fred Hutchinson Cancer Research Center, Univ Washington, Seattle, WA/ Aude Chapuis NCT00871481 | Autologous CD8 positive T Cells expressing a TCR targeting NY-ESO-1 administered with anti-CTLA-4 (Cyclophosphamide/IL-2) | Phase I/II -10 | Metastatic Melanoma [43] |
| Fred Hutchinson Cancer Research Center, Univ Washington, Seattle, WA/ Seth Pollack NCT01477021 | Autologous CD8 positive T Cells expressing a TCR targeting NY-ESO-1 (Cyclophosphamide/IL-2) | Phase I - 6 | Metastatic or Unresectable Sarcomas [43, 44] |
| Loyola University, Chicago, IL/ Michael Nishimura NCT01586403 | Autologous T cells expressing a TCR targeting Tyrosinase p368-376 | I - 18 | Metastatic Melanoma [45] |

*NCT is the identifier on www.clinicaltrials.gov

At the National Institutes of Health (NIH) in Bethesda, MD, the first 5 TCR and CAR T cell protocols listed in Table **1** are open for patients with melanoma, mesothelioma, pancreatic, renal and esophageal cancers. All NIH protocols have Phase I or II status that involve prior lymphodepletion regimens before adoptive cell transfer and are given with T cell supportive IL-2. Three trials use TCR and two use second or third generation CAR T cells. Memorial Sloan Kettering Cancer Center has a Phase I trial for prostate cancer that involves lymphodepletion with cyclophosphamide and uses a second generation CAR T cell directed to prostate specific membrane antigen. Roger Williams Medical Institute in Providence, RI has four Phase I or II trials for adenocarcinomas or prostate cancer that target either carcinoembryonic or prostate specific antigens. The University of California, Los Angeles Cancer Center has two Phase II trials with TCR targeting NY-ESO or MART-I antigens. The NY-ESO trial is for patients with advanced metastatic disease and the one with MART-1 is for melanoma patients. Both also involve prior lymphodepletion and IL-2 supplementation. At Washington University in Saint Louis, MO patients are being treated with TCR that are manufactured at the University of Pennsylvania. They target NY-ESO on metastatic melanoma. At the Baylor College of Medicine, Houston, TX, two Phase I CAR T cell trials are open for advanced cancer patients with breast, colon, esophageal, gastric, lung, and prostate cancers targeting the Her2/neu antigen. The Fred Hutchinson Cancer Research Center has two clinical trials using TCR targeting NY-ESO on metastatic melanoma and sarcoma. Interestingly, one of the trials employs the additional administration of antibody to CTLA-4 to inhibit immunosuppressive cells expressing this factor. Finally, Loyola University in Chicago, IL has a Phase I trial using TCR targeting a tyrosinase for metastatic melanoma.

## CARS FOR THE TREATMENT OF MALIGNANT GLIOMAS

Our research group has specific interests in TCR and CAR T cells for the therapy of primary malignant brain tumors. Thus, in our search on clinicaltrials.gov we substituted solid tumor for brain tumors in our search string and found that there are 3 CAR T cell protocols specific for gliomas, which we describe in Table **2**. Chimeric antigen receptors have been generated for glioma-associated antigens, including IL-13R$\alpha$2, HER2 and EGFRvIII.

**Table 2:** Clinical trials open for patient enrollment that involve CAR T cells for treatment of gliomas

| Center/Investigator/NCT* | Therapy/Protocol | Phase/Enrollment No. | Eligibility [References] |
|---|---|---|---|
| City of Hope, Duarte, CA/ Behnam Badie NCT 01082926 | Allogeneic T cells expressing a CAR against IL-13Rα2 (intratumoral administration) IL-2 by CED | I - 6 | Recurrent Grade III or IV Glioma [26, 46-48] |
| Baylor College of Medicine, Houston, TX/ Neil Ahmed NCT01109095 | Autologous CMV specific CTL expressing a CAR Targeting HER2 (Intravenous administration) IL-2 | I - 18 | Recurrent or Progressive Grade IV Glioma [40, 42, 49] |
| NIH Clinical Center, Bethesda, MD/Steven A. Rosenberg NCT01454596 | Autologous CTL Expressing a CAR Targeting EGFRvIII (intravenous administration) (Fludarabine + Cyclophosphamide/IL-2) | I/II - 160 | Recurrent Gliosarcoma or Grade IV Glioma [2, 50, 51] |

*NCT is the identifier on www.clinicaltrials.gov

A Phase I clinical study utilizing allogeneic T cells expressing IL-13Rα2- specific CAR is currently underway at the City of Hope in Duarte, CA [26]. Recurrent WHO grade III or IV glioma patients are eligible. The IL-13Rα2 is highly overexpressed in gliomas, but has little to no expression in normal tissue with the exception of the testes [48]. This is a first generation, high affinity CAR that uses a mutated portion of the IL-13 domain to bind to IL13Rα2, unlike other studies that employ CAR T cells that utilize specific antibody fragments to bind antigen [26, 46, 47]. The T cells are given with supportive IL-2 by convection enhanced delivery. The trial has a target enrollment of 6 patients with target completion date in late 2013. Although the primary endpoints are to assess the safety and toxicity of the zetakine given with IL-2, the trial also involves neuroimaging by positron emission tomography [46]. A thymidine kinase "kill switch" has been built into the T cell construct which provides a clinical safety measure designed to eliminate IL-13-zetakine expressing T cells by treatment with the prodrug, ganciclovir, which is converted by Herpes simplex virus thymidine kinase (HSV TK) to a lethal product in transduced cells if significant toxicities such as graft *versus* host disease or autoimmune effects are observed [26, 47].

A clinical trial at Baylor College of Medicine, Houston, TX is using a second generation anti-HER2 CAR that contains the intracellular signaling domains CD28 and CD3 zeta that is transduced into cytomegalovirus (CMV) specific autologous T cells to target WHO grade IV gliomas [40, 42]. Patients must have a HER2 positive glioblastoma and be CMV seropositive. Over 75% of gliomas have been shown to be positive for HER2/neu [49]. Anti-HER2 CAR T cells secreted IL-2 and IFNγ in response to HER2 positive targets [40, 42]. Interestingly, anti-HER2 CAR T cells lysed CD133 positive stem cell like tumor targets, which are considered to correlate with increased tumorigenicity, radio- and chemo-resistance [40]. Also, the T cells are administered systemically, so they must cross the blood brain barrier to have an effect.

The last Phase I/II trial for gliomas is being conducted at the NIH and uses a third generation CAR design based on the EGFRvIII target known to be expressed by about a third of glioblastomas [51]. The CAR T cells are given systemically with IL-2 after lymphodepletion [2]. The CAR design is based on a human monoclonal antibody 139 also termed PG13-139-CD8-CD28BBZ (F10) [2, 50]. It contains a single chain Fv fragment from the 139 antibody as well as an intracellular signaling domain CD28, CD137 (4-1BB), and CD3 zeta domains and a CD8 extracellular-transmembrane domain [2, 50].

## SUMMARY OF EXPERIENCE WITH AND ADVERSE EFFECT OBSERVATIONS WITH TCR/CAR T CELL ADOPTIVE TRANSFERS

The majority of trials open for the use of genetically engineered TCR and CAR T cells have been used to target CD19 or CD20 positive B cells in patients with refractory non-Hodgkins lymphomas, mantle cell lymphomas, chronic lymphocytic leukemias, or acute lymphoblastic leukemias [30-32, 52]. In some cases, CD20 CAR T cells were both safe and efficacious; responses were noted and toxicity profiles indicated minimal grades 1-2 toxicity, due in part to CD20 expression being limited to B cells and non-vital tissues [52]. In a recent study where two pediatric acute lymphocytic leukemia patients were treated with CD19 directed CAR T cells, complete responses were initially seen in both patients [32]. This treatment was accompanied by significant grade 3-4 adverse events in both patients, including B cell aplasia and cytokine release syndrome with resulting macrophage activation syndrome, respiratory and cardiovascular compromise requiring pressors and mechanical ventilation [32].

An early study treating melanoma patients with anti-MART-1 TCR T cells resulted in sustained engraftment of the TCR clones that were demonstrated to be in peripheral circulation for over a year [21]. Objective responses also occurred in these patients, who exhibited a reduction in metastatic tumor. Likewise, in a follow-on study using highly avid TCR targeting MART-1, improved objective responses were also noted [22]. However, this study described "on target, off organ" adverse effects due to low levels of MART-1 and gp100 melanoma-associated antigens in healthy tissues. In patients with melanoma, for instance, the T cells caused autoimmune destruction of melanocytes in the skin (vitiligo) or eye (anterior uveitis). This early observation of collateral damage due to normal tissue cell expression of target antigen(s) still remains a concern with any adoptive transfer of specific T cells.

Successful adoptive transfer of T cells expressing high-avidity anti-carcinoembryonic antigen TCR was performed with subsequent objective regression of metastases in treatment of refractory metastatic colorectal adenocarcinomas [53]. Clinical response in this study was complicated by severe transient (4-6 weeks) inflammatory colitis due to highly avid TCR targeting normal epithelial crypt cells [53]. In contrast, a variety of other cancer types have been targeted with NY-ESO-1 cancer testis antigen where limited toxicities have been observed in patients with synovial cell sarcomas, melanomas, prostate, breast, thyroid and ovarian cancers [34].

Impressive toxicity profiles were documented in a trial for patients with metastatic renal cell carcinomas [54]. In this study, the CAR T cells targeted carbonic anhydrase IX expression. Grades 2-4 liver toxicity, some with cholangitis, occurred likely as a result of carbonic anhydrase IX expression in bile duct epithelial cells. This is another example of "on-target, off-organ" toxicity due to antigen expression in normal tissues. Interestingly, the patients developed antibodies to the carbonic anhydrase, such that the investigators amended the protocol to include administration of an antibody to saturate liver tissue prior to administration of the genetically modified T cells to reduce toxicity [54].

In at least one instance, treatment with CAR T cells targeting Her2/neu resulted in the death of a patient with metastatic colon cancer. Within minutes post infusion of the CAR T cells, the patient developed pulmonary edema, severe hypotension and experienced multiple cardiac arrests consistent with acute respiratory disease syndrome due to cytokine storm and respiratory failure as a result of Her2/neu expression in lung epithelium. Autopsy showed ischemia with hemorrhagic microangiopathy and multiple organ failure, while serum analyses displayed marked increases in IL-6, IL-10, GM-CSF, TNFα and IFNγ [55].

## CURRENT PERSPECTIVES AND FUTURE DIRECTIONS

Safety and efficacy remain the main limitations to successful use of adoptive cell transfer for immunotherapy. Selection of proper TAA is important due to the ability of TCR/CAR to react to normal tissues, levels of expression and avidity affecting efficacy of tumor cell destruction and the side effect profiles of given therapies. It is possible that antigen specific T cells can be used to target antigens that are upregulated in response to pharmacologic treatments with demethylating agents, such as decitabine and TAA NY-ESO [56]. Graft *versus* host disease related complaints may be dealt with an inducible iCasp9system resulting in destruction of adoptively transferred cells upon administration of a dimerizer compound [57] or the build-in of a suicide gene such that innocuous prodrug [26, 27] can be given to keep the T cells in check. Also, separating CD3 zeta and costimulatory signals into separate CARs may create a more physiologic response [20]. While adverse events such as "on target, off organ" effects and the resulting "cytokine storm" may be reduced by local (*e.g.,* intratumoral or intraperitoneal) CAR T cell administration [58]. Finally, adoptive transfer of engineered T cells may become more widely applicable and clinically feasible because in cancers, such as metastatic melanoma, they share common antigens with gliomas [21, 22, 34, 59].

## ACKNOWLEDGEMENTS

Financial support for the study was supplied in part by NIH/NCATS UCLA CTSI Grant Number UL1TR000124, the Joan S. Holmes Memorial Research Fund, NIH R25 NS079198, R01 CA125244, and NIH R01CA154256.

## CONFLICT OF INTEREST

The author confirms that this chapter contents have no conflict of interest.

## REFERENCES

[1] Hall SS. A commotion in the blood: Life, death, and the immune system: Henry Holt New York; 1997.

[2] Rosenberg SA. Raising the bar: the curative potential of human cancer immunotherapy. Sci Transl Med 2012; 4: 127ps8.

[3] Hawkins RE, Gilham DE, Debets R, *et al.* Development of adoptive cell therapy for cancer: a clinical perspective. Hum Gene Ther 2010; 21: 665-72.

[4] Nagasawa DT, Fong C, Yew A, *et al.* Passive immunotherapeutic strategies for the treatment of malignant gliomas. Neurosurg Clinics No Am 2012; 23: 481-95.

[5] Gomez GG, Kruse CA. Mechanisms of malignant glioma immune resistance and sources of immunosuppression. Gene Ther Mol Biol 2006; 10: 133-46.

[6] Dudley ME, Yang JC, Sherry R, *et al.* Adoptive cell therapy for patients with metastatic melanoma: evaluation of intensive myeloablative chemoradiation preparative regimens. J Clin Oncol 2008; 26: 5233-9.

[7] Robbins PF, Dudley ME, Wunderlich J, *et al.* Cutting edge: persistence of transferred lymphocyte clonotypes correlates with cancer regression in patients receiving cell transfer therapy. J Immunol 2004; 173: 7125-30.

[8] Dudley ME, Wunderlich JR, Robbins PF, *et al.* Cancer regression and autoimmunity in patients after clonal repopulation with antitumor lymphocytes. Science 2002; 298: 850-4.

[9] Hofman FM, Stathopoulos A, Kruse CA, *et al.* Immunotherapy of malignant gliomas using autologous and allogeneic tissue cells. Anti-Cancer Agents in Medicinal Chemistry 2010; 10: 462-70.

[10] Kruse CA, Cepeda L, Owens B, *et al.* Treatment of recurrent glioma with intracavitary alloreactive cytotoxic T lymphocytes and interleukin-2. Cancer Immunol Immunother 1997; 45: 77-87.

[11] Kruse CA, Rubinstein D. Cytotoxic T lymphocytes reactive to patient major histocompatibility proteins for therapy of recurrent primary brain tumors. In: Liau LM, Cloughesy TF, Becker DP, *et al.*, editors. Brain Tumor Immunotherapy. Totowa: Humana Press; 2001. pp. 149-70.

[12] Hickey MJ, Malone CC, Erickson KL, *et al.* Combined alloreactive CTL cellular therapy with prodrug activator gene therapy in a model of breast cancer metastatic to the brain. Clin Cancer Res 2013; 19(15): 4137-48.

[13] Hickey MJ, Malone CC, Erickson KL, *et al.* Cellular and vaccine therapeutic approaches for gliomas. J Transl Med 2010; 8: 100-08.

[14] Maiers M, Gragert L, Klitz W. High-resolution HLA alleles and haplotypes in the United States population. Hum Immunol 2007; 68: 779-88.

[15] Noun G, Reboul M, Abastado JP, *et al.* Strong alloantigenicity of the alpha-helices residues of the MHC class I molecule. J Immunol 1998; 161: 148-53.

[16] van der Merwe PA, Dushek O. Mechanisms for T cell receptor triggering. Nat Rev Immunol 2011; 11: 47-55.

[17] Lombardi G, Barber L, Sidhu S, *et al.* The specificity of alloreactive T cells is determined by MHC polymorphisms which contact the T cell receptor and which influence peptide binding. Int Immunol 1991; 3: 769-75.

[18] Bjorkman PJ, Saper M, Samraoui B, *et al.* Structure of the human class I histocompatibility antigen, HLA-A2. Nature 1987; 329: 506-12.

[19] Jena B, Dotti G, Cooper LJ. Redirecting T-cell specificity by introducing a tumor-specific chimeric antigen receptor. Blood 2010; 116: 1035-44.

[20] Cartellieri M, Bachmann M, Feldmann A, *et al.* Chimeric antigen receptor-engineered T cells for immunotherapy of cancer. J Biomed Biotechnol 2010; 2010: 956304.

[21] Morgan RA, Dudley ME, Wunderlich JR, *et al.* Cancer regression in patients after transfer of genetically engineered lymphocytes. Science 2006; 314: 126-9.

[22] Johnson LA, Morgan RA, Dudley ME, *et al.* Gene therapy with human and mouse T-cell receptors mediates cancer regression and targets normal tissues expressing cognate antigen. Blood 2009; 114: 535-46.

[23] Cohen CJ, Li YF, El-Gamil M, *et al.* Enhanced antitumor activity of T cells engineered to express T-cell receptors with a second disulfide bond. Cancer Res 2007; 67: 3898-903.

[24] Rischer M, Pscherer S, Duwe S, *et al.* Human gammadelta T cells as mediators of chimaeric-receptor redirected anti-tumour immunity. Br J Haematol 2004; 126: 583-92.

[25] Hedfors IA, Beckstrom KJ, Benati C, *et al.* Retrovirus mediated gene transduction of human T-cell subsets. Cancer Immunol Immunother 2005; 54: 759-68.

[26] Kahlon KS, Brown C, Cooper LJ, *et al.* Specific recognition and killing of glioblastoma multiforme by interleukin 13-zetakine redirected cytolytic T cells. Cancer Res 2004; 64: 9160-6.

[27] Quintarelli C, Vera JF, Savoldo B, *et al.* Co-expression of cytokine and suicide genes to enhance the activity and safety of tumor-specific cytotoxic T lymphocytes. Blood 2007; 110: 2793-802.

[28] Sadelain M, Brentjens R, Rivière I. The basic principles of chimeric antigen receptor design. Cancer Discovery 2013; 3: 388-98.

[29] Kalos M, Levine BL, Porter DL, *et al.* T cells with chimeric antigen receptors have potent antitumor effects and can establish memory in patients with advanced leukemia. Sci Transl Med 2011; 3: 95ra73-95ra73.

[30] Porter DL, Levine BL, Kalos M, *et al.* Chimeric antigen receptor-modified T cells in chronic lymphoid leukemia N Engl J Med 2011; 365: 725-33.

[31] Savoldo B, Ramos CA, Liu E, *et al.* CD28 costimulation improves expansion and persistence of chimeric antigen receptor-modified T cells in lymphoma patients. J Clin Invest 2011; 121: 1822-6.

[32] Grupp SA, Kalos M, Barrett D, *et al.* Chimeric antigen receptor-modified T cells for acute lymphoid leukemia. N Engl J Med 2013; 368: 1509-18.

[33] Chinnasamy D, Yu Z, Theoret MR, *et al.* Gene therapy using genetically modified lymphocytes targeting VEGFR-2 inhibits the growth of vascularized syngenic tumors in mice. J Clin Invest 2010; 120: 3953-68.

[34] Robbins PF, Morgan RA, Feldman SA, *et al.* Tumor regression in patients with metastatic synovial cell sarcoma and melanoma using genetically engineered lymphocytes reactive with NY-ESO-1. J Clin Oncol 2011; 29: 917-24.

[35] Gade TP, Hassen W, Santos E, *et al.* Targeted elimination of prostate cancer by genetically directed human T lymphocytes. Cancer Res 2005; 65: 9080-8.

[36] Ma Q, DeMarte L, Wang Y, *et al.* Carcinoembryonic antigen-immunoglobulin Fc fusion protein (CEA-Fc) for identification and activation of anti-CEA immunoglobulin-T-cell receptor-modified T cells, representative of a new class of Ig fusion proteins. Cancer Gene Ther 2004; 11: 297-306.

[37] Ribas A, Comin-Anduix B, Chmielowski B, *et al.* Dendritic cell vaccination combined with CTLA4 blockade in patients with metastatic melanoma. Clin Cancer Res 2009; 15: 6267-76.

[38] Butterfield LH, Comin-Anduix B, Vujanovic L, *et al.* Adenovirus MART-1-engineered autologous dendritic cell vaccine for metastatic melanoma. J Immunother 2008; 31: 294-309.

[39] Linette GP, Stadtmauer EA, Maus MV, *et al.* Cardiovascular toxicity and titin cross-reactivity of affinity enhanced T cells in myeloma and melanoma. Blood 2013; 122(6): 863-71.

[40] Ahmed N, Salsman VS, Kew Y, *et al.* HER2-specific T cells target primary glioblastoma stem cells and induce regression of autologous experimental tumors. Clin Cancer Res 2010; 16: 474-85.

[41] Rainusso N, Brawley VS, Ghazi A, *et al.* Immunotherapy targeting HER2 with genetically modified T cells eliminates tumor-initiating cells in osteosarcoma. Cancer Gene Ther 2012; 19: 212-7.

[42] Ahmed N, Salsman VS, Yvon E, *et al.* Immunotherapy for osteosarcoma: genetic modification of T cells overcomes low levels of tumor antigen expression. Mol Ther 2009; 17: 1779-87.

[43] Chapuis AG, Thompson JA, Margolin KA, *et al.* Transferred melanoma-specific CD8+ T cells persist, mediate tumor regression, and acquire central memory phenotype. Proc Natl Acad Sci USA 2012; 109: 4592-7.

[44] Pollack SM, Jungbluth AA, Hoch BL, *et al.* NY-ESO-1 is a ubiquitous immunotherapeutic target antigen for patients with myxoid/round cell liposarcoma. Cancer 2012; 118: 4564-70.

[45] Roszkowski JJ, Lyons GE, Kast WM, *et al.* Simultaneous generation of CD8+ and CD4+ melanoma-reactive T cells by retroviral-mediated transfer of a single T-cell receptor. Cancer Res 2005; 65: 1570-6.

[46] Lazovic J, Jensen MC, Ferkassian E, *et al.* Imaging immune response *in vivo*: cytolytic action of genetically altered T cells directed to glioblastoma multiforme. Clin Cancer Res 2008; 14: 3832-9.

[47] Brown CE, Starr R, Aguilar B, *et al.* Stem-like tumor-initiating cells isolated from IL13Ralpha2 expressing gliomas are targeted and killed by IL13-zetakine-redirected T Cells. Clin Cancer Res 2012; 18: 2199-209.

[48] Mintz A, Gibo DM, Slagle-Webb B, *et al.* IL-13Rα2 is a glioma-restricted receptor for interleukin-13. Neoplasia (New York, NY) 2002; 4: 388-99.

[49] Liu G, Ying H, Zeng G, *et al.* HER-2, gp100, and MAGE-1 are expressed in human glioblastoma and recognized by cytotoxic T cells. Cancer Res 2004; 64: 4980-6.

[50] Morgan RA, Johnson LA, Davis JL, *et al.* Recognition of glioma stem cells by genetically modified T cells targeting EGFRvIII and development of adoptive cell therapy for glioma. Hum Gene Ther 2012; 23: 1043-53.

[51] Aldape KD, Ballman K, Furth A, *et al.* Immunohistochemical detection of EGFRvIII in high malignancy grade astrocytomas and evaluation of prognostic significance. J Neuropathol Exp Neurol 2004; 63: 700-7.

[52] Till BG, Jensen MC, Wang J, *et al.* Adoptive immunotherapy for indolent non-Hodgkin lymphoma and mantle cell lymphoma using genetically modified autologous CD20-specific T cells. Blood 2008; 112: 2261-71.

[53] Parkhurst MR, Yang JC, Langan RC, *et al.* T cells targeting carcinoembryonic antigen can mediate regression of metastatic colorectal cancer but induce severe transient colitis. Mol Ther 2011; 19: 620-6.

[54] Lamers CH, Sleijfer S, Vulto AG, *et al.* Treatment of metastatic renal cell carcinoma with autologous T-lymphocytes genetically retargeted against carbonic anhydrase IX: First clinical experience. J Clin Oncol 2006; 24: e20-2.

[55] Morgan RA, Yang JC, Kitano M, *et al.* Case report of a serious adverse event following the administration of T cells transduced with a chimeric antigen receptor recognizing ERBB2. Mol Ther 2010; 18: 843-51.

[56] Konkankit VV, Kim W, Koya RC, *et al.* Decitabine immunosensitizes human gliomas to NY-ESO-1 specific T lymphocyte targeting through the Fas/Fas Ligand pathway. J Transl Med 2011; 9: 1-13.

[57] Hoyos V, Savoldo B, Quintarelli C, *et al.* Engineering CD19-specific T lymphocytes with interleukin-15 and a suicide gene to enhance their anti-lymphoma/leukemia effects and safety. Leukemia 2010; 24: 1160-70.

[58] Parente-Pereira AC, Burnet J, Ellison D, *et al.* Trafficking of CAR-engineered human T cells following regional or systemic adoptive transfer in SCID beige mice. J Clin Immunol 2011; 31: 710-8.

[59] Zhang JG, Eguchi J, Kruse CA, *et al.* Antigenic profiling of glioma cells to generate allogeneic vaccines or dendritic cell-based therapeutics. Clin Cancer Res 2007; 13: 566-75.

# CHAPTER 7

# Therapeutic Antibody Engineering

**Anatoliy Markiv***

*University of Westminster, Faculty of Science and Technology, London, W1W 6UW, United Kingdom*

**Abstract:** For the past three decades monoclonal and recombinant antibodies have emerged as major therapeutic agents in the field of targeted therapy mainly in cancer and immunological disorders. To date, the United States Food and Drug Administration (FDA) as well as the European Medicines Agency (EMA) have approved more than 30 antibodies or antibody-based drugs for clinical applications. Many more are being developed for various therapeutic applications. This huge interest in antibody therapy is due to their specificity and affinity that allows for targeted therapy, as well as increased understanding of antibody sequence, structure and mechanism of action. With the development of hybridoma technology and the advancement of recombinant DNA technology and antibody engineering methods, novel antibody derived molecules have gained momentum due to their improved pharmacokinetics, increased selectivity and enhanced efficacy. Furthermore, modular antibody design permits careful engineering and development of the new generation therapeutics suitable for the personalized medicine. Many challenges still remain, to improve antibody recognition properties, to engineer their serum half-life, to improve their stability and to better control their immunogenicity and side effects.

In this chapter general principles of therapeutic antibody engineering will be addressed with the view to present the latest molecular engineering strategies for the production of next generation antibody-based therapeutics.

**Keywords:** Antibody-dependent cellular cytotoxicity, antibody-drug conjugates, antigen-binding site, bi-specific, bivalent, C1q binding, chimeric, complement-mediated lysis, complementarity determination region, engineering, Fab, Fc, FcRn, FcγR, heavy chain, humanised, light chain, monoclonal, multispecific, multivalent, recombinant antibody, scFv, therapeutics.

## INTRODUCTION

Antibodies are class of soluble glycoproteins that are found in the blood, extracellular space and in secretory body fluids. Antibodies have evolved to bind

***Corresponding author Anatoliy Markiv:** University of Westminster, Faculty of Science and Technology, London, W1W 6UW, United Kingdom; Tel: +44 (0) 20 7911 5000; E-mail: A.Markiv@westminster.ac.uk selectively to foreign substances and thus play an important role in the acquired immune response. The modular structure and biological characteristics of the antibody molecules makes them very useful in the prophylaxis, diagnostics and therapy of human diseases. Numerous approaches have been used to improve and optimise antibody:antigen binding site, antibody serum half-life and *in vivo* activities. These include making different antibody fragments and combining them with other molecules such as toxins, drugs and radioactive substances. Furthermore, increased understanding of the antibody amino acid sequence, structure and function have enabled redesigning their antigen binding and effector functions. Therefore, in the past 30 years, especially after development of the monoclonal antibody technology, antibody based drugs have made the transition from discovery to clinical practice and have become major therapeutic agents for the treatment of cancer, immunological disorders, transplant rejection and many others.

## ANTIBODY STRUCTURE AND CLASSES

### Immunoglobulin Structure

The basic antibody molecule is a modular Y-shaped protein molecule in which distinct functions are localised in different parts of the molecule (Fig. **1**). The immunoglobulin molecule is composed of four polypeptide sequences, two larger heavy (H) chains and two smaller light (L) chains. Each H chain is formed of four domains of about 110 amino acids in length and each L chain is formed of two domains of the similar size. Each H chain combines with one L chain and identical H chain through non-covalent bonding as well as the covalent inter-chain disulphide bridges, the number of which depends on the antibody type. The amino acid sequences of the H and L chains from different antibody classes are less conserved in the N-terminal antibody domain that is termed the variable domain, VH and VL respectively. The C-terminal domains are known as the constant (C) domains. There are three constant domains in the H chain (CH1, CH2 and CH3) and one constant domain in the L chain (CL) [1-4].

The stem region of the Y-shaped antibody molecules is formed by four constant domains of two H chains and is called the Fc region. The Fc region is responsible for the effector function of the antibody molecule because it interacts with complement and Fc receptors on the cells of the immune system [5].

Four domains, two from H and two from L chains, consisting one constant and one variable region each, form the Fab arms. Two variable domains, one from H chain and one from L chain form the antigen-binding site that is located at the tip of the two identical Fab arms. The interactions between the H and L chains in the Fab arm are stabilised by the disulphide bond between the two constant domains.

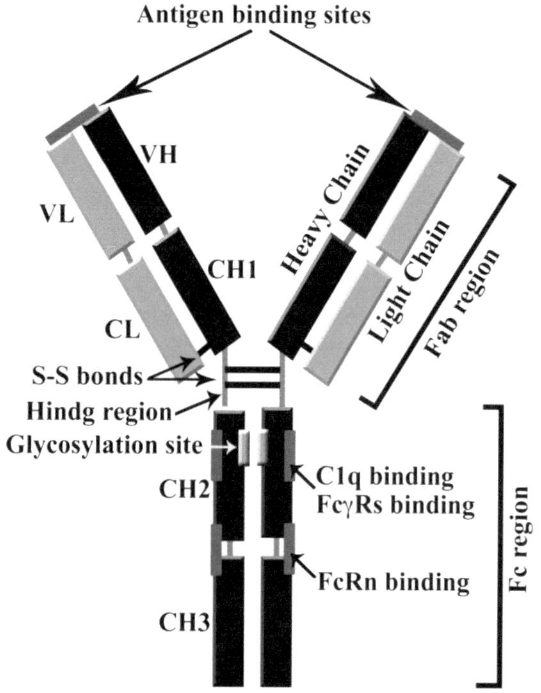


**Figure 1: The structure of the IgG molecule.** VL, light chain variable domain; VH, heavy chain variable domain; CH1, CH2, and CH3, heavy chain constant domain; Fab, antigen-binding fragment; Fc, constant region fragment; C1q, first component of complement; FcγRs, Fcγ receptor; FcRn, neonatal Fc receptor; S-S bonds, disulfide bonds.

A flexible hinge region links the Fab arm and the Fc region and the inter-chain disulphide bonds in these hinge regions link two heavy chains into the full-length immunoglobulin structure [6].

## Immunoglobulin Classes

The amino acid sequence of each heavy chain of the antibody molecule defines the immunoglobulin class. Thus, five H chains – α, γ, δ, ε and μ, make up five antibody classes IgA, IgG, IgD, IgE and IgM, respectively (Fig. **2**). Structurally IgG, IgE and IgD classes are closely related monomeric antibody molecules composed of two heavy and two light chains [7]. The IgA antibody molecule in addition to the two heavy chains and two light chains has a J chain and secretory component [8]. IgM is the largest of the five antibody classes and is composed of five antibody sub-units linked by disulphide bonds with one J-chain stabilising the overall antibody structure [9].

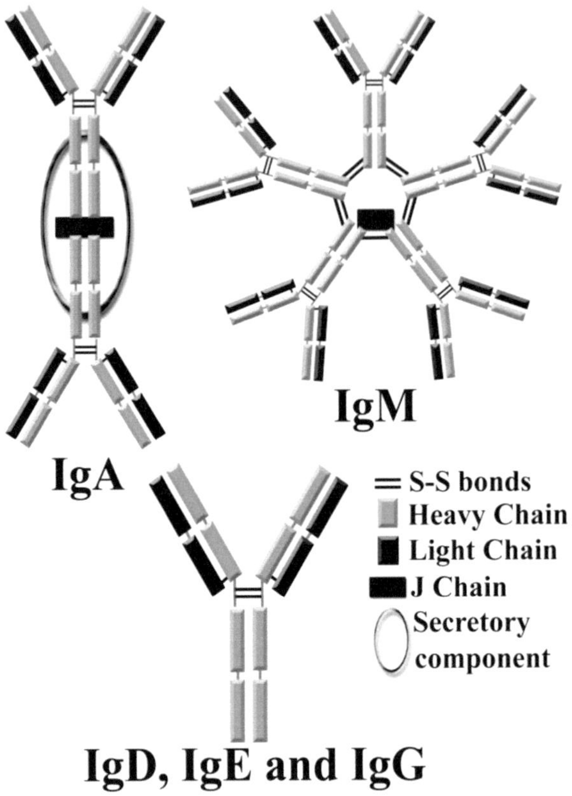


**Figure 2: General structure of the Immunoglobulin classes.** Five different immunoglobulin classes are based on the amino acid sequence of heavy chain that is designated by Greek letters mu (IgM), delta (IgD), gamma (IgG), epsilon (IgE) and alpha (IgA).

## Antigen Binding Site

Two variable domains form the antigen-binding site of the antibody molecule, one from each heavy and light chain. These variable domains contain regions that have considerable amino acid sequence variability that are adapted to recognise different antigens and are termed hyper variable regions (HRs). Other regions of relatively conserved stretches of the amino acid sequences, determine the overall 3D structure of the V domains and are termed framework region (FRs) [10]. These framework regions contribute to the formation of the β-sheet of the V domain secondary structure, while the variable regions contribute to the formation of polypeptide loops that connect β-strands at the top of the V domains. Loops that are involved in the formation of the antigen-binding site are also known as complementarity-determining regions (CDRs). There are three CDRs in each VH and VL domain. When VH and VL domains associate by non-covalent bonding to form heterodimeric quaternary structure they position the three CDRs from each H and L chains in the conformation that creates a cleft or pocket for antigen binding. Numerous amino acid sequence variations in the antigen-binding site contribute to the affinity of antigen binding [11, 12]. There are no fixed numbers of amino acids that are involved in the antigen binding for different antigens and in some cases when the antigen is a small molecule not all the CDRs are involved in binding process.

### Antibody Post-Translational Modification

Antibody molecules possess amino acid sequences that include sites for the post-translational modifications, one of which is a glycosylation [13]. Usually these N-linked glycosylation sites are present in the CH antibody domains, but their precise position is determined by the antibody isotype [14]. The addition of the carbohydrate chain contributes to the antibody structure, effector function, serum half-life and other biological properties. In the IgG class, the glycosylation site is located in the CH2 domain. The IgM and IgE have additional carbohydrate attachment sites in CH1, CH2 and CH3 domains are thus more glycosylated as compared to the IgG molecule [14, 15]. The IgA molecule is probably the most glycosylated of all immunoglobulin classes as it has in its hinge region additional five O-link glycosylation sites [15]. The presence of the carbohydrates on the Fab arm has been shown to influence the antigen-binding properties of the antibody molecule while absence of the carbohydrate moieties reduces antibody stability as well as the effector function and the serum half-life [16-18].

## ENGINEERING ANTIGEN BINDING ANTIBODY ACTIVITIES

### Antibody Humanisation

To engineer antibody with high antigen binding specificities and affinities for therapeutic usely it is important to isolate antigen-binding domains. This can be achieved either by isolating antibodies from the immune source or constructing them artificially using genetic modification methods. The choice of starting material is based on biological needs and technical possibilities. Classically, libraries of antibody candidates are generated and screened. To modulate the binding specificities or antibody biophysical properties, targeted or random mutagenesis, chain or CDR shuffling methods are used. If antibody structure is known from X-ray crystallography then either site-specific random mutagenesis or structure based computational design engineering approaches could be used.

Alternatively, the 3D structure of antibody molecule can be generated using homology-modelling methods, which can provide a good guide for the antibody optimisation experiments. Domain-based assembly of antibodies allows separation of different domains and also for genetic modifications to be made to any individual domain of the antibody. Thus antigen binding VH and VL domains can be separated from the Fc portion and can be linked to the Fc domains of human or non-human antibody origin. Furthermore the individual antigen binding loops from the antibody:antigen binding sites can be grafted on the antibody from different species. In this way chimeric or humanised antibody can be made using antigen binding specificities of a non-human antibody [19].

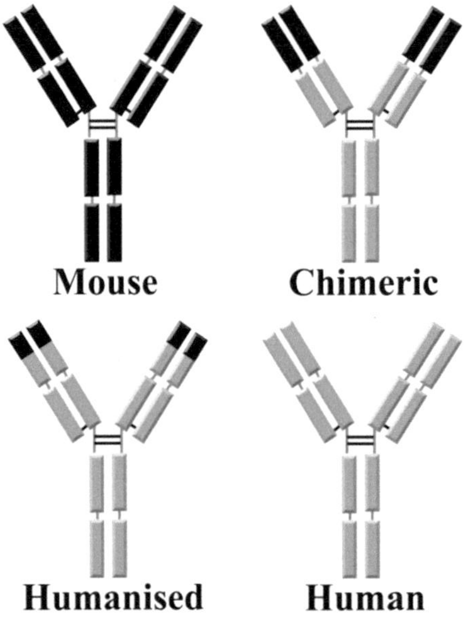


**Figure 3: Antibody humanisation.** Murine antibody parts are shown in black colour, human parts are shown in grey colour. Black colour lines indicate disulphide bonds.

For example, the first non-human monoclonal antibody made for human therapeutic use was anti-CD3 murine antibody Muromomab [20]. It was approved in 1986 for the treatment of transplantation rejection but soon failed as a good therapy because the Fc portion of the murine antibody had weak effector function in humans and also because of the high anti-murine antibody immune response. A new strategy was needed and, to reduce immunogenicity of these and other murine antibodies, chimeric antibodies were constructed and marketed (Fig. **3**). These new antibodies had murine antibody VH and VL domains and human constant antibody regions. Using the same approach, first in 1994, chimeric Fab antibody ReoPro as constructed [21, 22], then in 1997 Rituxan [23, 24], in 1998 Simulect [25, 26] and Remicade [27, 28], in 2004 Erbitux [29] and most recently in 2011 Adcetris [30]. However, although these antibody constructs were shown to be better than fully murine antibodies some patients developed an anti-chimeric immune response [31].

To further minimise the mouse component of the antibody fragments and prevent anti-antibody response, CDR grafting method was suggested to humanise the original murine antibodies [32, 33]. This method involves placing amino acids from the antigen binding regions (CDRs) and some key framework amino acids of the murine antibody onto the human antibody template. The aim of this method is to keep antigen-binding properties of the original murine antibody but introduce as many human antibody amino acids as possible to make them less immunogenic [34].

Humanised antibodies are made by genetic engineering technology in order to convert non-human antibody into fully human antibody [35]. There are several strategies to this approach all designed to transfer the antigen binding amino acids from non-human antibody into the library of human antigen binding domains and using many rounds of selection process to identify an antibody that will have desired specificity and affinity to the antigen of interest [36]. Examples of humanised antibody approved for clinical use are shown in Table **1**.

**Table 1:** Therapeutic humanised antibody approved for clinical use

| Generic name (Trade Name) | Description | Mode of action | Year first FDA approval and Therapeutic Indication |
|---|---|---|---|
| Daclizumab (Zenapax) | Humanized IgG1κ | Binds to IL-2Rα | 1997<br>Prophylaxis of acute organ rejection in renal transplants |
| Palivizumab (Synagis) | Humanized IgG1κ | Binds to RSV F protein | 1998<br>Respiratory syncytial virus infection |
| Trastuzumab (Herceptin) | Humanized IgG1κ | Binds to Her2 | 1998<br>Breast cancer |
| Alemtuzumab (Campath) | Humanized IgG1κ | Binds to CD52 | 2001<br>B-cell chronic lymphocytic leukemia |
| Omalizumab (Xolair) | Humanized IgG1κ | Binds to IgE | 2003<br>Moderate to severe persistent asthma |
| Efalizumab (Raptiva2) | Humanized IgG1κ | Binds to CD11a | 2003<br>Moderate to severe plaque psoriasis |
| Bevacizumab (Avastin) | Humanized IgG1κ | Binds to VEGF-A | 2004<br>Various solid tumours |

*Table 1: contd...*

| | | | |
|---|---|---|---|
| Natalizumab (Tysabri) | Humanized IgG4κ | Binds to α4-integrin | 2004 Multiple sclerosis and Crohn's disease |
| Ranibizumab (Lucentis) | Humanized Fab | Binds to VEGF-A | 2006 Age-related macular degeneration |
| Eculizumab (Soliris) | Humanized IgG2/4κ | Binds to C5 | 2007 Paroxysmal nocturnal hemoglobinuria |
| Tocilizumab (Actemra) | Humanized IgG1κ | Binds to IL-6R | 2010 Rheumatoid arthritis |

## Single Antigen Binding Domain Antibody Fragments

In camels, in comparison to murine or human antibody, antigen-binding properties are within a single antibody domain VH. This 14 kDa antibody domain has antigen-binding specificity and affinity similar to the multidomain human or murine antibodies. Structurally, in this single domain antibody the three CDR loops are longer and are stabilised by disulphide bridges [37]. Such small antibody constructs are useful when high tissue penetration and short serum half-life of an antibody are required [38]. To make human single domain antibody fragments using human VH, extensive genetic modifications to increase domain stability, antigen-binding specificity and affinity to the level found in two domain antibodies are needed [39, 40].

## Fv Fragments

The Fv antibody fragments are non-covalently linked heterodimers of the VH and VL domains with the molecular size of 25 kDa [41]. These small antibody fragments have been shown to retain antigen binding specificity and affinity of the original antibody, however, they have been shown to have tendency to dissociate into separate VH and VL domains and lose their antigen binding properties. This makes them less useful as therapeutic agents. To stabilise these Fv molecules, chemical crosslinking, intermolecular disulphide bonding or short peptide linkers between the VH and VL chains have been suggested [42-44].

## Single Chain Fv (scFv) Fragments

Joining VH and VL chains of an antibody amino acid sequence by a flexible peptide linker enables transcription and translation of the VH and VL domains together as one protein molecule and creates a single chain (scFv) antibody with the binding specificity and affinity similar to the original antibody [45, 46]. These linker sequences are typically made using Gly and Ser amino acids in the format

(Gly4Ser)n [46]. The antigen binding properties of such antibody fragments are influenced by the domain orientation and linker length [47]. Thus the optimal length of the linker sequence was found to be 20-25 amino acids for a VL-linker-VH constructs and 15-20 amino acids for the VH-linker-VL constructs. These calculations were based on the X-ray structural analysis of the distances between the C-terminus of the VL and the N-terminus of the VH and also between the C-terminus of the VH and the N-terminus of the VL, that have been determined to be 39-43 and 32-34 Å, respectively [47]. Single chain Fv antibody fragments have only antigen binding properties, but no Fc region, no effector function and as a consequence are not able to activate complement or initiate cell-mediated cytotoxicity. On the other hand, they have excellent tissue penetration due to their small molecular size of 26 kDa, but on the other hand, they have short serum half-life and are cleared rapidly by kidney [48]. Possible therapeutic applications of these scFv fragments are in those conditions that require deep tissue penetration, do not need complement activation and do not need the extended intravascular half-life, as for example, in case of solid tumours [49].

In addition to the monovalent scFv fragments, shortening linker length can generate bi- and multivalent scFv antibody. These bivalent scFv fragments have been shown to have higher avidity to the antigen and also exhibit an extended serum half-life as compared to the monovalent scFv fragments. Several approaches are employed to engineer these bi- and multivalent scFv antibody fragments. The first approach, for example, is to reduce linker length between VH and VL domains. If linker length is less than 10 amino acids stable dimers of two scFv fragments are formed with two antigen-binding sites [50, 51]. If VH and VL domains are joined in a single protein chain without a linker, scFv trimers are formed with three antigen-binding sites. The second approach is to link two scFv fragments into one amino acid sequence by a flexible linker to allow bending and rotation [52]. These antibody constructs have been termed mini-antibodies. The third approach is to combine scFv and core-streptavidin. This approach will create stable tetrameric antibody complexes.

Another interesting approach is to create bi- and multivalent and multispecific antibody fragments by combining scFv fragments with different antigen specificities [53]. These antibodies have useful therapeutic properties, as they are able to bind and join two or more antigens together.

## Fab Fragments

The Fab fragments are antibody fragments that are made of the first two domains from the heavy and light antibody chains, an antigen binding Fv-part (VH and VL domains) plus the first constant domains of the antibody heavy chain (CH1) and the light chain (CL). Addition of the constant domains to the Fv fragments is known to contribute to the higher stability of the Fab in comparison to the Fv-fragments, since CL and CH1 domains extend the heavy and light chain binding interface and are stabilised by the disulphide bond. This also increases molecular size of the Fab fragments to 50 kDa [54].

The Fab antibodies have similar antigen binding specificity and affinity to the full-length antibody, but are smaller in size since they do not have any of the Fc regions and therefore are not able to activate complement or initiate cell-mediated cytotoxicity. Compared to the Fv-fragments, Fab antibodies have reduced tissue penetration but longer serum half-life. These properties of Fab fragments make them ideally suited in therapeutic applications when extended intravascular half life is require without the need for the effector function or deep tissue penetration, for example, to block some blood or endothelial cell receptors or serum antigens. A range of these antibody drugs has been successfully used in clinics. For example, Reopro (anti GPIIb/IIIa receptor antibody) has been approved for prevention of cardiac ischemic complication, Lucentis (anti-VEGF-A antibody) for age-related macular degeneration and Cimzia (anti-TNFα antibody) for Crohn's disease and rheumatoid arthritis [55, 56, 57].

## Fab' and $F(ab)_2$ Fragments

Fab' fragments are derivatives of Fab in which a single cysteine amino acid hinge is introduced at the C-terminus of the protein chain. The Fab' are expressed and then chemically crosslinked using a thio-ether linkage to provide the monovalent, bispecific antibody [58]. In this way a therapeutic antibody can target two antigens from two different cells, for example, the CD3 receptor present on human T cells and the Her2 receptor on the cancer cell. The $F(ab)_2$ fragments are derivatives of the Fab that consist of two Fab-fragments connected by a flexible linker making them bivalent antibody molecules. The $F(ab)_2$ fragments can be made to be monospecific or bi-specific by linking two identical or two different Fab fragments. $F(ab)_2$ fragments have a size of 100 kDa and a serum half life, the antigen binding specificity, affinitiy and avidity similar to those of the original full-length antibody molecule, but as in the case of Fab fragments they have no effector function and therefore will not activate either complement, or Fc-receptors [59]. Therapeutically, the $F(ab)_2$ fragments are ideally suited to clinical applications when the dual antigen binding properties and a long serum half-life are required.

# ENGINEERING EFFECTOR FUNCTION OF ANTIBODY

The Fc portion of the antibody chain, that in the IgG comprises the CH2 and CH3 domains as well as the antibody hinge region, confers antibody effector functions. Four different human subclasses of the IgG molecule can interact with either the complement system or the Fc receptors of the immune cells (cytotoxic T cells, natural killer cells, monocytes, granulocytes and macrophages) with varying degree of affinity and specificity. These interactions are based on the variations in the amino acid sequences of the Fc portion of the antibody subclass, hinge length, flexibility and the glycosylation patterns of the CH2 domain. Differences in the amino acid sequence of the Fc portion of the antibody subclass confer different ability to activate complement and to initiate complement-mediated lysis (CML) as well as the antibody-dependent cellular cytotoxicity (ADCC). Post-translational modification of the Fc portion of the IgG molecule by glycosylation and the composition of the carbohydrate chain also influences the antibody effector function. From a therapeutic stand point, antibody effector function can be manipulated by genetic modifications and by changes to the post-translational glycosylation of the antibody molecule to tailor antibody for necessary effector function. This is particularly relevant for an antibody designed to treat cancer and inflammatory disorders [60, 61].

## Improving Complement Activation Properties

The classical complement pathway is triggered by the interaction of the first complement protein complex, composed of C1q, C1r and C1s, with the antibody-antigen complex. The multivalent C1q subcomponent of human complement protein complex is the first complement protein that interacts with the second heavy chain domain (CH2) of the IgG molecule. Different IgG subclasses have different complement activation activities, for example, the IgG3 subclass is the most effective at complement activation, followed by the IgG1 and IgG2, while the IgG4 is completely ineffective in the complement activation. Furthermore, it has been observed that multimeric antibody or antibody complexes are better in complement activation than monomeric antibody. Thus, in therapeutic applications, when complement activation properties are important, it is suggested that either, the CH2 domain and the hinge region of the IgG1 or the IgG3 are used, or chimeric IgG1/IgG3 Fc are constructed [62, 63].

## Improving FcγR and FcRn Receptors Binding

Human FcγRI (CD64) receptor preferential binds to the monomeric human IgG1 and IgG3. The IgG4 antibody subclass binds to this receptor with 10-fold lower affinity and IgG2 antibodies do not bind at all. The binding site for the FcγRI is localised on the antibody chain between the hinge disulphide region and the N-terminal region of the CH2 domain [64, 65]. Another receptor molecules, the FcγRII (CD32) preferentially binds antibody complexes, especially those of IgG1 and IgG3. The FcγRII binding site is localised in the CH2 antibody domain and overlaps the binding site for the FcγRI. The third receptor has low affinity for the monomeric immunoglobulin, but binds well to the polymeric IgG1 and IgG3. Thus, in therapeutic applications when FcγRI, FcγRII or FcγRIII activation is important, the preference will be antibodies for the IgG1 or the IgG3 subclass [66, 67].

Increased knowledge of the amino acids in IgG1 that are involved in the FcγR interactions has led to the generation and testing of the antibody mutants with enhanced or reduced affinities of the IgG molecule to the FcγR [68]. Thus, to increase the FcγR affinities the following amino acid positions on the IgG1 molecule have to be modified: Gly236, Ser 239, Phe 243, Pro247, Asp280, Lys290, Arg292, Ser298, Thr299, Tyr300, Val305, Lys326, Ala330, Ile332, Glu333, Lys334, Ala339 and Pro396. Also, the triple IgG1 mutants of Leu234Phe, Leu235Glu and Pro331Ser, the tetra mutants of His268Gln, Val309Leu, Ala330Ser and Pro331Ser, or the penta IgG1 variants of Cys226Ser, Cys229Ser, Glu233Pro, Leu234Val and Leu235Ala can achieve decrease in the FcγR affinities.

In therapeutic applications the ADCC can be exploited using antibody drugs to link target cell to the CD3 antigen of the cytotoxic T cells or the CD16 FcγRIII receptor on the natural killer cells [69, 70]. Such an approach has shown encouraging anti-tumour effects in clinics.

In addition to the FcγR binding and the effector functions, Fc antibody domains can bind to the neonatal Fc receptors (FcRn). Enhancement of the FcRn binding leads to the increased antibody serum half-life. Thus, when extended serum half-life is desired, the FcRn binding region of the Fc antibody fragment could be modified to increase the FcRn affinities [71-76].

## Engineering Antibody Glycosylation

The carbohydrate chain attached to the CH2 domain plays an important role in the regulation of the antibody serum half-life and the effector function. Human IgG molecules normally survive in the blood circulation longer than any other serum proteins. For example, serum half-life for the IgG1, IgG2 and IgG4 subclasses is about 3 weeks. Only the IgG3 subclass that has a long hinge region has a relatively short half-life of about 1 week [76].

The carbohydrate chain attached to the conserved aspargine 297 (Asn297) on the CH2 domain comprises of a core heptasacharide of the N-acetylglucosamine (GlcNAc) and mannose, followed by the addition of the galactose, fucose, sialic acid and the bisecting GlcNAc residues [77]. It has been shown that, although the Fc carbohydrates have no direct contact with the FcγRs [78], the aglycosylated or deglycosylated antibody molecules have reduced binding affinities to the C1q or FcγRs and as consequence have no Fc-mediated effector function [79]. Therefore, the effector functions of the antibody molecule can be fine-tuned by the modification of the Fc glycosylation patterns. For example, the bisecting GlcNAc residue on the antibody glycoform leads to the increase in the antibody dependent cell cytotoxicity effector function [80]. Furthermore, removal of the core fucose increases antibody-binding affinity to the FcγRIII and thus enhances the ADCC both *in vitro* [81] and *in vivo* [82]. These changes to the antibody effector function by modifying carbohydrate moieties have been shown to play a significant role in anti-cancer therapy [83, 84]. Thus, the next generation of the anti-cancer antibodies could be glycoengineered to have desired afucosylated carbohydrates [85].

### Bi- and Multi-Specific Antibody Formats

Bi-specific and multi-specific antibody formats [86] offer potential novel opportunities and therapeutic possibilities in many applications targeting disease by blocking infection with bi-specific domain antibody, directing a cytotoxic agent to a cancer cell and activating cellular cytotoxic effects [87, 88]. These bi- and multi-specific antibody formats can be generated by making the same antigen-binding site with the dual specificity, for example Her2 and VEGF [89], dual-variable domain IgG with bivalent binding abilities to the double targets [90] or the linked pair of the antibody molecules that selectively recognize distinct epitopes on the target antigen [91]. Several approaches exist to create an antibody with the multiple specificities, for example, chemical crosslinking [92], tandem fusion of the scFv or the single domain antibodies [93], fusion of the heavy chains [94], hybrid hybridomas (quadromas) [95], knob-in-hole CH3 engineering [96] and the SEEDbodies technology [97].

## ANTIBODY FUSION PROTEINS

### Antibody:Antigen Binging Domain Fusion Proteins

Antibody:antigen binding domain fusion proteins are very attractive molecules for the anti-cancer therapy. One of the approaches is to link the binding site from an anti-tumour antibody to an inflammatory cytokine at the gene level with expression of the engineered molecule in suitable hosts. Cytokines can be attached either immediately after the last codon of the hinge, replacing CH2 and CH3 domains, or after the CH2 or CH3 domains. For example, fusions with IL-2 [98], IL-8 [99], granulocyte/macrophage colony-stimulating factor (GMCSF) [100] and the tumour necrosis factor TNFα and TNFβ have been generated and used in clinics [101].

Another approach is to fuse antigen-binding part of an antibody molecule and an immunotoxin. Some highly potent toxins, such as the plant toxins ricin and abrin, diphtheria toxin and others have been analysed and several such molecules are in clinical development [102]. A potential problem with the use of the non-human toxins is the risk of generation of the immune responses to the antibody-toxin fusion protein. The degree of retention of cytotoxic activity and antibody antigen-binding affinity has also been shown to vary in such fusions.

## Fc-Fusion Proteins

In the therapeutic antibody molecule the CH2 and CH3 domains provide an immune effector function. Functional properties of the Fc portion of the four IgG isoforms are well known and their diversities allow a choice of the strength of interaction of the antibody with the components of complement or with the cells of the immune system [103, 104]. It is also now possible to manipulate the strength of the interaction of the various IgG isotopes with the Fc receptors by defined point mutations in the amino acid sequence of the Fc fragment as explained earlier in this chapter. Expression hosts are also an important factor, as the Fc portion is normally glycosylated and the presence and the type of the carbohydrates are important for the activation of the complement or the cell-mediated cytotoxicity. Engineering Fc containing molecules permits generation of the monovalent antibody-like molecules useful when the antibody-binding to the antigen surfaces is undesirable but where the effector Fc function is still required. However, currently the primary reason for the Fc fragment fusion protein generation is the extension of the serum half-life of such proteins. The Fc domain prolongs the half-life of such Fc-fusion proteins due to pH-dependent binding to the neonatal Fc receptor (FcRn), which protects protein from being degraded by endosomes. An additional advantage of the Fc-fusion protein is that the Fc-domain helps protein solubility and purification can be achieved using protein A-affinity purification. Several Fc-fusion proteins have been approved for clinical use as shown in Table **2**.

**Table 2:** Therapeutic Fc-fusion proteins

| Generic name (Trade Name) | Description | Mode of action | Year first FDA approval and Therapeutic Indication |
|---|---|---|---|
| Etanercept (Enbrel®) | 75 kDa soluble extracellular domain (ECD) of tumour necrosis factor (TNF) receptor II fused to human IgG1 Fc | Binds membrane-bound and soluble forms of TNF, thereby reducing concentrations of inflammatory cytokines | 1998<br>Rheumatoid arthritis |
| Alefacept (Amevive®) | First ECD of lymphocyte function-associated antigen 3 (LFA-3) fused to human IgG1 Fc | Binds CD2; blocks the interactions between LFA on APCs with CD2 on T cells, thereby inhibiting T-cell activation | 2003<br>Plaque psoriasis |
| Abatacept (Orencia®) | ECD of human cytotoxic T lymphocyte associated molecule-4 (CTLA-4) fused to human IgG1 Fc | Blocks the interactions between CD80 or CD86 on APCs and CD28 on T cells, thereby inhibiting T-cell activation | 2005<br>Rheumatoid arthritis |
| Rilonacept (Arcalyst®) | Two chains, each comprising the C-terminus of the IL-1R accessory protein ligand binding region fused to the N-terminus of the IL-1RI ECD, fused to human IgG1 Fc | Binds IL-1, thereby preventing interaction with endogenous cell-surface receptors | 2008<br>Plaque psoriasis |
| Romiplostim (Nplate®) | Peptide thrombopoietin (TPO) mimetic fused to the C-terminus of aglycosylated human IgG1 Fc | Binds and agonizes the TPO receptor; Fc functionality minimized due to lack of glycosylation | 2008<br>Thrombocytopenia |
| Belatacept (Nulojix®) | ECD of CTLA-4 fused to human IgG1 Fc; differs from abatacept by two amino acid substitutions (L104E, A29Y) in the CTLA-4 region | Blocks the interactions between CD80 or CD86 on APCs and CD28 on T cells, thereby inhibiting T-cell activation | 2011<br>Prophylaxis of organ rejection in adult kidney transplant recipients |
| Aflibercept (Eylea™) | ECDs of VEGF receptors 1 and 2 fused to human IgG1 Fc | Binds all forms of VEGF-A, as well as placental growth factor, thereby inhibiting angiogenesis | 2011<br>Neovascular Age-Related Macular Degeneration |
| Ziv-Aflibercept (Zaltrap™) | ECDs of VEGF receptors 1 and 2 fused to human IgG1 Fc | Binds all forms of VEGF-A, as well as placental growth factor, thereby inhibiting angiogenesis | 2012<br>Metastatic Colorectal Cancer |

## Chemoimmunoconjugates

In circumstances where genetically encoded function of antibody may be insufficient to have a desired therapeutic effect, post-translational conjugation of cytotoxic agents may be employed. Antibodies in this case will specifically target the therapeutic agent directly to cells when targeted agents can be either directly toxic to cells or can be converted into toxic agents at the site of delivery. Such antibody conjugates can also be used to extend the half-life of the antibody drug.

The major limitation of the systemic chemotherapy in cancer patients is a lack of tumour specificity. Since antibodies can specifically target cancer cells the idea of antibody:toxin conjugate is to eliminate unwanted function of the toxic molecule on the cancer-surrounding cells and to tailor-make cancer therapy molecules with well-defined anti-tumour activity function. Several antibody-drug conjugates have been constructed and proposed as a novel group of the anti-tumour agents. These include antibody-anti metabolites (aminopterin, cytosine arabinoside, metotrexan, 5-fluorouracil and 5-fluorodeoxyuridine), anti-mitotic agents (vinca alkaloids, colchicine and podophyllotoxin), anthracyclines (melphalan, chlorambucil, mitomycin C and Cis-platimun), and others [105, 106].

## Radioimmunoconjugates

Antibody-radioisotope conjugates are mainly used for tumour imaging and therapy [107]. The most important requirements for this type of antibody molecules are high specificity to the tumour, high tissue penetration for solid tumours and rapid clearance from the other tissues to minimise radiation dose, particularly to the bone marrow [108]. For antibody-radioisotope conjugation Fab' or scFv molecules are expressed with a hinge peptide containing a single cysteine to facilitate cross-linking. Examples of the antibody radioimmunoconjugates approved for clinical use are shown in Table **3**. Furthermore, many new radioimmunoconjugates are in the development for cancer diagnostic imaging and other therapeutic applications [109-111].

## PEGylated Antibodies and Antibody Fragments

It has been known for some time that conjugation of the antibody molecule with the polyethylene glycol (PEGylation) reduces the immunogenicity of the therapeutic antibodies. This chemical addition of polyethylene glycol (PEG) to the antibody also increases the size of the antibody fragments, prolongs circulating serum half-life and may also enhance targeting by antibody, and thus antibody therapeutic effect. An example of the clinically approved PEGylated antibody conjugate is the anti-TNFα PEGylated Fab fragment (Certolizumab Pegol) for patients with the Crohn's disease [112].

**Table 3:** Therapeutic radioimmunoconjugates

| Generic name (Trade Name) | Description | Mode of action | Year first FDA approval and Therapeutic Indication |
|---|---|---|---|
| Ibritumomab Tiuxetan (Zevalin) | $Y^{90}$-murine IgG1κ | Binds to CD20 | 2002<br>B-cell<br>Non-Hodgkin's lymphoma |
| Tositumomab (Bexxar) | $I^{131}$-murine IgG2aλ | Binds to CD20 | 2003<br>Non-Hodgkin's lymphoma |
| $I^{131}$-TNT (Cotara4) | $I^{131}$-chimeric IgG1 | Binds DNA | 2003 in China<br>Lung cancer |

## CONCLUSION

Antibody based therapy is an established therapeutic modality that has gained much the interest in recent time. The construction and the reconstruction of the antibody domains has been enhanced by recombinant DNA and hybridoma technologies. These have enabled the creation of a large variety of antibody forms, which can be further individually tailored to the specific therapeutic needs. Desired pharmacological properties, such as low immunogenicity, good serum half-life and tissue penetration, as well as required binding and effector functions can now be grafted into the antibody molecule. The binding site can be optimised and made in different formats to create desired affinity and valencies. Currently antibody-based drugs have two major therapeutic mechanisms. One is mediated by the antigen binding properties of the Fab portion of the antibody molecule and includes binding and neutralisation of other functional proteins, such as cytokines and angiogenic factors, as well as antibody mediated cell signalling and targeted drug delivery. The second mechanism is mediated by the Fc portion of the antibody and includes recruitment of the effector cells *via* FcγR and FcRn interactions and also binding to the C1q and thus, complement activation.

More and more antibodies are being approved for therapeutic use and even more are currently in clinical development, making this category of biologics one of the fastest growing therapeutic sectors. Despite substantial progress in antibody engineering, there still challenges remaining, for example, to improve antibody design and the therapeutic affordability. It is important to keep in mind that post-translational glycosylation of full-length antibody molecules impacts on their intrinsic immunogenicity and effector function. Therefore designing better controlled and less expensive expression systems is one of the most important challenges to help to expand the use of the recombinant antibodies in the clinic.

## ACKNOWLEDGEMENT

Declared None.

## CONFLICT OF INTEREST

The authors confirm that this chapter contents have no conflict of interest.

## REFERENCES

[1] Labeta MO, Margni RA, Leoni J, Binaghi RA. Structure of asymmetric non-precipitating antibody: presence of a carbohydrate residue in only one Fab region of the molecule. Immunology 1986; 57(2): 311-7.

[2] Ruban E, Staroscik K, Janusz M, Kratzin H, Hilschmann N. [Rule of antibody structure: the primary structure of a human monoclonal IgA1-immunoglobulin (myeloma protein Tro), II. Cleavage of the monomer IgA-molecule and the reduced and alkylated H- and L-chains by cyanogen bromide (author's transl)]. Hoppe-Seyler's Zeitschrift fur physiologische Chemie 1978; 359(12): 1689-95.

[3] Murakami K, Nakamura H. Flexible structure of immunoglobulin G molecule. Fluorescence depolarization studies on hapten-antihapten antibody interactions using arylnaphthalenesulfonates as the ligands. Jpn J Exp Med 1976; 46(1): 59-70.

[4] Colman PM, Deisenhofer J, Huber R. Structure of the human antibody molecule Kol (immunoglobulin G1): an electron density map at 5 A resolution. J Mol Biol 1976; 100(3): 257-78.

[5] Wardlaw AC. The antibody molecule: structure and function. Canadian journal of medical technology 1969; 31(5): 177-87.

[6] Braden BC, Goldman ER, Mariuzza RA, Poljak RJ. Anatomy of an antibody molecule: structure, kinetics, thermodynamics and mutational studies of the antilysozyme antibody D1.3. Immunol Rev 1998; 163: 45-57.

[7] Collins AM, Jackson KJ. A Temporal Model of Human IgE and IgG Antibody Function. Frontiers in Immunology 2013; 4: 235

[8] Snoeck V, Peters IR, Cox E. The IgA system: a comparison of structure and function in different species. Vet Res 2006; 37(3): 455-67.

[9] Wiersma EJ, Collins C, Fazel S, Shulman MJ. Structural and functional analysis of J chain-deficient IgM. J Immunol 1998; 160(12): 5979-89.

[10] Vargas-Madrazo E, Lara-Ochoa F, Almagro JC. Canonical structure repertoire of the antigen-binding site of immunoglobulins suggests strong geometrical restrictions associated to the mechanism of immune recognition. J Mol Biol 1995; 254(3): 497-504.

[11] Segal DM, Padlan EA, Cohen GH, Rudikoff S, Potter M, Davies DR. The three-dimensional structure of a phosphorylcholine-binding mouse immunoglobulin Fab and the nature of the antigen binding site. Proc Natl Acad Sci U S A 1974; 71(11): 4298-302.

[12] Zikan J, Draber P, Vojtiskova M. Monoclonal IgG3 (kappa) antibodies against murine Thy-1.2 antigen produced by murine hybridomas. Differences in the specificity of the antigen binding site and in the structure of the hinge region. Folia Biologica 1982; 28(6): 377-94.

[13] Radaev S, Sun PD. Recognition of IgG by Fcgamma receptor. The role of Fc glycosylation and the binding of peptide inhibitors. J Biol Chem 2001; 276(19): 16478-83.

[14] Butler M, Quelhas D, Critchley AJ, Carchon H, Hebestreit HF, Hibbert RG, *et al.* Detailed glycan analysis of serum glycoproteins of patients with congenital disorders of glycosylation indicates the specific defective glycan processing step and provides an insight into pathogenesis. Glycobiology 2003; 13(9): 601-22.
[15] Krapp S, Mimura Y, Jefferis R, Huber R, Sondermann P. Structural analysis of human IgG-Fc glycoforms reveals a correlation between glycosylation and structural integrity. J Mol Biol 2003; 325(5): 979-89.
[16] Ferrara C, Brunker P, Suter T, Moser S, Puntener U, Umana P. Modulation of therapeutic antibody effector functions by glycosylation engineering: influence of Golgi enzyme localization domain and co-expression of heterologous beta1, 4-N-acetylglucosaminyltransferase III and Golgi alpha-mannosidase II. Biotechnol Bioeng 2006; 93(5): 851-61.
[17] Arnold JN, Wormald MR, Sim RB, Rudd PM, Dwek RA. The impact of glycosylation on the biological function and structure of human immunoglobulins. Annu Rev Immunol 2007; 25: 21-50.
[18] Jefferis R. Recombinant antibody therapeutics: the impact of glycosylation on mechanisms of action. Trends in Pharmacological Sciences 2009; 30(7): 356-62.
[19] Morrison SL, Johnson MJ, Herzenberg LA, Oi VT. Chimeric human antibody molecules: mouse antigen-binding domains with human constant region domains. Proc Natl Acad Sci U S A 1984; 81(21): 6851-5.
[20] Perens G, Levi DS, Alejos JC, Wetzel GT. Muronomab-CD3 for pediatric acute myocarditis. Pediatric Cardiology 2007; 28(1): 21-6.
[21] Brezina K, Murphy M, Stonner T. Care of the patient receiving ReoPro following angioplasty. J Invasive Cardiol 1994; 6 Suppl A: 38A-42A; discussion 54A-6A.
[22] Tcheng JE. Dosing and administration of ReoPro (c7E3 Fab). J Invasive Cardiol 1994; 6 Suppl A: 29A-33A; discussion 51A-4A.
[23] Lee EJ, Kueck B. Rituxan in the treatment of cold agglutinin disease. Blood 1998; 92(9): 3490-1.
[24] Jonas C. Rituxan: the new kid on the block. Oncology Nursing Forum 1998; 25(4): 669.
[25] Kovarik JM, Kahan BD, Rajagopalan PR, Bennett W, Mulloy LL, Gerbeau C, *et al.* Population pharmacokinetics and exposure-response relationships for basiliximab in kidney transplantation. The U.S. Simulect Renal Transplant Study Group. Transplantation 1999; 68(9): 1288-94.
[26] Mulloy LL, Wright F, Hall ML, Moore M. Simulect (basiliximab) reduces acute cellular rejection in renal allografts from cadaveric and living donors. Transplant Proc 1999; 31(1-2): 1210-3.
[27] D'Haens GR. Infliximab (Remicade), a new biological treatment for Crohn's disease. Italian Journal of Gastroenterology and Hepatology 1999; 31(6): 519-20.
[28] Reddy P. Infliximab (Remicade). Connecticut Medicine 1999; 63(7): 413-6.
[29] Yang B, Wang JJ. Industry Analysis: Erbitux and targeted therapies for cancer. Discovery Medicine 2004; 4(20): 15-7.
[30] Katz J, Janik JE, Younes A. Brentuximab Vedotin (SGN-35). Clin Cancer Res 2011; 17(20): 6428-36.
[31] Chan AC, Carter PJ. Therapeutic antibodies for autoimmunity and inflammation. Nat Rev Immunol 2010; 10(5): 301-16.
[32] Kettleborough CA, Saldanha J, Heath VJ, Morrison CJ, Bendig MM. Humanization of a mouse monoclonal antibody by CDR-grafting: the importance of framework residues on loop conformation. Protein Eng 1991; 4(7): 773-83.
[33] Daugherty BL, DeMartino JA, Law MF, Kawka DW, Singer, II, Mark GE. Polymerase chain reaction facilitates the cloning, CDR-grafting, and rapid expression of a murine monoclonal antibody directed against the CD18 component of leukocyte integrins. Nucleic Acids Res 1991; 19(9): 2471-6.
[34] Kim JH, Hong HJ. Humanization by CDR grafting and specificity-determining residue grafting. Methods Mol Biol 2012; 907: 237-45.
[35] Lewis AP, Crowe JS. Immunoglobulin complementarity-determining region grafting by recombinant polymerase chain reaction to generate humanised monoclonal antibodies. Gene 1991; 101(2): 297-302.
[36] Stewart LM, Young S, Watson G, Mather SJ, Bates PA, Band HA, *et al.* Humanisation and characterisation of PR1A3, a monoclonal antibody specific for cell-bound carcinoembryonic antigen. Cancer Immunol Immunother 1999; 47(6): 299-306.

[37] Desmyter A, Transue TR, Ghahroudi MA, Thi MH, Poortmans F, Hamers R, *et al.* Crystal structure of a camel single-domain VH antibody fragment in complex with lysozyme. Nature Structural Biology 1996; 3(9): 803-11.

[38] Hattori T, Umetsu M, Nakanishi T, Sawai S, Kikuchi S, Asano R, *et al.* A high-affinity gold-binding camel antibody: antibody engineering for one-pot functionalization of gold nanoparticles as biointerface molecules. Bioconjug Chem 2012; 23(9): 1934-44.

[39] Baral TN, Chao SY, Li S, Tanha J, Arbabi-Ghahroudi M, Zhang J, *et al.* Crystal structure of a human single domain antibody dimer formed through V(H)-V(H) non-covalent interactions. PLoS One 2012; 7(1): e30149.

[40] Rouet R, Dudgeon K, Christ D. Generation of human single domain antibody repertoires by Kunkel mutagenesis. Methods Mol Biol 2012; 907: 195-209.

[41] Skerra A, Pluckthun A. Assembly of a functional immunoglobulin Fv fragment in Escherichia coli. Science 1988; 240(4855): 1038-41.

[42] Guo L, Yan X, Qian S, Meng G. Selecting and expressing protective single-chain Fv fragment to stabilize L-asparaginase against inactivation by trypsin. Biotechnology and applied biochemistry 2000; 31 (Pt 1): 21-7.

[43] Benhar I, Pastan I. Identification of residues that stabilize the single-chain Fv of monoclonal antibodies B3. J Biol Chem 1995; 270(40): 23373-80.

[44] Glockshuber R, Malia M, Pfitzinger I, Pluckthun A. A comparison of strategies to stabilize immunoglobulin Fv-fragments. Biochemistry 1990; 29(6): 1362-7.

[45] Jager M, Pluckthun A. Domain interactions in antibody Fv and scFv fragments: effects on unfolding kinetics and equilibria. FEBS Lett 1999; 462(3): 307-12.

[46] Worn A, Pluckthun A. Different equilibrium stability behavior of ScFv fragments: identification, classification, and improvement by protein engineering. Biochemistry 1999; 38(27): 8739-50.

[47] Carmichael JA, Power BE, Garrett TP, Yazaki PJ, Shively JE, Raubischek AA, *et al.* The crystal structure of an anti-CEA scFv diabody assembled from T84.66 scFvs in V(L)-to-V(H) orientation: implications for diabody flexibility. J Mol Biol 2003; 326(2): 341-51.

[48] Evans L, Hughes M, Waters J, Cameron J, Dodsworth N, Tooth D, *et al.* The production, characterisation and enhanced pharmacokinetics of scFv-albumin fusions expressed in Saccharomyces cerevisiae. Protein Expression and Purification 2010; 73(2): 113-24.

[49] Ahmad ZA, Yeap SK, Ali AM, Ho WY, Alitheen NB, Hamid M. scFv antibody: principles and clinical application. Clinical & Developmental Immunology 2012; 2012: 980250.

[50] Olafsen T, Sirk SJ, Betting DJ, Kenanova VE, Bauer KB, Ladno W, *et al.* ImmunoPET imaging of B-cell lymphoma using 124I-anti-CD20 scFv dimers (diabodies). Protein Eng Des Sel 2010; 23(4): 243-9.

[51] Dolezal O, Pearce LA, Lawrence LJ, McCoy AJ, Hudson PJ, Kortt AA. ScFv multimers of the anti-neuraminidase antibody NC10: shortening of the linker in single-chain Fv fragment assembled in V(L) to V(H) orientation drives the formation of dimers, trimers, tetramers and higher molecular mass multimers. Protein Eng 2000; 13(8): 565-74.

[52] Wang R, Xiang S, Feng Y, Srinivas S, Zhang Y, Lin M, *et al.* Engineering production of functional scFv antibody in E. coli by co-expressing the molecule chaperone Skp. Frontiers in Cellular and Infection Microbiology 2013; 3: 72.

[53] Muller KM, Arndt KM, Strittmatter W, Pluckthun A. The first constant domain (C(H)1 and C(L)) of an antibody used as heterodimerization domain for bispecific miniantibodies. FEBS Lett 1998; 422(2): 259-64.

[54] Rodrigues ML, Snedecor B, Chen C, Wong WL, Garg S, Blank GS, *et al.* Engineering Fab' fragments for efficient F(ab)2 formation in Escherichia coli and for improved *in vivo* stability. J Immunol 1993; 151(12): 6954-61.

[55] Johnson D, Sharma S. Ocular and systemic safety of bevacizumab and ranibizumab in patients with neovascular age-related macular degeneration. Curr Opinion in Ophthalmology 2013; 24(3): 205-12.

[56] Lang L. FDA approves Cimzia to treat Crohn's disease. Gastroenterology 2008; 134(7): 1819.

[57] Connock M, Tubeuf S, Malottki K, Uthman A, Round J, Bayliss S, *et al.* Certolizumab pegol (CIMZIA(R)) for the treatment of rheumatoid arthritis. Health Technology Assessment 2010; 14(Suppl. 2): 1-10.

[58] Rodrigues ML, Shalaby MR, Werther W, Presta L, Carter P. Engineering a humanized bispecific F(ab')2 fragment for improved binding to T cells. Int J Cancer Suppl 1992; 7: 45-50.

[59] Covell DG, Barbet J, Holton OD, Black CD, Parker RJ, Weinstein JN. Pharmacokinetics of monoclonal immunoglobulin G1, F(ab')2, and Fab' in mice. Cancer Res 1986; 46(8): 3969-78.

[60] Cartron G, Dacheux L, Salles G, Solal-Celigny P, Bardos P, Colombat P, *et al.* Therapeutic activity of humanized anti-CD20 monoclonal antibody and polymorphism in IgG Fc receptor FcgammaRIIIa gene. Blood 2002; 99(3): 754-8.

[61] Lejeune J, Thibault G, Ternant D, Cartron G, Watier H, Ohresser M. Evidence for linkage disequilibrium between Fcgamma RIIIa-V158F and Fcgamma RIIa-H131R polymorphisms in white patients, and for an Fcgamma RIIIa-restricted influence on the response to therapeutic antibodies. J Clin Oncol 2008; 26(33): 5489-91; author reply 91-2.

[62] Horton HM, Bernett MJ, Pong E, Peipp M, Karki S, Chu SY, *et al.* Potent *in vitro* and *in vivo* activity of an Fc-engineered anti-CD19 monoclonal antibody against lymphoma and leukemia. Cancer Res 2008; 68(19): 8049-57.

[63] Natsume A, In M, Takamura H, Nakagawa T, Shimizu Y, Kitajima K, *et al.* Engineered antibodies of IgG1/IgG3 mixed isotype with enhanced cytotoxic activities. Cancer Res 2008; 68(10): 3863-72.

[64] Liu X-y, Pop LM, Vitetta ES. Engineering therapeutic monoclonal antibodies. Immunol Rev 2008; 222: 9-27.

[65] Strohl WR. Optimization of Fc-mediated effector functions of monoclonal antibodies. Curr Opin Biotechnol 2009; 20(6): 685-91.

[66] Desjarlais JR, Lazar GA, Zhukovsky EA, Chu SY. Optimizing engagement of the immune system by anti-tumour antibodies: an engineer's perspective. Drug Discovery Today 2007; 12(21-22): 898-910.

[67] Lazar GA, Desjarlais JR, Jacinto J, Karki S, Hammond PW. A molecular immunology approach to antibody humanization and functional optimization. Mol Immunol 2007; 44(8): 1986-98.

[68] Shields RL, Namenuk AK, Hong K, Meng YG, Rae J, Briggs J, *et al.* High resolution mapping of the binding site on human IgG1 for Fc gamma RI, Fc gamma RII, Fc gamma RIII, and FcRn and design of IgG1 variants with improved binding to the Fc gamma R. J Biol Chem 2001; 276(9): 6591-604.

[69] Kipriyanov SM, Cochlovius B, Schafer HJ, Moldenhauer G, Bahre A, Le Gall F, *et al.* Synergistic antitumour effect of bispecific CD19 x CD3 and CD19 x CD16 diabodies in a preclinical model of non-Hodgkin's lymphoma. J Immunol 2002; 169(1): 137-44.

[70] Kipriyanov SM, Moldenhauer G, Strauss G, Little M. Bispecific CD3 x CD19 diabody for T cell-mediated lysis of malignant human B cells. Int J Cancer 1998; 77(5): 763-72.

[71] Dall'Acqua WF, Kiener PA, Wu H. Properties of human IgG1s engineered for enhanced binding to the neonatal Fc receptor (FcRn). J Biol Chem 2006; 281(33): 23514-24.

[72] Oganesyan V, Damschroder MM, Woods RM, Cook KE, Wu H, Dall'acqua WF. Structural characterization of a human Fc fragment engineered for extended serum half-life. Mol Immunol 2009; 46(8-9): 1750-5.

[73] Yeung YA, Wu X, Reyes AE, 2nd, Vernes JM, Lien S, Lowe J, *et al.* A therapeutic anti-VEGF antibody with increased potency independent of pharmacokinetic half-life. Cancer Res 2010; 70(8): 3269-77.

[74] Zalevsky J, Chamberlain AK, Horton HM, Karki S, Leung IW, Sproule TJ, *et al.* Enhanced antibody half-life improves *in vivo* activity. Nat Biotechnol 2010; 28(2): 157-9.

[75] Hinton PR, Johlfs MG, Xiong JM, Hanestad K, Ong KC, Bullock C, *et al.* Engineered human IgG antibodies with longer serum half-lives in primates. J Biol Chem 2004; 279(8): 6213-6.

[76] Hinton PR, Xiong JM, Johlfs MG, Tang MT, Keller S, Tsurushita N. An engineered human IgG1 antibody with longer serum half-life. J Immunol 2006; 176(1): 346-56.

[77] Jefferis R. Glycosylation of recombinant antibody therapeutics. Biotechnology Progress 2005; 21(1): 11-6.

[78] Sondermann P, Huber R, Oosthuizen V, Jacob U. The 3.2-A crystal structure of the human IgG1 Fc fragment-Fc gammaRIII complex. Nature 2000; 406(6793): 267-73.

[79] Jefferis R, Lund J. Interaction sites on human IgG-Fc for FcgammaR: current models. Immunol Lett 2002; 82(1-2): 57-65.

[80] Fukuta K, Abe R, Yokomatsu T, Omae F, Asanagi M, Makino T. Control of bisecting GlcNAc addition to N-linked sugar chains. J Biol Chem 2000; 275(31): 23456-61.

[81] Shields RL, Lai J, Keck R, O'Connell LY, Hong K, Meng YG, *et al.* Lack of fucose on human IgG1 N-linked oligosaccharide improves binding to human Fcgamma RIII and antibody-dependent cellular toxicity. J Biol Chem 2002; 277(30): 26733-40.

[82] Nimmerjahn F, Ravetch JV. Divergent immunoglobulin g subclass activity through selective Fc receptor binding. Science 2005; 310(5753): 1510-2.

[83] Umana P, Jean-Mairet J, Moudry R, Amstutz H, Bailey JE. Engineered glycoforms of an antineuroblastoma IgG1 with optimized antibody-dependent cellular cytotoxic activity. Nat Biotechnol 1999; 17(2): 176-80.

[84] Shinkawa T, Nakamura K, Yamane N, Shoji-Hosaka E, Kanda Y, Sakurada M, *et al.* The absence of fucose but not the presence of galactose or bisecting N-acetylglucosamine of human IgG1 complex-type oligosaccharides shows the critical role of enhancing antibody-dependent cellular cytotoxicity. J Biol Chem 2003; 278(5): 3466-73.

[85] Yamane-Ohnuki N, Satoh M. Production of therapeutic antibodies with controlled fucosylation. MAbs 2009; 1(3): 230-6.

[86] Carter P. Bispecific human IgG by design. J Immunol Methods 2001; 248(1-2): 7-15.

[87] Huston JS. Engineering antibodies for the 21st century. Protein Eng Des Sel 2012; 25(10): 483-4.

[88] Merchant AM, Zhu Z, Yuan JQ, Goddard A, Adams CW, Presta LG, *et al.* An efficient route to human bispecific IgG. Nat Biotechnol 1998; 16(7): 677-81.

[89] Bostrom J, Yu SF, Kan D, Appleton BA, Lee CV, Billeci K, *et al.* Variants of the antibody herceptin that interact with HER2 and VEGF at the antigen binding site. Science 2009; 323(5921): 1610-4.

[90] Wu C, Ying H, Grinnell C, Bryant S, Miller R, Clabbers A, *et al.* Simultaneous targeting of multiple disease mediators by a dual-variable-domain immunoglobulin. Nat Biotechnol 2007; 25(11): 1290-7.

[91] Robinson MK, Hodge KM, Horak E, Sundberg AL, Russeva M, Shaller CC, *et al.* Targeting ErbB2 and ErbB3 with a bispecific single-chain Fv enhances targeting selectivity and induces a therapeutic effect *in vitro*. Br J Cancer 2008; 99(9): 1415-25.

[92] Brennan M, Davison PF, Paulus H. Preparation of bispecific antibodies by chemical recombination of monoclonal immunoglobulin G1 fragments. Science 1985; 229(4708): 81-3.

[93] De Bernardis F, Liu H, O'Mahony R, La Valle R, Bartollino S, Sandini S, *et al.* Human domain antibodies against virulence traits of Candida albicans inhibit fungus adherence to vaginal epithelium and protect against experimental vaginal candidiasis. The Journal of Infectious Diseases 2007; 195(1): 149-57.

[94] Shen J, Vil MD, Jimenez X, Iacolina M, Zhang H, Zhu Z. Single variable domain-IgG fusion. A novel recombinant approach to Fc domain-containing bispecific antibodies. J Biol Chem 2006; 281(16): 10706-14.

[95] Milstein C, Cuello AC. Hybrid hybridomas and their use in immunohistochemistry. Nature 1983; 305(5934): 537-40.

[96] Ridgway JB, Presta LG, Carter P. 'Knobs-into-holes' engineering of antibody CH3 domains for heavy chain heterodimerization. Protein Eng 1996; 9(7): 617-21.

[97] Davis JH, Aperlo C, Li Y, Kurosawa E, Lan Y, Lo KM, *et al.* SEEDbodies: fusion proteins based on strand-exchange engineered domain (SEED) CH3 heterodimers in an Fc analogue platform for asymmetric binders or immunofusions and bispecific antibodies. Protein Eng Des Sel 2010; 23(4): 195-202.

[98] Hombach AA, Abken H. Antibody-IL2 fusion proteins for tumour targeting. Methods Mol Biol 2012; 907: 611-26.

[99] Holzer W, Petersen F, Strittmatter W, Matzku S, von Hoegen I. A fusion protein of IL-8 and a Fab antibody fragments binds to IL-8 receptors and induces neutrophil activation. Cytokine 1996; 8(3): 214-21.

[100] Hornick JL, Khawli LA, Hu P, Lynch M, Anderson PM, Epstein AL. Chimeric CLL-1 antibody fusion proteins containing granulocyte macrophage colony-stimulating factor or interleukin-2 with specificity for B-cell malignancies exhibit enhanced effector functions while retaining tumour targeting properties. Blood 1997; 89(12): 4437-47.

[101] Christ O, Matzku S, Burger C, Zoller M. Interleukin 2-antibody and tumour necrosis factor-antibody fusion proteins induce different antitumour immune responses *in vivo*. Clin Cancer Res 2001; 7(5): 1385-97.

[102] Kreitman RJ, Pastan I. Antibody fusion proteins: anti-CD22 recombinant immunotoxin moxetumomab pasudotox. Clin Cancer Res 2011; 17(20): 6398-405.

[103] Stuart SG, Simister NE, Clarkson SB, Kacinski BM, Shapiro M, Mellman I. Human IgG Fc receptor (hFcRII; CD32) exists as multiple isoforms in macrophages, lymphocytes and IgG-transporting placental epithelium. The EMBO J 1989; 8(12): 3657-66.

[104] Seki T. Identification of multiple isoforms of the low-affinity human IgG Fc receptor. Immunogenetics 1989; 30(1): 5-12.

[105] Pietersz GA, Rowland A, Smyth MJ, McKenzie IF. Chemoimmunoconjugates for the treatment of cancer. Adv Immunol 1994; 56: 301-87.

[106] Schrappe M, Bumol TF, Apelgren LD, Briggs SL, Koppel GA, Markowitz DD, *et al.* Long-term growth suppression of human glioma xenografts by chemoimmunoconjugates of 4-desacetylvinblastine-3-carboxyhydrazide and monoclonal antibody 9.2.27. Cancer Res 1992; 52(14): 3838-44.

[107] Cornelissen B, Waller A, Able S, Vallis KA. Molecular radiotherapy using cleavable radioimmunoconjugates that target EGFR and gammaH2AX. Mol Cancer Ther 2013; 12(11): 2472-82.

[108] Rauch C, Seidl C, Schlapschy M, Skerra A, Morgenstern A, Bruchertseifer F, *et al.* High molecular mass radioimmunoconjugates are promising for intraperitoneal alpha-emitter immunotherapy due to prolonged retention in the peritoneum. Nucl Med Biol 2012; 39(5): 617-27.

[109] Razumienko EJ, Scollard DA, Reilly RM. Small-animal SPECT/CT of HER2 and HER3 expression in tumour xenografts in athymic mice using trastuzumab Fab-heregulin bispecific radioimmunoconjugates. J Nucl Med 2012; 53(12): 1943-50.

[110] Razumienko E, Dryden L, Scollard D, Reilly RM. MicroSPECT/CT imaging of co-expressed HER2 and EGFR on subcutaneous human tumour xenografts in athymic mice using (1)(1)(1)In-labeled bispecific radioimmunoconjugates. Breast Cancer Research and Treatment 2013; 138(3): 709-18.

[111] Pickhard A, Piontek G, Seidl C, Kopping S, Blechert B, Misslbeck M, *et al.* (2)(1)(3)Bi-anti-EGFR radioimmunoconjugates and X-ray irradiation trigger different cell death pathways in squamous cell carcinoma cells. Nucl Med Biol 2014; 41(1): 68-76.

[112] Blick SK, Curran MP. Certolizumab pegol: in Crohn's disease. BioDrugs: Clinical Immunotherapeutics, Biopharmaceuticals and Gene Therapy 2007; 21(3): 195-201; discussion 2-3.

CHAPTER 8

# Interferon-Alfa as a Vaccine Adjuvant

**Megan C. Duggan and William E. Carson III***

*Comprehensive Cancer Center, The Ohio State University, Columbus, OH 43210, USA*

**Abstract:** Colorectal cancers are the third leading cause of cancer-associated deaths in the United States. Carcinoembryonic antigen (CEA) is a glycoprotein which is over-expressed in all adenocarcinomas of the colon and rectum and is extensively used as a serologic marker of colon cancer. Its presence in the normal fetal colon, as well as in gut crypts and healing intestinal mucosa of adults makes it a challenging immunologic target, as cytotoxic T lymphocytes (CTL) must overcome tolerance and be directed towards CEA-expressing cancer cells while sparing normal CEA-expressing cells. CAP1-6D, a unique 9-mer peptide of the CEA protein with a single amino acid mutation has been identified as a tumor specific antigen that can induce a stronger immune response than the wild type CEA peptide. Costimulatory signals, such as B7.1 are also critically important in the generation of an effective T cell response to any antigen. The cytokine GM-CSF is a useful vaccine adjuvant for its ability to increase antigen-presenting cells and enhance the antigen-specific anti-tumor response. Additionally, interferon-alpha as an adjuvant can enhance the expression of tumor antigens, such as CEA. This chapter describes the rationale for a clinical trial in which two virus-based CEA vaccines encoding the CAP1-6D peptide as well as costimulatory molecules (B7.1, ICAM-1, and LFA-3) were administered along with the vaccine adjuvants interferon-alpha and GM-CSF.

**Keywords:** Carcinoembryonic antigen, Clinical trial, Colorectal cancer, ELISPOT assay, Interferon-alfa, Recombinant vaccines, Tumor immunotherapy, Viral vector.

## INTRODUCTION

Our group has investigated the use of interferon-alfa as a vaccine adjuvant. This approach to the vaccine therapy of cancer was evaluated in the context of a clinical trial in which a vaccine against the carcinoembryonic antigen (CEA) was combined with subcutaneous injections of interferon-alfa. Two virus-based CEA vaccines were employed in this trial: vaccinia-CEA(6D)-TRICOM and fowlpox-CEA(6D)-TRICOM. These viruses are able to infect professional antigen

***Corresponding author William E. Carson III:** Comprehensive Cancer Center, The Ohio State University, Columbus, OH 43210, USA; Tel: (614) 293-6306; E-mail: william.carson@osumc.edu

**Jianxun Song (Ed)**

presenting cells which then present the CEA gene, including a modified 9-MER CEA peptide, to CD8+ T cells in the context of HLA class I. These viral vectors also induce the expression of several co-stimulatory molecules (B7.1, ICAM-1, and LFA-3) which further provide activating signals to antigen-specific T cells.

In the clinical trial, the safety and efficacy of the vaccine regimen are being evaluated for its combination with interferon-alpha 2B (IFN-α-2b). Previous investigations have demonstrated that IFN-α-2b upregulates CEA expression on established tumor cell lines and isolated tumor cells. A phase I study by Roselli *et al.* found considerable increases in tumor CEA levels in patients with colorectal cancer who received IFN-α-2b at a dose of $3 \times 10^6$ per day three times per week. Also, several studies have shown that the expression of HLA-class I molecules can be upregulated in response to exogenous IFN. Taken together, it appears that the administration of interferon might be a useful vaccine adjunct. Thus, it was hypothesized that the administration of IFN-α-2b would significantly increase the prevalence of CEA: MHC complexes on carcinoma cells and that this would enhance the activation of CEA-specific cytotoxic T cells. Hopefully, the ultimate result of this immune manipulation would be an increased clearance of tumor cells.

## METASTATIC COLORECTAL CANCER

The majority of colorectal cancer cells express CEA and for this reason there is great interest in vaccines that could target this disease entity. In the United States, colorectal cancers are the third leading cause of cancer-associated mortality [1]. Each year, approximately 150,000 new cases of colorectal cancer are identified in the United States [2]. Locally advanced tumors and tumors associated with lymph node involvement frequently recur even after successful surgery and the administration of adjuvant chemotherapy [3]. The five-year survival rate for patients with advanced disease is typically around 20%. However, improvements in systemic therapy are leading to improvements in this figure. Surgical resection may benefit the small fraction of patients with limited metastatic disease, but the majority of patients with distant disease require systemic chemotherapy [4-6]. 5-fluorouracil (5-FU) has served as the cornerstone of therapy for patients with metastatic or locally advanced colorectal cancer [7]. There have been several attempts to maximize the efficacy of 5-FU through biochemical modulation [8-9]. Newer chemotherapeutic drugs have been approved for use in this disease (*e.g.*, irinotecan and oxaliplatin) that employ mechanisms of action different from those of 5-FU and when these are utilized in combination with 5-FU (usually with leucovorin), investigators have witnessed improved response rates, increased periods of response, and improvements in overall survival. Irinotecan (CPT-11) combined with 5-FU/leucovorin is currently the standard first-line regimen for clinical trials [10]. Additionally, several randomized studies have produced results indicating that there is a role for irinotecan as second line therapy for selected patients who have failed first-line therapy with fluorouracil and leucovorin [5]. Despite these advances, the search for novel therapies that make use of alternate anti-tumor mechanisms is ongoing [11]. A monoclonal antibody specific for the pro-angiogenic factor VEGF (vascular endothelial growth factor) known as bevacizumab and a monoclonal antibody for HER1 known as cetuximab are now often utilized in patients who are suffering from metastatic disease.

## CEA VACCINES

### Rationale for CEA as Target

Carcinoembryonic antigen (CEA) is a glycoprotein which is found in greatest abundance in the normal fetal colon. CEA has a molecular weight of 180,000. In adult humans, CEA and other members of its family are normally found in the colonic mucosa [12]. However, CEA over-expression can be found in virtually all adenocarcinomas of the colon and rectum. CEA is also usually present on adenocarcinomas of the breast, lung, and pancreas [13-15]. In colorectal carcinomas, CEA is produced at such high levels that it can be detected in the circulation [16]. As a result, CEA is extensively used as a serologic marker of colorectal cancer. The over-expression of CEA in colon and rectal cancers has led to intensive research on vaccine strategies based on this protein.

Normally, CEA is thought to function as an intercellular recognition and adhesion molecule. It is a member of the immunoglobulin superfamily [17]. These molecules are important determinants of cell to cell and cell to substrate interactions. As such, their over-expression is felt to play a role in the invasiveness of colorectal cancer cells. However, the exact mechanisms by which CEA promotes malignant behavior are unknown, as the expression of CEA has not been found to reliably predict tumor aggressiveness or correlate with cell growth [18, 19]. Thus, the role of CEA in mediating the progression of colon cancer remains controversial. While CEA is over-expressed in most adenocarcinomas, it is still a normal antigen that is expressed during the course of fetal development. CEA is also found in low levels in the gut crypts of adults and healing intestinal mucosa. As a result, there is a minimal immune response to CEA when it appears at high levels on the surface of tumor cells. In fact, very high levels of CEA in the circulation are well tolerated by cancer patients [20].

The creation of an effective immunologic therapy directed towards CEA could result in paradigm-shift in terms of treatment. The first use for an effective CEA vaccine would be in the treatment of advanced, metastatic cancers arising from the colon, stomach, pancreas, breast and lung. If a CEA vaccine were effective in the metastatic setting then it would ultimately be applied to patients who had been rendered disease-free *via* surgery so that the incidence of recurrences might be reduced. Potentially, an effective CEA vaccine could be used as a means of prevention in high-risk populations. Widespread usage of a successful vaccine preparation is the expected outcome of research in this area. An immediate goal is the identification of the optimal vaccination strategies for the current preparation. A long-term goal is to see CEA-based vaccines become a standard therapy with confirmed survival benefits.

CEA as an immunologic target has been the focus of several research groups [21, 22-26]. However, using CEA as a target in immunologic-based therapies has two potential problems. First, given that CEA is a protein that is normally expressed in the human body, tolerance to this protein is likely to exist. Tolerance has been difficult to overcome in many vaccine research programs. Secondly, if one were successful in generating an immune response, autoimmune disease could result which would be an intolerable toxicity. Severe autoimmune events could limit the effectiveness and acceptance of an immune-based treatment. Thus, the goal is that an effective anti-CEA immunotherapy would initiate an immune response against CEA-expressing cancer cells by producing cytotoxic T-lymphocytes (CTL) that lyse CEA-expressing cancer cells while sparing normal CEA-expressing cells in the gastrointestinal tract [18].

## Peptide *vs.* Vector Encoded Tumor

Utilization of a live recombinant pox vector (such as the vaccinia virus) to accomplish the immunization process allows for the expression of foreign antigens which are encoded by a transgene in a variety of host cells. Expression of exogenous genetic material within professional antigen-presenting cells (APC) would be especially desirable. This approach is not an uncommon one in vaccine research. This type of immunization process would enable APC to process and present antigenic peptides in the context of host histocompatibility antigens and selected co-stimulatory molecules.

Multiple researchers have shown that recombinant vaccinia viruses can be used to deliver immunogenic peptides. Importantly, presentation of the recombinant protein in the context of vaccinia infection is a great deal more immunogenic than the simple injection of the purified protein in combination with an adjuvant [27-29]. It was shown in one study that two injections of CEA protein in adjuvant stimulated a minimal anti-CEA immune response in a CEA transgenic mouse [28]. It is understood that the transgenic mouse model has advantages and disadvantages. In contrast, when a recombinant vaccinia virus containing the CEA transgene (designated rV-CEA) was administered, it generated a very strong T cell response against the CEA protein [28]. The improved results with the vaccinia-based approach may be the result of the significant inflammatory response that the host mounts against vaccinia proteins. This inflammatory environment is characterized by high levels of stimulatory cytokines that enhance T cell proliferation and the overall T cell response to antigen. This is the presumed mechanism of action, but there are likely multiple reasons for the effectiveness of viral vectors. Since the recombinant vaccinia virus replicates rapidly in the host over a short period of time, large amounts of the transgene antigen will be presented to the immune system. Higher levels of antigen are thought to correlate with an enhanced possibility of immune activation. Notably, the host immune response to the vaccinia vector will result in elimination of the virus.

## Diversified Prime and Boost Strategies

The use of a priming vaccination with recombinant vaccinia and a subsequent boost vaccination with recombinant avipox appears to be superior to the prolonged use of either vector by itself [25, 30]. A clinical trial in patients with metastatic CEA-expressing carcinomas showed a clinical benefit of priming with rV-CEA followed by a number of boosts with avipox-CEA vaccine. Patients were randomized to two different vaccination strategies. In one arm, patients received a priming vaccination with vaccinia-CEA (V) followed by 3 monthly boosting vaccinations with avipox-CEA (A). This regimen was designated as the VAAA regimen. The alternative regimen consisted of 3 monthly avipox-CEA vaccinations followed by a fourth vaccination with rV-CEA vaccine. This regimen was designated as the AAAV regimen. Patients that exhibited clinical benefit from the vaccinations (stable disease or tumor shrinkage) were permitted to receive additional vaccinations over time. This is a common approach in vaccine studies. The immunologic response to each regimen was assessed using an ELISPOT assay. As a group, these patients had a median survival of about 12 months. However, after two years of follow-up, two-thirds of patients randomized to the VAAA arm exhibited stable disease with certain patients receiving up to 24 monthly vaccinations. In contrast, all of the patients enrolled in the AAAV arm exhibited progressive disease. Notably, patients in the VAAA arm of this trial had a median survival of 24 months *vs*. 9 months for the AAAV arm (p=0.05). In addition, the level of the CEA-specific immune response correlated with improved survival after controlling for disease status (p=0.03) [31]. This data is highly supportive of the original hypothesis. Thus, the strategy of priming with vaccinia followed by boosting with an avian vector seems to be more effective than the use of either vaccine alone. Consequently, the current trial utilized rVaccinia-CEA(6D)/TRICOM as a priming vaccination and rFowlpox-CEA(6D)-TRICOM as a booster vaccination.

## Tolerance

CEA present in the circulation of patients with colon cancer could have dichotomous effects. If the circulating antigen is processed by professional APC then there is the possibility that an anti-tumor immune response could be produced. In this scenario, the patient might actually develop an anti-tumor response in the absence of active immunization. However, in most patients the presence of high levels of CEA and other tumor-associated antigens actually leads to anergy to the antigens. Consequently, in these patients the immune system ends up not being able to develop an anti-tumor response in the setting of a vaccination protocol. This theoretical problem may not be an issue in clinical practice. In a clinical trial of a CEA-based vaccine HLA-A2+ in patients with advanced CEA-expressing cancers, it was found that high circulating levels of CEA did not appear to have an effect on the induction of CEA-specific T cells as measured by ELISPOT. In fact, the CEA-specific immune response to the vaccine did not appear to be affected by CEA in the circulation [32]. Indeed, in multiple pre-clinical studies and now in clinical trials CEA vaccine regimens have demonstrated the ability to overcome tolerance.

## TRICOM

The immunologic destruction of tumor targets necessitates the presentation of antigenic peptides in the context of MHC molecules present on APC. These peptides must then be recognized by the T cell receptor. The acquisition of additional costimulatory signals by the T cell is critically important in the generation of an effective T cell response to any antigen. The initiation of T cell immunity requires that the naïve T cell receive at least two stimulatory signals. The antigen specific signal may be considered the first signal and it occurs when the T cell receptor is engaged by the appropriate peptide/MHC complex. This event will cause the T cell to enter the cell cycle. A second "costimulatory", signal is required in order for the T cell to engage in cytokine production and embark on a proliferative program. The proper induction of T cell cytokine production is critical for optimal T cell immune responses. A critical costimulatory molecule is B7.1 which is also known as CD80. B7.1 is expressed on APCs such as dendritic cells, activated B cells, and monocytes and interacts with CD28 and CTLA4 on the T cell [33-36]. Engagement of CTLA4 provides a negative signal to T cells, whereas interaction of B7.1 with CD28 provides an important stimulus to the T cell that has seen specific antigen. Recent clinical advances have shown the importance of this pathway. Importantly, several other costimulatory molecules on APCs have been identified. One of these is the intercellular adhesion molecule-1 (ICAM-1) whose ligand on the T cell is LFA-1. Leukocyte function associated antigen-3 (LFA-3), is another important costimulatory factor that binds to CD2 on the surface of T cells [37]. It is thought that the inability of tumor cells to express adequate levels of costimulatory molecules, resulting in a failure to induce T cell responses is a major reason for poor host immunity to tumor targets. The generation of costimulation at the level of the tumor microenvironment is a major goal of vaccine researchers. The importance of stimulation of T cells by multiple pathways is highlighted by the fact that tumor cells appear to escape detection and elimination by the immune system by way of the low expression of costimulatory molecules on APCs that have been exposed to the tumor microenvironment and similar low expression by tumor cells [38-41]. Consequently, it was hypothesized that the introduction of costimulatory molecules into tumor cells that expressed unique tumor associated antigens should aid in the generation of a T cell-based anti-tumor immune response. This theory has been proven in several instances. In fact, a potent immune response against tumor targets can be generated by transfecting tumor cells with B7.1. Moreover, the resulting immune response is subsequently able to target both modified and unmodified tumor cells *via* a by-stander effect [42, 43]. B7.1-transfected tumors were able to induce protective immunity to subsequent re-challenge with untransfected tumor cells. Expression of ICAM-1 and LFA-3 by tumor cells is also an effective way to improve T cell anti-tumor immune responses in murine models [44, 45]. The evidence in humans is supportive of this approach as well. Tumor cells expressing ICAM as the result of infection with a recombinant vaccinia vector (rV-ICAM-1) were rejected by mice with competent immune systems. Similarly, murine colon adenocarcinoma tumor cells that had been treated with rV-LFA-3 failed to grow when introduced into a murine host.

Dual expression of cognate antigen and costimulatory molecules on the same cell is necessary for the appropriate engagement of the T cell receptor and costimulatory receptor on the effector cell. In order to achieve this, the Schlom group has devised a recombinant vaccinia vector that provides for co-expression of costimulatory molecules in order to provide for optimal activation of T cells. This elegant work has been conducted in a logical and stepwise fashion over many years. Several pre-clinical studies have been conducted that provide evidence that this is a valid approach. Immunization of mice with a mixture of two recombinant vaccinia viruses, one encoding for B7.1 (rV-B7.1) and the other encoding for CEA (rV-CEA) led to a significant improvement in the specific immune response to CEA and enhanced protection against challenge with CEA-expressing tumor cells, as compared with immunization with either vector alone [46]. Co-expression of CEA and B7.1 in a single recombinant vaccinia virus was even more effective in generating specific immunity against the CEA protein than was an admixture of the rV-CEA and rV-B7.1 single gene vectors [47]. These results suggested that further modification of the viral vector might pay dividends. Additional evidence of the utility of the combined approach was provided by murine studies using a recombinant virus encoding the MUC-1 antigen (rV-MUC-1) and rV-B7.1 which showed a similar enhancement of antigen-specific anti-tumor immunity [48]. Investigators have created constructs using poxviral vectors (avipox and vaccinia) that contain multiple genes. A construct containing the transgenes encoding for the costimulatory molecules B7.1, ICAM-1, and LFA-3 was created and was given the designation TRICOM. A recombinant vaccinia-based vector (rV-TRICOM) and a recombinant avipox-based vector (rF-TRICOM) have been created. The TRICOM constructs were employed in pre-clinical studies and were shown to be superior to constructs which contained only one or two of the costimulatory molecules [25, 33, 49]. The recombinant vaccinia virus co-expressing murine TRICOM induced greater T cell proliferation and led to enhanced anti-tumor immunity as compared to recombinant vaccinia vectors that expressed only the single costimulatory molecules. A CEA-TRICOM vector subsequently exhibited the ability to induce enhanced immune and anti-tumor responses when compared to vectors that encoded CEA or CEA plus B7.1 [49].

## Agonist Epitopes

The identification of tumor specific antigens to be used in the immunization process has been a major hurdle in the drive to develop anti-tumor vaccines. Most tumor antigens that have been described for human cancers are expressed at high levels in the cancer cell, but these same antigens are usually found at one or more sites in normal tissues. Tissues may or may not be highly accessible to circulating immune cells. There are many barriers to the generation of immune responses to such antigens. Research into methods to overcoming these barriers may be the key to the development of a successful immune response directed toward "self" proteins. In an attempt to increase the immune response directed against "self" antigens a unique CEA protein has been created.

CAP-1 is a 9-mer peptide (YLSGANLNL) of the CEA protein that binds to HLA-A2. This peptide is able to induce antigen-specific CTLs from peripheral blood mononuclear cells (PBMCs) obtained from cancer patients that have been immunized with rV-CEA and ALVAC-CEA. Several laboratories have generated CAP-1 specific CTLs *in vitro* and *in vivo* utilizing dendritic cells (DCs) as APC and pulsing them with peptide [50]. Investigations into the gp100 melanoma antigen and the papilloma virus tumor antigen E6 have demonstrated that enhanced immunogenicity can be obtained in response to modified peptide sequences. Even very slight modifications of peptide antigens can markedly affect the immune response that is generated. Peptide modifications may either inhibit or augment the immune response. The exact response to these modifications is not always easy to predict. Modifications that result in increased binding of peptides to the major histocompatibility complex (MHC) will generally lead to an improved immune response. Zaremba *et al.* have defined a mutation in CAP-1 termed CAP1-6D (arginine at position 6 being replaced by aspartic acid) which appears to be considerably more effective in the induction of an immune response when compared to the wildtype CEA peptide. Several pre-clinical studies have documented the ability of CAP1-6D to produce a more potent immune response than CAP-1 [51-53]. In the context of a clinical trial, CAP-1 pulsed DC elicited very little immune and anti-tumor activity whereas CAP1-6D elicited clinical responses that correlated with the induction of anti-CEA immune responses [54]. The results of these DC studies were relatively conclusive. Another study showed that Cap1-6D induced distinct cytotoxic T cells with different functional capacities than those induced by Cap-1 in human CTL lines further confirming that this altered peptide ligand can alter immune response [110].

The advantage of agonist epitopes has been demonstrated in clinical trials. In patients with metastatic melanoma, objective clinical responses were obtained when patients were vaccinated with agonist epitopes to the gp-100 melanoma associated antigen [55]. Similarly, CAP1-6D was of clinical benefit in patients with tumors that express CEA at high levels [54]. In one study, patients received vaccinations with DC that had been loaded with a CEA agonist peptide. Two patients out of a total of 12 experienced a complete response (CR), one patient developed a mixed response, and two exhibited stable disease (SD). The clinical response in this trial was found to correlate with the induction of a CEA-specific T cell response.

## CEA TRICOM Vaccines

Marshall *et al.* have evaluated the concept of four sequential vaccinations with rFowlpox-CEA(6D)-TRICOM alone, in combination with rVaccinia-CEA (6D)-TRICOM, and in combination with GM-CSF. These vaccines were administered to patients with CEA-expressing carcinomas. The Fowlpox-CEA(6D)-TRICOM vaccine was administered at a dose of 4 x $10^8$ pfu (plaque forming unts) *via* the subscutaneous (s.c.) route. The rVaccinia-CEA(6D)-TRICOM vaccine was administered at a dose of 1.2 x $10^8$ pfu *via* the s.c. route. The point of combining the vaccine with GM-CSF was to induce greater numbers of DC [32]. The trial employed a phase I dose escalation schema of the vaccine component of the vaccine regimen. This approach was felt to be a valid means of testing the vaccine at doses that could potentially be effective. CEA-specific T cell responses were compared between treatment groups and evaluated in the context of clinical response and survival. The patients who entered this study all had late stage CEA-expressing cancers, acceptable performance status, and good organ function. These patients had failed all standard therapies. No dose limiting toxicities were observed among the 58 patients who were enrolled. ELISPOT analysis was used to measure CEA-specific T cell responses. Of the HLA-2 positive patients, in the different cohorts, 10 out of 13 mounted CEA-specific T cell responses with two-fold or greater increase after four vaccinations *versus* before vaccination. In some cases, there was the ability to perform additional studies of patient tissues. One patient with lung disease had a complete response after receiving monthly injections of rFowlpox-CEA(6D)-TRICOM. The patient died of accidental causes 15 months after vaccine initiation, but autopsy results reported no evidence of cancer. Stable disease was achieved at four months in 40% of patients (23 patients), with 14 of these patients having prolonged stable disease (greater than six months). Since dose-limiting toxicity was not observed, the maximal doses employed in this study have been used in subsequent trials, including the described herein where interferon-alpha was employed in combination with GM-CSF. Higher doses may also be safe and their efficacy is currently unknown.

### Construct and Verification of Vaccine

The clinical grade vaccines that were used in prior studies and in the current clinical trial were manufactured by Therion Biologics Corporation as part of a cooperative research agreement. The parental virus used for the generation of rVaccinia-CEA(6D)-TRICOM vaccine was derived from the Wyeth (New York City Board of Health) strain of vaccinia. This strain was used for the preparation of the Dryvax® Smallpox Vaccine. The parental virus for the generation of rFowlpox- CEA(6D)-TRICOM was a plaque-purified isolate from the Poxvac-TC vaccine strain of fowlpox virus. Homologous recombination between the parental pox viral DNA and a plasmid vector containing the CEA(6D) and TRICOM genes was used in the construction of both recombinant viruses. The viruses have been plaque purified and tested extensively. These recombinant viruses were used to create master stocks and also working virus stocks. After extensive characterization, these stocks were used for manufacturing the clinical grade vaccines.

## SAFETY OF THE RECOMBINANT POX-VIRUS VACCINES

### Pox-Based Vaccines in Clinical Trials

Phase I and phase II clinical trials have been conducted in order to test the components of the CEA(6D)-TRICOM vaccine (the vaccinia and fowlpox vectors, the CEA antigen, and the TRICOM costimulatory molecules B7.1, ICAM-1, and LFA-3) [32, 34, 56-59]. These studies were sponsored by the NCI through the Cancer Therapy Evaluation Program (CTEP), Division of Cancer Treatment and Diagnosis (DCTD). Over 500 cancer patients have been treated with pox-virus–based vaccines, and the majority of these had advanced cancers. A great deal of important safety data has been acquired during the course of these studies. Notably, vaccinia- and/or fowlpox-based vaccines have been administered safely *via* various routes. These included the intradermal (by injection or scarification), intramuscular, subcutaneous, intravenous, and intratumoral routes. There is still discussion as to the best route for the administration of virus-based vaccines. Doses up to 2 x $10^9$ pfu have been achieved for the vaccinia-based vaccines and doses up to 6 x $10^9$ pfu have been achieved for the fowlpox-based vaccines. Importantly, vaccinia-based and fowlpox-based vaccines containing costimulatory molecules have been given alone and in combination with CEA antigen without any severe adverse effects.

### Safety of Poxvirus-Expressing TRICOM

A pair of studies was conducted in a mouse model in order to determine the safety of recombinant vaccinia and fowlpox viruses that express the combination of B7.1, LFA-3 and ICAM-1 (TRICOM). In the first, murine TRICOM (B7.1, LFA-3, and ICAM-1) was administered to C57BL/6 mice. Mice were sacrificed at approximately 6 months and one year following the first vaccination. These mice were carefully studied in several ways. Extensive histopathologic analyses and blood chemistries were conducted. This testing showed that TRICOM treatment had no biologically significant effect on body weight, hematologic parameters, clinical chemistries, or gross organ structure/function as compared to the vehicle control group. Additionally, there was no evidence of treatment-related stimulation of autoimmunity.

A second study utilized transgenic mice that express the human CEA molecule as a self-antigen. The tissue distribution of the CEA antigen was found to be quite comparable to that of humans [109]. Mice received immunizations with $10^8$ pfu of rFowlpox-CEA, rFowlpox-CEA/muTRICOM, rVaccinia-CEA or rVaccinia-CEA/muTRICOM. Control vaccinations consisted of the non-recombinant vaccinia and fowlpox viruses (1 x $10^8$ pfu). Vaccinia-based constructs were given by scarification on days 0 and 21. The fowlpox-based recombinant cosntructs were administered intramuscularly on days 0, 21 and 35. Animals were harvested at 35 weeks after the first vaccination and evaluated as described above. These tests showed that there were no biologically significant test article–related effects on body weight, hematology, clinical chemistry, or organ function. Analysis of over 30 different organs and tissues revealed no microscopic differences between the test group and the control groups.

## Safety in Non-Human Primates of a Recombinant Vaccinia Virus Expressing CEA

The safety and immunogenicity of a human CEA-expressing recombinant vaccinia virus (rV-CEA) in rhesus monkeys was tested by Kantor *et al.* [20]. These studies provide important safety information in primates. In the study, a cohort of eight monkeys was vaccinated three or four times with the recombinant CEA vaccine while four monkeys received wild-type vaccinia as control. Both groups showed the symptoms typically seen in humans following vaccinia administration, including skin irritation at the vaccination site, regional lymphadenopathy and low-grade fevers. In the rV(NYC)-CEA monkeys, hematologic parameters, clinical chemistries, and gross organ function remained normal following vaccination and stayed within the normal range for up to 1 year following the initiation of treatment. Thus, the rV-CEA vaccine appears to have a favorable safety profile in primates. Moreover, rV-CEA group exhibited a strong response to human CEA at the humoral and cellular levels.

Given the results of these toxicology studies, four Phase I clinical trials with recombinant pox viruses expressing human TRICOM (rV-TRICOM, and rF-TRICOM or human TRICOM plus CEA (rV-CEA(6D)/TRICOM and rF-CEA(6D)/TRICOM) have been conducted. At the conclusion of these studies, no Grade 3 or higher adverse reactions to these vaccines have been identified.

## EFFECTS OF IFN-α ON TUMOR CELL EXPRESSION OF CEA AND MHC MOLECULES

The effects of IFN-α on the expression of tumor antigens such as CEA and TAG-72 have been evaluated by several investigators. IFN-α also has effects on the expression of HLA class I and II molecules. The CEA protein is encoded by a gene family located on chromosome 19q. Post-transcriptional modifications consisting of various patterns of glycosylation are thought to contribute to some of the immunologic heterogeneity that has been observed [60]. IFN-α, IFN-β, and IFN- γ can all mediate the increased expression of CEA on human cell lines. Also, treatment of tumor cells isolated from malignant ascites with interferons can lead to significant increases in CEA expression [61-73]. These actions of IFN-α occur at concentrations that are easily attainable in the clinic *via* the infusion or injection of IFN-α. Moreover, these effects continue well past the time of exposure to IFN [62]. Careful analysis of IFN-treated tumor cells reveals that this cytokine actually leads to increased production and stability of the transcript for IFN-α [74].

The effectiveness of monoclonal antibody (mAb)-based treatments are significantly enhanced by IFN-α pre-treatments in experimental tumor models. The mechanism for this seems to depend on the ability of IFN-α to enhance the expression of tumor antigens [64, 75-78]. Similar findings have been observed in the context of clinical trials. The IM administration of IFN-α at a dose of $3 \times 10^6$ U on a daily basis significantly increased the localization of an anti-melanoma Ab to tumor deposits in melanoma patients with metastatic disease [79]. Similar results were obtained in a study in which patients with metastatic breast cancer received either IFN-α at a dose of $3 \times 10^6$ U daily by SC injection or no treatment [80]. Tumor tissues were sampled prior to treatment and again at 48 hours following the injection of IFN-α. Quantitative immunohistochemistry was performed on biopsy specimens and this showed that IFN administration led to an increase the expression of a tumor-associated glycoprotein (known as TAG-72) as compared to patients that received no treatment. Administration of either IFN-γ or IFN-βser to patients with advanced cancer led to increased levels of serum CEA in almost two-thirds of patients. Similar results have been obtained using a variety of IFN schedules and dosages. These results support the applicability of this approach to multiple clinical situations [81]. Increases in the expression of CEA and TAG-72 on malignant cells have also been achieved *via* the intra-peritoneal administration of IFN-γ to patients suffering from malignant ascites [82]. The effects of IFN-α administration on CEA expression on tumor cells appear to be fairly persistent. This assertion is supported by the work of Mahvi *et al.* who showed that the effects of an intravenous dose of 1 x $10^6$ U of IFN-α lasted for up to 48 hours [83]. These results were confirmed in a subsequent study in patients with ovarian cancer. Peak elevations in serum CA125 levels occurred nearly three days following the subcutaneous administration of IFN-α at a dose of 6 x $10^6$ U [84]. Roselli *et al.* evaluated the expression of CEA on tumors of patients with gastrointestinal malignancies following the systemic administration of IFN-α under the assumption that this manipulation could lead to enhanced levels of cancer antigens on malignant cells [85]. Patients underwent endoscopic biopsy of the primary tumor and then received two or three doses of IFN-α prior to definitive surgery. Two different doses (3 or 6 x $10^6$ U IV) of IFN-α were employed with each of these schedules. A carefully defined system of tumor sampling was employed to insure that representative biopsies were collected from a variety of sites within the tumor. At least four different areas from each tumor were sampled. Tumor levels of CEA and TAG-72 within the tumor specimens were assessed by both immunohistochemistry and radioimmunoassay. As expected, tumor levels of CEA and TAG-72 were consistently elevated in patients receiving three doses of IFN-α, as compared to those receiving two doses, regardless of the IFN dose that was employed. Importantly, the expression of these antigens in normal colonic mucosa was not affected [85]. Guadagni *et al.* have demonstrated that the cell surface expression of CEA and MHC antigens on freshly isolated tumor cells is significantly enhanced following exposure to type I interferons [86]. Based on these studies, it is logical to assume that the levels of CEA peptide:MHC complexes on carcinoma cells would increase significantly if humans were exposed to IFN-α at the doses employed by Roselli *et al.* in their study [87]. Optimal activation of the TCR on effector T lymphocytes is ultimately dependent upon the prevalence of sufficient levels of cognate antigens on the surface of the target cell bound to MHC class I molecule [88, 89]. Consequently, it is reasonable to suggest that upregulation of carcinoma cell CEA expression by IFN-α would lead to enhanced activation of antigen-specific T cells in subjects receiving the IFN-α in combination with a vaccine regimen. The effects of antigen expression on the success of anti-CEA vaccines have been investigated in animal models. Mizobata *et al.* demonstrated that CEA-specific T cell clones were better able inhibit tumor growth *in vivo* if CEA tumor cells expressed CEA at high levels on their surface [90]. This hypothesis is supported by the work of Grosenbach *et al.* They employed CEA transgenic mice that express high levels of CEA in their tumor tissues to evaluate the effectiveness of various CEA vaccine strategies. These studies showed that the anti-tumor activity of antigen-specific CTL was dependent upon the density of CEA expression on the tumor cell [30].

It has been observed that many tumors express low levels of MHC molecules [91-94]. This deficiency can be caused by a mutation in any of the genes that take part in the assembly and expression of these molecules [91, 92]. Low levels of MHC expression can lead to impaired recognition by specific immune effector cells. Notably, low levels of MHC class I on colon cancer cell lines tend to favor NK cells as effectors since these cells are activated in the absence of MHC stimulation. Conversely, high levels of MHC class I expression on tumor cells favor the induction of T cells as anti-tumor effectors [95]. Overall, IFN-α exerts its anti-tumor effects through multiple mechanisms, some of which are direct (*i.e.*, anti-proliferative) and others which are indirect (*i.e.*, *via* the stimulation of MHC class I and leukocyte adhesion molecules such as ICAM-1) [96-98]. MHC class I and II as well as ICAM-1 are critically important to effector cell recognition of cancer cells [95-99]. The potentially favorable effects of IFN-α on MHC class I and II expression in adenocarcinoma cells are well documented [100-102]. One might think of IFN-α treatments as having the ability to alter the topographic quality of the colon cancer cell by increasing the density of MHC class I and ICAM-1 proteins on the cell surface [99]. Indeed, treatment of human tumor cells with IFN renders them more susceptible to lysis by a CEA-specific CD8+ T-cell line [52].

## Timing of IFN-α-2b Administration

Despite interferon's ability to increase tumor antigen expression, it is also known to be responsible for enhancing the efficacy of the adaptive immune response to viral infections and for inhibiting viral replication. To minimize this potential effect for the Vaccinia-based vector, the three injections of IFN-α-2b were given eight days following the administration of the rV-CEA(6D)-TRICOM vaccine. Avipox viruses, such as fowlpox, infect mammalian cells and express their transgene product for 14 – 21 days preceding the death of the cell and then don't go on to infect other cells [98]. Consequently, IFN-α-2b could be given alongside the rF-CEA(6D)-TRICOM vaccine. This schedule of therapy attempted to minimize the influence of IFN-α-2b on the viral infection induced by the vaccine vectors. The proposed schedule allowed for the administration of IFN on an every other day basis (for a total of three doses) during the week *following* the administration of the rV CEA(6D)-TRICOM vaccine. For the rF-CEA(6D)-TRICOM vaccine, the IFN-α-2b was administered *during* the week of vaccination. Thus, for both vaccines, the hypothesized upregulation of CEA expression was induced just after the injection of vaccine.

In summary, there is a large body of research to suggest that IFN-α administration is an effective means of increasing tumor cell expression of antigens and MHC molecules. The clinical studies performed to date support this conclusion. Based on the detailed studies conducted by Roselli *et al.* a regimen of IFN-α-2b consisting of the administration of three doses of 1, 3, 6 or 9 x $10^6$ U IFN-α-2b *via* the subcutaneous route following vaccine administration represents a highly effective schedule.

## GM-CSF (SARGRAMOSTIM) AS A VACCINE ADJUVANT

An important area of focus in vaccine research is the use of cytokines as adjuvants. Laboratory and clinical studies have shown that sargramostim (GM-CSF) may be a useful vaccine adjuvant. Levels of antigen-specific T cells may be expected to be low in unvaccinated individuals. The induction of a significant population of antigen-specific T cells is necessary in order to develop an effective immune response and develop long-lasting immunological memory. The best method to achieve this induction is the subject of significant research. To achieve this goal, cancer immunologists have often employed adjuvants for use with the vaccine. These agents can often increase the immunogenicity of weak antigens. Adjuvants may act in multiple ways: to change the character and number of APC in the area of vaccine administration. One approach is for the adjuvant to act as a repository for the vaccine, thus prolonging the time it is presented to APC. Another approach is to alter the manner in which the protein is presented or processed. The use of cytokine adjuvants is of particular interest because they may be useful in determining the immune compartment that is engaged by the vaccine.

GM-CSF is a cytokine that can stimulate the activation, development, and migration of APC such as DC and macrophage. Importantly, it is quite effective in stimulating their expression of class II MHC molecules [103]. Disis *et al.* have shown that GM-CSF functioned in a manner similar to complete Freund's adjuvant in its ability to boost the immune response to both tetanus toxoid and a peptide sequence from rat neu (c-erbB-2) [26]. In a separate study it was shown that GM-CSF was able to enhance the response of CD8 cytotoxic T cells to various melanoma-associated peptide antigens [104]. GM-CSF has been used in a large number of vaccine studies. Increased tumor immunogenicity was also accomplished in experiments where irradiated tumor cells were injected along with a microsomal preparation of GM-CSF [26]. Indeed, antigen-specific anti-tumor immune responses were markedly enhanced when tumor cells transfected with the gene for GM-CSF gene was administered to mice [105]. GM-CSF also increased the effectiveness of vaccinia-CEA in a murine model of melanoma [106].

## TRIAL DESIGN

The present trial employs two novel anti-CEA vaccines; recombinant (r) Vaccinia-CEA(6D)-TRICOM and recombinant Fowlpox-CEA(6D)-TRICOM. These viruses are capable of infecting professional antigen presenting cells which in turn present part of the CEA gene (a modified 9-MER CEA peptide) in the context of HLA class I to CD8+ T cells. These viral vectors also direct the expression of three co-stimulatory molecules (B7-1, ICAM-1, and LFA-3) each of which is capable of providing a critical second activating signal to antigen-specific T cells. In this trial we have evaluated the safety and efficacy of the vaccine regimen when combined with interferon-alpha-2b (IFN-α-2b). Interferon alfa-2b suppresses cancer cellular proliferation and possesses immunomodulatory properties. It also appears to enhance lymphocyte cytotoxicity for cancer cells. These actions are believed to be important in the suppression of certain malignancies, including CEA-positive cancers. It has been previously demonstrated that IFN-α-2b also upregulates CEA expression on established tumor cell lines and tumor cells isolated from malignant ascites. As was noted above, a phase I study by Roselli *et al.* revealed that administration of IFN-α-2b at a dose of $3 \times 10^6$ U/d thrice weekly (TIW) to patients with colorectal cancer led to significant increases in tumor CEA levels. Numerous studies have also shown that IFNs upregulate the expression of HLA-class I molecules. It has also been shown that treatment of human tumor cells with IFN renders them more susceptible to lysis by a CEA-specific CD8+ T-cell line [52]. The potential for severe complications to develop following administration of this regimen might be increased in immunocompromised individuals. Thus, the myelosuppressive effects of IFN-α-2b are of concern in this population of solid tumor patients that will have been heavily pre-treated with first and second line chemotherapeutic regimens. The administration of GM-CSF will promote the development of granulocytes and thereby lessen the possibility of adverse events related to the interferon therapy. In addition, it has been shown that the combination of IFN-α-2b and GM-CSF induces a surprisingly rapid maturation of monocytes into dendritic cells that are functionally superior to those induced by treatment with IL-4 plus GM CSF. The vaccine containing the viral vector will be administered on day 1 followed by GM-CSF on days 1-4 (Table **1**). In Cycle 1 patients receive thrice weekly injections of IFN-α-2b *via* the subcutaneous (s.c.) route the week after the rVaccinia-CEA(6D)-TRICOM vaccine is administered. Seven days will have to pass since vaccination so that the IFN-α-2b does not inhibit replication of the vaccinia virus. In Cycles 2-4 patients receive three s.c. injections of IFN-α-2b

**Table 1:** Treatment schema. In cycle one, recombinant Vaccinia-CEA(6D)-TRICOM vaccine (V) was administered at 1.2 x $10^8$ pfu subcutaneously (s.c.). 100 mcg GM-CSF (G) was given s.c. at the injection site on days 1-4. IFNα-2b (I) was administered s.c. away from the vaccination site at 1, 3, 6 or 9 MU on days 9, 11 and 13 to coincide with induction of CTLs, and to ensure that the IFN did not inhibit replication of the vaccinia virus. On day 15, a mandatory tumor biopsy (Bx) was performed for CEA and MHC Class I immunohistochemistry. Patients in cohort zero did not undergo biopsy. Pre-study biopsies were also performed as necessary to determine the CEA status of tumors. In cycles 2-4, recombinant Fowlpox-CEA(6D)-TRICOM vaccine (F) was administered at 4 x $10^8$ pfu s.c. on day 1. GM-CSF (G) was given s.c. at the injection site at 100 mcg on days 1-4 of each cycle. IFN-α-2b (I) was administered on days 1, 3, and 5 at the injection site since IFN-α-2b can augment dendritic cell maturation and will not inhibit the activity of the Fowlpox vector

| | | | | | | | | |
|---|---|---|---|---|---|---|---|---|
| **Cycle 1:** | | | | | | | | |
| Week 1: | Day | 1 | 2 | 3 | 4 | 5 | 6 | 7 |
| | Treatment | V/G | G | G | G | | | |
| | | | | | | | | |
| Week 2: | Day | 8 | 9 | 10 | 11 | 12 | 13 | 14 |
| | Treatment | | I | | I | | I | |
| | | | | | | | | |
| Week 3: | Day | 15 | 16 | 17 | 18 | 19 | 20 | 21 |
| | Treatment | Bx | | | | | | |
| | | | | | | | | |
| Week4: | Day | 22 | 23 | 24 | 25 | 26 | 27 | 28 |
| | Treatment | | | | | | | |
| | | | | | | | | |
| **Cycles 2-4:** | | | | | | | | |
| Week 1: | Day | 1 | 2 | 3 | 4 | 5 | 6 | 7 |
| | Treatment | F/G/I | G | G/I | G | I | | |
| | | | | | | | | |
| Week 2: | Day | 8 | 9 | 10 | 11 | 12 | 13 | 14 |
| | Treatment | | | | | | | |
| | | | | | | | | |
| Week 3: | Day | 15 | 16 | 17 | 18 | 19 | 20 | 21 |
| | Treatment | | | | | | | |
| | | | | | | | | |
| Week4: | Day | 22 | 23 | 24 | 25 | 26 | 27 | 28 |
| | | | | | | | | |
| | | | | | | | | |
| COHORT 0: V –F –F –F + G (no IFN-α-2b) | | | | | | | | |
| COHORT 1: V –F –F –F + G + IFN-α-2b (1 x $10^6$ U). | | | | | | | | |

***Table 1: contd....***

| | | | | |
|---|---|---|---|---|
| COHORT 2: V –F –F –F + G + IFN-α-2b (3 x $10^6$ U). | | | | |
| COHORT 3: V –F –F –F + G + IFN-α-2b (6 x $10^6$ U). | | | | |
| COHORT 4: V –F –F –F + G + IFN-α-2b (9 x $10^6$ U). | | | | |

at the same time that the rFowlpox-CEA(6D)-TRICOM vaccine and GM-CSF are being administered, since IFN-α-2b can augment dendritic cell maturation and should not inhibit the activity of the Fowlpox vector. We hypothesized that this treatment will increase levels of CEA and HLA Class I expression on patient tumor cells and lead to an improved anti-CEA immune response. Clinical correlates were performed to determine the effect of IFN-α-2b administration on tumor expression of CEA. An initial 6 patient cohort (Cohort 0) received no IFN-α-2b. Following this, dose escalation of the IFN-α-2b component of therapy took place in cohorts of three patients. There was no intra-patient dose escalation of IFN-α-2b. IFN-α-2b was administered s.c. at rotating sites located away from the vaccination site during Cycle 1. In Cycles 2-4 the IFN-α-2b was given along with the GM-CSF at the vaccination site. There were at least three patients in each of the four cohorts. HLA-A2 status was determined for these patients, but HLA-A2 positivity was not a requirement for entry into the study. In the process of determining the MTD, one cohort was expanded with an additional 6 patients. These additional 6 patients were all HLA-A2 positive.

Patients who did not progress and did not have unacceptable toxicity after completing the initial phase of vaccinations were offered additional vaccinations of rFowlpox-CEA(6D)-TRICOM (in combination with GM-CSF and IFN-α-2b). Patients received the same dose of vaccine and IFN-α–2b as per the treatment arm on which they were enrolled every 28 days up through vaccination #6 and then every 3 months thereafter for up to two years. Off-study criteria and clinical/immunologic monitoring continued unchanged for these patients. Patients were re-staged every two months. The final results of this study will be published in the near future.

## IMMUNE ASSAYS AND CORRELATIVE STUDIES

The ELISPOT assay for T cell production of IFN-γ is highly quantitative and reproducible in the setting of vaccine therapy [57, 107-109]. The sustained use of one reproducible assay is useful in the evaluation of the patients' immune response to experimental strategies. The ELISPOT assay will be used to evaluate the patients' T cell response to the CEA(6D)-TRICOM vaccines when used in combination with GM-CSF and IFN-α. Peripheral blood mononuclear cells obtained pre-study and prior to each vaccination on patients that are HLA-A2 positive will be utilized for the assay.

## COHORT ZERO

In order to gain a sense of the immune effects of the rVaccinia-CEA(6D)-TRICOM vaccine when it is used in the absence of interferon, an initial cohort of 6 patients received the vaccine, but did not receive IFN-α-2b. Patient tumors will be evaluated for expression of the CEA antigen pre- and post-therapy *via* immunohistochemistry. Since tumor expression of CEA was unlikely to be altered by administration of the vaccine alone, these initial 6 patients did not undergo tumor biopsy on day 15 of Cycle 1.

## CONCLUSION

Tumor associated antigens (TAAs), such as CEA, are by definition either inadequately immunogenic or functionally non-immunogenic in the tumor-bearing host. Both pre-clinical and clinical experience indicates that T cells are primarily responsible for the inhibition of growth and/or eradication of established tumors in the setting of most immune-based anti-tumor approaches. Vaccines and vaccine strategies that can enhance T cell responses to TAAs should result in more vigorous anti-tumor responses, as established by pre-clinical and recent clinical studies. This CEA-based vaccine trial incorporated five different strategies to improve host-immune responses to CEA, and thus to CEA-expressing colon tumors: (1) the insertion of the CEA gene into poxvirus vectors (recombinant vaccinia and recombinant avipox vectors), (2) the use of a prime and boost vaccination regimens, (3) the use of a vector containing CEA and multiple costimulatory molecules (*i.e.*, CEA-TRICOM vectors), (4) the modification of an epitope of CEA to render it more highly immunogenic in patients possessing the HLA-A2 allele, and (5) the administration of IFN-α-2b as a way to enhance the expression of CEA and HLA class I by tumor cells, thus rendering them more vulnerable to destruction by cytolytic T cells (due to enhanced prevalence of CEA-MHC peptide complexes on the tumor surface).

## ACKNOWLEDGEMENTS

The authors would like to thank the members of the Carson Lab, past and present, at The Ohio State University Comprehensive Cancer Center.

# CONFLICT OF INTEREST

The authors confirm that this chapter contents have no conflict of interest.

# REFERENCES

[1] American Cancer Society. Cancer Facts & Figures 2013. Atlanta: American Cancer Society; 2013.

[2] Schoen RE. The case for population-based screening for colorectal cancer. Nat Rev Cancer 2002; 2(1): 65-70.

[3] Demols A, Van Laethem JL. Adjuvant chemotherapy for colorectal cancer. Curr Gastroenterol Rep 2002; 4(5): 420-6.

[4] Van Cutsem E, Verslype C, Demedts I. The treatment of advanced colorectal cancer: where are we now and where do we go? Best Pract Res Clin Gastroenterol 2002; 16(2): 319-30.

[5] Ragnhammar P, Hafstrom L, Nygren P, Glimelius B. A systematic overview of chemotherapy effects in colorectal cancer. Acta Oncol 2001; 40(2-3): 282-308.

[6] Mulcahy MF, Benson AB 3rd. Recent and ongoing clinical trials for treating colorectal cancer. Expert Opin Investig Drugs 2002; 11(6): 871-80.

[7] Chau I, Cunningham D. Chemotherapy in colorectal cancer: new options and new challenges. Br Med Bull 2002; 64: 159-80.

[8] Rustum YM. Clinical implications of 5-FU modulation. Oncology (Huntingt) 1999; 13(7 Suppl 3): 22-5.

[9] Hobday TJ, Erlichman C. Adjuvant therapy of colon cancer: a review. Clin Colorectal Cancer 2002; 1(4): 230-6.

[10] Saltz LB, Cox JV, Blanke C, Rosen LS, Fehrenbacher L, Moore MJ, *et al.* Irinotecan plus fluorouracil and leucovorin for metastatic colorectal cancer. Irinotecan Study Group. N Engl J Med 2000; 343(13): 905-14.

[11] Midgley R, Kerr D. Conventional cytotoxic and novel therapeutic concepts in colorectal cancer. Expert Opin Investig Drugs 2001; 10(6): 1011-9.

[12] Rogers GT. Carcinoembryonic antigens and related glycoproteins: Molecular aspects and specificity. Biochim Biophys Acta 1983; 695(3-4): 227-249.

[13] Muraro R, Wunderlich D, Thor A, *et al.* Definition by monoclonal antibodies of a repertoire of epitopes on carcinoembryonic antigen differentially expressed in human colon carcinomas *versus* normal human adult tissues. Cancer Res 1985; 45(11 pt 2): 5769-5780.

[14] Steward AM, Nixon D, Zamcheck N, *et al.* Carcinoembryonic antigen in breast cancer patients: Serum levels and disease progress. Cancer 1974; 33(5): 1246-1252.

[15] Vincent RG, Chu TM: Carcinoembryonic antigen in patients with carcinoma of the lung. J Thorac Cardiovasc Surg 1978; 66(2). 320-328.

[16] Ladenson JH, McDonald JM, Landt M, *et al.* Colorectal carcinoma and carcinoembryonic antigen (CEA). Clin Chem 1980; 26(8): 1213-1220.

[17] Benchimol S, Fuks A, Jothy S, *et al.* Carcinoembryonic antigen, a human tumor marker, functions as an intercellular adhesion molecule. Cell 1989; 57(2): 327-334.

[18] Schlom J. Carcinoembryonic Antigen (CEA) Peptides and Vaccines for Carcinoma, in Kast M (ed): Peptide-Based Cancer Vaccines. Austin, TX, Landes Bioscience, 2000, p. 90-105.

[19] Kantor J, Irvine K, Abrams S, *et al.* Anti-tumor activity and immune responses induced by a recombinant vaccinia-carcinoembryonic antigen (CEA) vaccine. J Natl Cancer Inst 1992; 84(14): 1084-1091.

[20] Kantor J, Irvine K, Abrams S, *et al.* Immunogenicity and safety of a recombinant vaccinia virus vaccine expressing the carcinoembryonic antigen gene in a nonhuman primate. Cancer Res 1992; 52(24): 6917-6925.

[21] Tsang KY, Zaremba S, Nieroda CA, *et al.* Generation of human cytotoxic T cells specific for human carcinoembryonic antigen epitopes from cancer patients immunized with recombinant vaccinia-CEA vaccine. J Natl Cancer Inst 1995; 87(13): 982-990.

[22] McAneny D, Ryan CA, Beazley RM, Kaufman HL: results of phase I trial of a recombinant vaccinia virus that expresses carcinoembryonic antigen in patients with advanced colorectal cancer. Ann Surg Oncol 1996; 3(5): 495-500.

[23] Tsang KY, Zhu MZ, Nieroda CA, *et al*. Phenotypic stability of a cytotoxic T-cell line directed against an immunodominant epitope of human carcinoembryonic antigen. Clin Cancer Res 1997; 3(12 pt 1): 2439-2449.

[24] Marshall JL, Hawkins MJ, Tsang KY, *et al*. Phase I study in cancer patients of a replication-defective avipox recombinant vaccine that expresses human carcinoembryonic antigen. J Clin Oncol 1999; 17(1): 332-337.

[25] Hodge JW, McLaughlin JP, Kantor JA, *et al*. Diversified prime and boost protocols using recombinant vaccinia virus and recombinant nonreplicating avian pox virus to enhance T-cell immunity and antitumor responses. Vaccine 1997; 15(6-7): 759-768.

[26] Disis ML, Bernhard H, Shiota FM, *et al*. Granulocyte-macrophage colony-stimulating factor: an effective adjuvant for protein and peptide-based vaccines. Blood 1996; 88(1): 202-10.

[27] Irvine K, *et al*. Comparison of a CEA-recombinant vaccinia virus, purified CEA, and an anti-idiotype antibody bearing the image of a CEA epitope in the treatment and prevention of CEA-expressing tumors. Vaccine Res 1993; 2: 79-94.

[28] Kass E, Schlom J, Thompson J, *et al*. Induction of protective host immunity to carcinoembryonic antigen (CEA), a self-antigen in CEA transgenic mice, by immunizing with a recombinant vaccinia-CEA virus. Cancer Res 1999; 59(3): 676-683.

[29] Bernards R, Destree A, McKenzie S, Gordon E, Weinberg RA, and Panicali D. Effective tumor immunotherapy directed against an oncogene-encoded product using a vaccinia virus vector. Proc. Natl. Acad. Sci. USA 1987; 84(19): 6854- 8

[30] Grosenbach DW, Barrientos JC, Schlom J, Hodge JW. Synergy of vaccine strategies to amplify antigen-specific immune responses and anti-tumor effects. Cancer Res 2001; 61(11): 4497-505.

[31] Slack R, Ley L, Chang P, *et al*. Association between CEA-specific T cell responses (TCR) following treatment with vaccinia-CEA(V) and Alvac-CEA(A) and survival in patients (Pts) with CEA-bearing tumors. Abstract No. 1086, Proceedings of the 37th Annual Meeting of the American Society of Clinical Oncology 2001, San Francisco, CA, May 12-15, 2001, Vol. 20, Pt I, p. 272a

[32] Marshall JL, Arlen PM, Gulley J *et al*. Phase I study of sequential vaccinations with fowlpox-CEA(6D)-TRICOM alone, and sequentially with vaccinia-CEA(6D)-TRICOM, with and without granulocyte-macrophage colony-stimulating factor, in patients with carcinoembryonic antigen-expressing carcinomas. Journal of Clin Onc 2005; 23(4).

[33] Schwartz RH. Costimulation of T lymphocytes: the role of CD28, CTLA-4, and B7/BB1 in interleukin-2 production and immunotherapy. Cell 1992; 71(7): 1065-8.

[34] Chen L, Ashe S, Brady WA, *et al*. Costimulation of antitumor immunity by the B7 counterreceptor for the T lymphocyte molecules CD28 and CTLA-4. Cell 1992; 71(7): 1093-102.

[35] Freeman GJ, Freedman AS, Segil JM, *et al*. B7, a new member of the Ig superfamily with unique expression on activated and neoplastic B cells. J. Immunol 1989; 143(8): 2714-22.

[36] Freeman GJ, Gray GS, Gimmi CD, *et al*. Structure, expression, and T cell costimulatory activity of the murine homologue of the human B lymphocyte activation antigen B7. J. Exp. Med 1991; 174(3): 625-31.

[37] Springer, TA. Adhesion receptors of the immune system. Nature 1999; 346(6283): 425-34.

[38] Hellstrom KE, Hellstrom I, Linsley P, and Chen L. On the role of costimulation in tumor immunity. Ann NY Acad Sci 1993; 690: 225-30.

[39] Hellstrom I, Hellstrom KE. Tumor immunology: an overview. Ann NY Acad Sci 1993; 690: 24-31.

[40] Gregory CD, Murray RJ, Edwards CF, and Rickinson AB. Down-regulation of cell adhesion molecules LFA-3 and ICAM-1 in Epstein-Barr virus-positive Burkitt's lymphoma underlies tumor cell escape from virus-specific T cell surveillance. J Exp Med 1988; 167(6): 1811-24.

[41] Damle NK, Klussman K, Linsley PS, *et al*. Differential costimulatory effects of adhesion molecules B7, ICAM-1, LFA-3, and VCAM-1 on resting and antigen-primed CD4+ T lymphocytes. J Immunol 1992; 148(7): 1985-92.

[42] Townsend SE, Allison JP. Tumor rejection after direct costimulation of CD8+ T cells by B7-transfected melanoma cells. Science 1993; 259(5093): 368-70.

[43] Chen L, Linsley PS, and Hellstrom KE. Costimulation of T cells for tumor immunity. Immunol. Today 1993; 14(10): 483-6.

[44] Lorenz MG, Kantor JA, Schlom J, *et al.* Induction of anti-tumor immunity elicited by tumor cells expressing a murine LFA-3 analog *via* a recombinant vaccinia virus. Hum Gene Ther 1999; 10(4): 623-31.

[45] Uzendoski K, Kantor JA, Abrams SI, Schlom J, and Hodge JW. Construction and characterization of a recombinant vaccinia virus expressing murine intercellular adhesion molecule-1: induction and potentiation of antitumor responses. Hum Gene Ther 1997; 8(7): 851-60.

[46] Hodge JW, McLaughlin JP, Abrams S, *et al.* Admixture of a recombinant vaccinia virus containing the gene for the costimulatory molecule B7 and a recombinant vaccinia virus containing a tumor-associated antigen gene results in enhanced specific T-cell responses and antitumor immunity. Cancer Res. 1995; 55(16): 3598-603.

[47] Kalus, R.M., Kantor JA, Gritz L, *et al.* The use of combination vaccinia vaccines and dual-gene vaccinia vaccines to enhance antigen-specific T-cell immunity *via* T-cell costimulation. Vaccine 1999; 17(7-8): 893-903.

[48] Akagi J, Hodge JW, McLaughlin JP, *et al.* Therapeutic antitumor response after immunization with an admixture of recombinant vaccinia viruses expressing a modified MUC1 gene and the murine T-cell costimulatory molecule B7. J Immunother 1997; 20(1): 38-47.

[49] Hodge JW, Sabzevari H, Yafal AG, *et al.* A triad of costimulatory molecules synergize to amplify T-cell activation. Cancer Res 1999; 59(22): 5800-7.

[50] Morse MA, Deng Y, Coleman D, *et al.* A phase 1 study of active immunotherapy with carcinoembryonic antigen peptide (CAP-1)-pulsed, autologous human cultured dendritic cells in patients with metastatic malignancies expressing CEA. Clin Cancer Res 1999; 5(6): 1331-1338.

[51] Palena C, Schlom J, and Tsang K-Y. Differential gene expression profiles in a human T-cell line stimulated with a tumor-associated "self" peptide *vs.* an enhancer agonist peptide. Clin Cancer Res 2003; 9(5): 1616-27.

[52] Zaremba S, Barzaga E, Zhu MZ, Soares N, Tsang KY, and Schlom J. Identification of an enhancer agonist cytotoxic T lymphocyte peptide from human carcinoembryonic antigen. Cancer Res 1997; 57(20): 4570-4577.

[53] Salazar E, Zaremba S, Tsang KY, Arlen P, and Schlom J. Agonist peptide from a cytotoxic T lymphocyte epitope of human carcinoembryonic antigen stimulates production of Tc1-type cytokines and increases tyrosine phosphorylation more efficiently than cognate peptide. Int J Cancer 2000; 85(6): 829-838.

[54] Fong L, Hou Y, Rivas A, Benike C, Yuen A, Fisher GA, Davis MM, Engleman EG. Altered peptide ligand vaccination with Flt3 ligand expanded dendritic cells for tumor immunotherapy. Proc Natl Acad Sci USA 2001; 98(15): 8809-14.

[55] Rosenberg SA, Yang JC, Schwartzentruber DJ, *et al.* Immunologic and therapeutic evaluation of a synthetic peptide vaccine for the treatment of patients with metastatic melanoma. Nat Med 1998; 4(3): 321-7.

[56] Eder JP, Kantoff PW, Roper K, Xu GX, Bubley GJ, Boyden J, *et al.* A phase I trial of a recombinant vaccinia virus expressing prostate-specific antigen in advanced prostate cancer. Clin. Cancer Res 2000; 6(5): 1632-8.

[57] Gulley J, Chen AP, Dahut W, Arlen PM, Bastian A, Steinberg SM, *et al.* A Phase I study of a vaccine using recombinant vaccinia virus expressing PSA (rV-PSA) in patients with metastatic androgen-independent prostate cancer. The Prostate 2002; 53(2): 109-117.

[58] Sanda MG, Smith DC, Charles LG, Hwang C, Pienta KJ, Schlom J, *et al.* Recombinant vaccinia-PSA (PROSTVAC) can induce a prostate-specific immune response in androgen-modulated human prostate cancer. Urology 1999; 53(2): 260-6.

[59] Marshall JL, Hoyer RJ, Toomey MA, *et al.* Phase I study in advanced cancer patients of a diversified prime-and-boost vaccination protocol using recombinant vaccinia virus and recombinant nonreplicating avipox virus to elicit anti-carcinoembryonic antigen immune responses. J Clin Oncol 2000; 18(23): 3964-73.

[60] Cournoyer D, Beauchemin N, Boucher D, Benchimol S, Fuks A, Stanners CP. Transcription of genes of the carcinoembryonic antigen family in malignant and nonmalignant human tissues. Cancer Res 1988; 48(11): 3153-3157.

[61] Attallah AM, Needy CF, Noguchi PD, Elisberg BL. Enhancement of carcinoembryonic antigen expression by interferon. Int J Cancer 1979; 24(1): 49-52.

[62] Greiner JW, Hand PH, Noguchi P, Fisher PB, Pestka S, Schlom J. Enhanced expression of surface tumor-associated antigens on human breast and colon tumor cells after recombinant human leukocyte alpha-interferon treatment. Cancer Res 1984; 44(8): 3208-14.

[63] Greiner JW, Fisher PB, Pestka S, Schlom J. Differential effects of recombinant human leukocyte interferons on cell surface antigen expression. Cancer Res 1986; 46(10): 4984-90.

[64] Greiner JW, Guadagni F, Noguchi P, Pestka S, Colcher D, Fisher PB, Schlom J. Recombinant interferon enhances monoclonal antibody-targeting of carcinoma lesions *in vivo*. Science. 1987; 235(4791): 895-8.

[65] Guadagni F, Witt PL, Robbins PF, Schlom J, Greiner JW. Regulation of carcinoembryonic antigen expression in different human colorectal tumor cells by interferon-gamma. Cancer Res 1990; 50(19): 6248-55.

[66] Guadagni F, Kantor J, Schlom J *et al*. Regulation of tumor antigen expression by recombinant interferons. Ed: Fisher PB. In: Mechanisms of Differentiation, vol 2. Boca Raton, FL, CRC 1990; pp 57-80.

[67] Hauck W, Stanners CP. Control of carcinoembryonic antigen gene family expression in a differentiating colon carcinoma cell line, Caco-2. Cancer Res 1991; 51(13): 3526-33.

[68] Yamaguchi N, Kawai K. Factors affecting the CEA secretion of human adenocarcinoma cell lines into the spent medium. Gastroenterol Jpn 1983; 18(5): 428-35.

[69] Toth CA, Thomas P. The effect of interferon treatment on 14 human colorectal cancer cell lines: growth and carcinoembryonic antigen secretion *in vitro*. J Interferon Res 1990; 10(6): 579-88.

[70] Leon JA, Mesa-Tejada R, Gutierrez MC, Estabrook A, Greiner JW, Schlom J, *et al*. Increased surface expression and shedding of tumor associated antigens by human breast carcinoma cells treated with recombinant human interferons or phorbol ester tumor promoters. Anticancer Res 1989; 9(6): 1639-47.

[71] Esposito G, Bombardieri E, Lindi C, Valtolina M, Marciani P, Cocciolo MG, Gioria MR. Effects of cholesterol and alfa-2-recombinant interferon on cell growth and cell antigen production in the HT 29 cells, an established cell line of human colon adenocarcinoma. J Biol Regul Homeost Agents 1987; 1(4): 166-72.

[72] De Filippi R, Prete SP, Giuliani A, Silvi E, Yamaue H, Nieroda CA, *et al*. Differential effects of recombinant interferon-alpha and 5-fluorouracil against colon cancer cells or against peripheral blood mononuclear cells. Anticancer Res 1994; 14(5A): 1767-73.

[73] Guadagni F, Roselli M, Schlom J, Greiner JW. *In vitro* and *in vivo* regulation of human tumor antigen expression by human recombinant interferons: a review. Int J Biol Markers 1994; 9(1): 53-60.

[74] Kantor J, Tran R, Greiner JW, *et al*. Modulation of carcinoembryonic antigen messenger RNA levels in human colon carcinoma cells by recombinant human gamma-interferon. Cancer Res 1989; 49(10): 2651-2655.

[75] Guadagni F, Schlom J, Pothen S, Pestka S, Greiner JW. Parameters involved in the enhancement of monoclonal antibody targeting *in vivo* with recombinant interferon. Cancer Immunol Immunother 1988; 26(3): 222-30.

[76] Kuhn JA, Beatty BG, Wond JY, Esteban J, Wanek PM, Wall F, *et al*. Interferon enhancement of radioimmunotherapy for colon carcinoma. Cancer Res 1991; 51(9): 2335-2339.

[77] Greiner JW, Ullmann CD, Nieroda C, Qi CF, Eggensperger D, Shimada S, *et al*. Improved radioimmunotherapeutic efficacy of an anticarcinoma monoclonal antibody (131I-CC49) when given in combination with gamma-interferon. Cancer Res 1993; 53(3): 600-8.

[78] Nieroda CA, Milenic DE, Carrasquillo JA, Scholm J, Greiner JW. Improved tumor radioimmunodetection using a single-chain Fv and gamma-interferon: potential clinical applications for radioimmunoguided surgery and gamma scanning. Cancer Res 1995; 55(13): 2858-65.

[79] Rosenblum MG, Lamki LM, Murray JL, Carlo DJ, Gutterman JU. Interferon-induced changes in pharmacokinetics and tumor uptake of 111In-labeled antimelanoma antibody 96.5 in melanoma patients. J Natl Cancer Inst 1988; 80(3): 160-5.

[80] Murray JL, Macey DJ, Grant EJ, Rosenblum MG, Kasi LP, Zhang HZ, *et al*. Enhanced TAG-72 expression and tumor uptake of radiolabeled monoclonal antibody CC49 in metastatic breast cancer patients following alpha-interferon treatment. Cancer Res 1995; 55(23 Suppl): 5925s-5928s.

[81] Greiner JW, Guadagni F, Goldstein D, Borden EC, Ritts RE Jr, Witt P, *et al.* Evidence for the elevation of serum carcinoembryonic antigen and tumor-associated glycoprotein-72 levels in patients administered interferons. Cancer Res 1991; 51(16): 4155-63.

[82] Greiner JW, Guadagni F, Goldstein D, Smalley RV, Borden EC, Simpson JF, *et al.* Intraperitoneal administration of interferon-gamma to carcinoma patients enhances expression of tumor-associated glycoprotein-72 and carcinoembryonic antigen on malignant ascites cells. J Clin Oncol 1992; 10(5): 735-46.

[83] Mahvi DM, Madsen JA, Witt PL, Sondel PM. Interferon alpha enhances expression of TAG-72 and carcinoembryonic antigen in patients with primary colorectal cancer. Cancer Immunol Immunother 1995; 40(5): 311-4.

[84] Gebauer G, Jaeger W, Thiel G, Lang N. Increase of serum tumor marker concentrations by interferon-alpha. Eur J Gynaecol Oncol 1998; 19(4): 363-7.

[85] Roselli M,Guadagni F, Buonomo O, Belardi A, Vittorini V, Mariani-Costantini R, *et al.* Systemic administration of recombinant interferon alfa in carcinoma patients upreguates the expression of the carcinoma-associated antigens tumor-associated glycoprotein-72 and carcinoembryonic antigen. J of Clin Oncol 1996; 14(7): 2031-2042.

[86] Guadagni F, Schlom J, Johnston WW, Szpak CA, Goldstein D, Smalley R, *et al.* Selective interferon-induced enhancement of tumor-associated antigens on a spectrum of freshly isolated human adenocarcinoma cells. J Natl Cancer Inst 1989; 81(7): 502-12.

[87] Pamer E, Cresswell P. Mechanisms of MHC class I--restricted antigen processing. Annu Rev Immunol 1998; 16: 323-58.

[88] Watts TH, McConnell HM. Biophysical aspects of antigen recognition by T cells. Annu Rev Immunol 1987; 5: 461-75.

[89] Kaech SM, Wherry EJ, Ahmed R. Effector and memory T-cell differentiation: implications for vaccine development. Nature Rev Immunol 2002; 2(4): 251-62.

[90] Mizobata S, Tompkins K, Simpson JF, Shyr Y, Primus FJ. Induction of cytotoxic T cells and their antitumor activity in mice transgenic for carcinoembryonic antigen. Cancer Immunol Immunother 2000; 49(6): 285-95.

[91] Garrido F, Ruiz-Cabello F, Cabrera T, Perez-Villar JJ, Lopez-Botet M, Duggan-Keen M, *et al.* Implications for immunosurveillance of altered HLA class I phenotypes in human tumours. Immunol Today 1997; 18(2): 89-95.

[92] Marincola FM, Jaffee EM, Hicklin D, Ferrone S. Escape of human solid tumors from T cell recognition: molecular mechanisms and functional significance. Adv Immunol 2000; 74: 181-273.

[93] Koopman LA, Corver WE, van der Slik AR, Giphar MJ, Fleuren GJ. Multiple genetic alterations cause frequent and heterogeneous human histocompatibility leukocyte antigen class I loss in cervical cancer. J Exp Med 2000; 191(6): 961-965.

[94] Elsner HA, Drabek J, Rebmann V, Ambruzova Z, Grosse-Wilde H, Blasczyk R. Non-expression of HLA-B*5111N is caused by an insertion into the cytosine island at exon 4 creating a frameshift stop codon. Tissue Antigens 2001; 57(4): 369-72.

[95] Imboden M, Murphy KR, Rakhmilevich AL, Neal ZC, Xiang R, Reisfeld RA, *et al.* The level of MHC class I expression on murine adenocarcinoma can change the antitumor effector mechanism of immunocytokine therapy. Cancer Res 2001; 61(4): 1500-7.

[96] Basham TY, Bourgeade MF, Creasey AA, Merigan TC. Interferon increases HLA synthesis in melanoma cells: interferon-resistant and -sensitive cell lines. Proc Natl Acad Sci USA 1982; 79(10): 3265-9.

[97] Gastl G, Marth C, Leiter E, Gattringer C, Mayer I, Daxenbichler G, *et al.* Effects of human recombinant alpha 2 arg-interferon and gamma-interferon on human breast cancer cell lines: dissociation of antiproliferative activity and induction of HLA-DR antigen expression. Cancer Res 1985; 45(7): 2957-61.

[98] van de Stolpe A, van der Saag PT. Intercellular adhesion molecule-1. J Mol Med 1996; 74(1): 13-33.

[99] Bacso Z, Bene L, Damjanovich L, Damjanovich S. INF-gamma rearranges membrane topography of MHC-I and ICAM-1 in colon carcinoma cells. Biochem Biophys Res Commun 2002; 290(2): 635-40.

[100] Bander NH, Yao D, Liu H, Chen YT, Steiner M, Zuccaro W, Moy P. MHC class I and II expression in prostate carcinoma and modulation by interferon-alpha and-gamma. Prostate 1997; 33(4): 233-9.

[101] Makridis C, Juhlin C, Akerstrom G, Oberg K, Rastad J. MHC class I and II antigen expression and interferon alpha treatment of human midgut carcinoid tumors. World J Surg 1994; 18(4): 481-6.
[102] Angus R, Collins CM, Symes MO. The effect of alpha and gamma interferon on cell growth and histocompatibility antigen expression by human renal carcinoma cells *in vitro*. Eur J Cancer 1993; 29A(13): 1879-85.
[103] Jones T, Stern A, Lin R. Potential role of granulocyte-macrophage colony-stimulating factor as vaccine adjuvant. Eur J Clin Microbiol Infect Dis 1994; 13 Suppl 2: S47-53.
[104] Jager E, Ringhoffer M, Dienes HP, *et al.* Granulocyte-macrophage-colony-stimulating factor enhances responses to melanoma-associated peptides *in vivo*. Int J Cancer 1996; 67(1): 54-62.
[105] Gerloni M, Lo D, Ballou WR and Zanetti M. Immunological memory after somatic transgene immunization is positively affected by priming with GM-CSF and does not require bone marrow-derived dendritic cells. Eur J Immunol 1998; 28(6): 1832-1838.
[106] Unpublished data from JW Hodge.
[107] Provinciali M, Di Stefano G, Colombo M, *et al.* Adjuvant effects of low dose interleukin-2 on antibody response to influenza virus vaccination in healthy elderly subjects. Mech Aging Dev 1994; 77(2): 75-82.
[108] Arlen P, Tsang KY, Marshall JL, Chen A, Steinberg SM, Poole D, *et al.* The use of a rapid ELISPOT assay to analyze peptide-specific peptide-specific immune responses in carcinoma patients to peptide *vs.* recombinant poxvirus vaccines. Cancer Immunol Immunother 2000; 49(10): 517-29.
[109] Jeff Schlom, personal communication.
[110] Hou Y, Kavanagh B, Fong L. Distinct CD8+ T cell repertoires primed with agonist and native peptides derived from a tumor-associated antigen. J Immunol 2008; 180(3): 1526-34.

CHAPTER 9

# Targeting T Cell Costimulation

**Yangbing Zhao***

*Department of Pathology and Laboratory Medicine, Abramson Family Cancer Research Institute, Perelman School of Medicine, University of Pennsylvania, Philadelphia, PA 19104, USA*

**Abstract:** T lymphocytes can be modified by gene transfer to enhance their anti-tumor activities for the cancer treatment. Yet to further improve this therapeutic approach, current efforts are being made to define and generate better T cells, manipulate the tumor microenvironment, and develop broad-spectrum tumor-reactive T cells. As a key element in T cell activation, differentiation, survival, and effector activity, costimulation signals have been widely incorporated in T cell modification, chimeric antigen receptor (CAR) design and T cell manufacture to directly boost the antitumor activities of T cell, or to counteract tumor suppressive microenvironment. Tumors are able progress in immunocompetent hosts for the reason they could handle to avoid from the immune system, for which they have used multiple mechanisms. Nearly all components of the immune system and all stages of immune response can be interfered by cancers. Selectively providing costimulation signals and cytokines during T cell stimulation and expansion process can dramatically influence the phenotype and T cells function *in vitro/in vivo*, which have strong impacts on the therapeutic antitumor efficacy. Therefore, the inclusion of costimulatory signals in the design of CAR would elicit enhanced anti-tumor activities compared with signaling *via* CD3-ζ alone. Direct introducing of costimulatory molecular ligands into the T cells delivers costimulatory signals and so offsets the costimulatory deficit of tumor antigen reactive $CD4^+$ or $CD8^+$ T cells. Also, manipulating other molecule, such as Cbl-b, that regulates T cell costimulation function is a promising strategy in designing cancer immunotherapy.

**Keywords:** 4-1BB, Adoptive cell therapy, B7, Cbl-b, CD28, Chimeric antigen receptor, Costimulation, CTLA-4, Gene therapy, IL12, IL-15, IL-2, IL-7, Immunotherapy, PD-1, PD-L1, PD-L2, T cell receptor, T lymphocytes, Tumor immune evasion.

## INTRODUCTION

T lymphocytes are essential regulators of *in vivo* immune responses, which are crucial in the body against infectious agents and malignancy. T cell mediated immune response is started through the contact of TCR/CD3 complex by a foreign

***Corresponding author Yangbing Zhao:** Department of Pathology and Laboratory Medicine, Abramson Family Cancer Research Institute, Perelman School of Medicine, University of Pennsylvania, Philadelphia, PA 19104, USA; Tel: (215) 746-7618; E-mail: Yangbing@exchange.upenn.edu

**Jianxun Song (Ed)**

peptide epitope presented on MHC, the major histocompatibility complex, which gives antigen specificity and signals that are needed for optimal stimulation. While a T lymphocyte fate is largely determined by other signals received during TCR engagement and activation. It was first found in the late 80s that TCR engagement with the complex of MHC-II/peptide without other motions is not able to stimulate the CD4 T cells, not resulting in T cell responses to further antigenic stimulus. As a result, the T cells become anergic [1, 2]. Furthermore, it is verified that additional, non-MHC restricted signals provided by professional APCs, the antigen presenting cells, which are critical for clonal expansion, then development of effector phenotype of T cells [3, 4]. Since then, T lymphocyte activation has been described by a ''two-signal hypothesis'' in which co-stimulation provided the second signal that is needed on behalf of the optimal T cell stimulation. This process is further evidenced by the discovery of CD28 as a costimulatory molecule, and it is shown that both TCR and costimulatory signaling are essential for a full T cell activation [5, 6]. T cell co-signaling receptors have been generally described as membrane-bound molecules that positively (costimulatory receptors) or negatively (coinhibitory receptors) transduce signals in T cells to modulate TCR signaling. These co-signaling (both costimulatory and coinhibitory) molecules are usually divided into two major family members: the IgSF (immunoglobulin) superfamily and the TNFR (tumor necrosis factor receptor)/TNF superfamily. The magnitude of the T cell response is significantly enhanced in the presence of costimulatory molecules, although TCR engagement alone is able to trigger the activation of a number of signaling pathways. The engagement of costimulatory molecules can induce not only quantitative but also qualitative changes in T cell signaling pathways [7].

## CD28/B7 IG SF

CD28 is the primarily known member of the IgSF family, also called the B7 family [8]. Now the IgSF family includes cytotoxic T lymphocyte-associated antigen 4 (CTLA-4 or CD152) [9], inducible co-stimulator (ICOS or CD278) [10], programmed death receptor 1 (PD-1 or CD279) [11] and B- and T-lymphocyte attenuator (BTLA, CD272) [12]. T cells constitutively express CD28 on the cell surface, which provides a critical costimulatory signal upon ligation to B7-1 (CD80) and B7-2 (CD86) mainly expressed on APCs [13]. Costimulation of CD28 on T cells with B7-1 or B7-2 on APCs has varied plus intense consequences. For example, CD28 signaling can enhance the T cell sensitivity to antigen stimulation, and induce T cell proliferation at otherwise submitogenic concentrations of antigen [14-16] and the production of cytokines; especially IL-2 is greatly increased [5, 17]. Interestingly, CD28 signaling is found resistant to cyclosporine-mediated suppression [18, 19]. In addition, CD28 costimulation promotes cell survival through the induction of anti-apoptotic genes, such as bcl-xL and c-FLIPs [20, 21] and the decreased expression of CD95L, which is important for preventing the activation induced death (AIDC) to protect activated T cells from cell death. Also, CD28 is essential for an appropriate PKCθ segregation during the immunological synapse; the failure to properly localize PKCθ will result in a weak activation of the NF-κB pathway and following IL-2 gene transcription [22, 23]. A number of studies demonstrated that the level of CD28 expression is important for the outcome of TCR engagement [24].

ICOS is an induced receptor on T cell and binds to B7-H2 (ICOSL, CD275), which is largely expressed in lymphoid tissue following the engagement of either TCR with MHC/antigen complex or CD28 to B7 ligand. The ICOS/B7H2 signaling provides a positive costimulation of the T cells, which it is clearly different from the CD28/B7 signaling. ICOS/B7H2 pathway is not involved in a direct IL-2 release, however, is associated with the differentiation of T helper (TH) cell subtypes [25]. ICOS signaling induced the expression of IL-4, IL-10 and IL-21 that is critical to the expansion of Th subsets (Th1, Th2, Th17 and TFH) and Tregs mediated by ICOS [25-28]. B7H2 also can bind to CD28 and CTLA4, however, compared to CD28 or CTLA4, ICOS binds to B7H2 with a higher affinity [29], which suggests a possible crosstalk between CD28 and ICOS costimulatory pathways.

CTLA4 is upregulated on the effector T cells and functions as a coinhibitor that suppresses the responses of T cells after the binding with CD80 and/or CD86 [30, 31]. The exprcssion of CTLA4 is induced 1-2 days later, after T cell activation; Compared with CD28, CTLA4 has a greater affinity with CD80 and CD86 [32]. CTLA4 is an important molecule in the induction of peripheral tolerance by directly restraining CD28 signaling or down-regulating cofactors that are required for TCR-mediated signaling. The co-inhibitory function of CTLA4 was shown in CTLA4-deficient animals that had a lethal impairment initiated through the unrestrained proliferation and infiltration of lymphocytes [33, 34]. In naive or resting state of T cells, CTLA-4 is not expressed, however, it is up regulated when cells become activated [35, 36]. In contrast, Tregs constitutively express CTLA-4 on the surface, which is a marker of this cell subset [37, 38]; indicating CTLA-4 is involved in the generation of Tregs, as well as the governing of Treg functions. PD-1 on T cell is inducibly expressed by TCR signaling and remains high during persistent stimulation. Of note, PD-1 was highly expressed on non-functional, exhausted T cells throughout chronic viral infection [39, 40]. The engagement of PD-1 with PD-L1 (B7-H1; CD274) or PD-L2 (B7-DC; CD273) mediates suppressive signals in T cells, inducing tolerance as well as immune-facilitated tissue destruction [41, 42]. PD-1/PD-L1 (or PD-L2) interaction can induce PD-1 tyrosine phosphorylation, which will recruit tyrosine phosphatases to control the signal transduction mediated by TCR and CD28. T cell activation induces the up-regulation of PD1 and the effects of PD-1 ligation in two hours [43]. Furthermore, PD-1 engagement during T cell activation blocks cytokine secretion, proliferation, effector function and survival [44]. The PD-1 inhibition relies on the intensity of the TCR signaling, having an additional inhibition in weak TCR stimulation, however, CD28 co-stimulation or IL-2 overrides PD-1-mediated inhibition [45, 46]. PD-1 engagement can also prevent the induction of a number of transcription factors that are related to the activity of effector cells, such as Eomes, GATA-3, and T-bet as well as bcl-xL [43, 47]. Meanwhile, PD-1 engagement can reduce the phosphorylation of CD3ζ-associated protein of 70 kDa (ZAP70), and protein kinase C θ (PKC-θ) [48]. PD-1 signaling also restrains the activation of Erk, which could be overcome by cytokine receptor signaling through activating STAT5, including IL-2, IL-7, and IL-15 [49]. Gene expression profiling showed that PD-1 has a greater capability to inhibit T-cell activation than CTLA-4 [48].

CD80 and CD86 as costimulatory molecules expressed on APCs are well characterized. Current studies have indicated that B7 on T cells may serve to down regulate responses and deliver signals in T cells [50, 51]. There are studies showed a substantially bidirectional inhibitory interaction between PD-L1 and CD80, which adds an extra immunoregulatory function of the B7/CD28 family [52, 53]. The binding affinity of CD80 to PD-L1 is intermediate to that of CD80 with CD28 and CD80 with CTLA-4. Functional studies indicated that CD80/PD-L1 interaction suppresses proliferation and cytokine production of T cells. Ligation of PD-L1 with CD80 expressed on T cells could result in an inhibitory signal in T cells. Conversely, interaction of PD-L1 of expressed T cells with CD80 can give rise to an inhibitory signal in T cells [52].

## TNFR SF

TNFR superfamily consists of approximately 50 membrane-bound and soluble members that are able to modulate cellular function [54]. Costimulatory molecules of TNFR superfamily that are commonly used for studying T cell based therapeutic approaches are OX40 (CD134), 4-1BB (CD137), and CD27.

OX40 is largely expressed on activated T cells [55]. Its ligand OX40L is mostly found on DCs, B cells, macrophages, T cells, and endothelial cells [56-58]. OX40 is a late costimulatory molecular on T cells, and ligation to OX40L on APCs leads to proliferation, cytokine production, and survival. The expression of OX40 is independent on CD28, however, CD28 augments the expression of OX40 [59, 60], indicating that these two molecules can cooperate. OX40 signals can act in a sequential way after CD28 signals, which support effector T cell survival and proliferation [61]. OX40 signaling perhaps also inhibits the generation and function of CD4+Foxp3+ Tregs [62, 63]. Working together with CD28, CD27 and 4-1BB, OX40 can modulate memory T cell development [59, 64, 65] by up-regulating of a number of bcl-2 family members, such as bcl-xL, bcl-2, and bfl-1 [59, 66], as well as survivin [67] and aurora B [68].

4-1BB was discovered in 1989 in activated T cell lines [69]. With the exception of DCs and Tregs, on which the 4-1BB is constitutively expressed, the expression of 4-1BB is activation- dependent. 4-1BB has a wide pattern of inducible expression in both hematopoietic system and non-hematopoietic cells [70]. Signaling *via* 4-1BB in the presence of TCR engagement results enhanced T-cell cytokine induction, expansion and upregulation of anti-apoptotic genes which aim to prevent activation-induced cell death (AICD) [71-73]; The 4-1BB ligand (4-1BBL or CD137L) is mainly shown on DCs, macrophages, and B cells [71, 74]. The engagement of 4-1BB, when coupled with TCR has the ability to induce CD28 independent IL-2 production [75]. 4-1BB signaling can regulate not only innate but also adaptive immune responses. In adaptive immune responses, 4-1BB promotes T cell proliferation, induces cytokine production, enhances the CTL cytotoxicity, and protects T cells from AICD with a TCR signal [76]. 4-1BB also stimulates expansion of memory T cells without cognate antigens which dramatically enhances survival of memory T cells [77]. In addition, 4-1BB plays a role in promoting DC activation by enhancing production of cytokines, including IL-6 and IL-12, as well as up-regulating B7 costimulation [78].

CD27 (also known as TNFRSF7) is constitutively expressed on human T cells, NKT cells, NK-cell subsets, and hematopoietic progenitors. CD27 is inducible in B-cell subsets [73, 79]. It is down regulated in effector T cells following the repetitive stimulus, and CD27 down-regulation is related to improved effector functions. CD27 ligand, CD70, is briefly expressed on activated T cells, B cells, and mature DCs. Engagement of CD27 with CD70 or agonistic monoclonal antibodies (mAbs) can stimulate T cell proliferation and the production of cytokine. CD27 mainly promotes survival of T cells rather than inducing cell cycle progression [80]. CD27 signaling co-stimulates T-cell activation but appears to be dispensable for immune development because CD27-/- mice are immunocompetent, lack overt autoimmune symptoms, and respond to viral infection. However, T-cell memory responses in these mice are impaired in different aspects such as formation, response kinetics, and cell number, which has been attributed to the impact of CD27 on survival of activated T-cell [80, 81]. Similarly, T-cell priming in the absence of CD70:CD27 interaction results in abortive clonal expansion, dysfunctional anti-tumor response, and failed CD8 T-cell memory formation [82].

Costimulatory molecules CD28 and CD27 expressed on naive T cells are critical initiators of cell activation with TCR signaling, while most coinhibitory receptors are undetectable in naive stage. The further expansion of such T cells requires signals through ICOS, 4-1BB, and OX40. Co-inhibitory molecules are often induced or up-regulated upon T cell activation to ensure T cell responses are firmly regulated to control or prevent excess normal tissues damage [83]. Down or up regulation of costimulatory and coinhibitory molecules is likely to be a method for tumors to avoid immune surveillance. Anergic T cells could be induced in the tumor microenvironment because of the lack of costimulation, which leads to the absence of a proper antitumor immune response [32].

## A THIRD SIGNAL (SIGNAL 3) FROM CYTOKINES FOR T CELL ACTIVATION

Without cytokine signaling, TCR and co-stimulatory signals could initiate the activation of naïve T cells, but the cell survives poorly, fails to acquire optimal effector functions and cannot generate a durable memory population. As a result, the cytokines perform as a 'switch', which determines TCR and costimulatory signals, leading to whether tolerance, or optimal effector functions, survival, and memory formation. Therefore, the cytokine signal is considered as 'signal 3', because it is required for an immune response with "signal 1" by TCR and "signal 2" through costimulatory signals. *In vitro* studies employing artificial APC (aAPC) showed that IL-12 and IFN$\alpha/\beta$ acted as a critical third signal and increased the CTL clonal expansion as well as enhanced the effector-function development [84]. IL-12 and IL-1 provide very important costimulation to CD8 T and CD4 T cells, respectively [85, 86]. In a study of CD8 T cells in TCR-transgenic mouse, Ag challenge in the absence of adjuvant induces an Ag-specific CD8 T cell tolerance. In contrast, IL-12 administration along with peptide leads massive clonal expansion, effector function development, and a long-lasting memory population establishment. This result provides solid support for a three-signal model for *in vivo* activation of naive CD8 T cells by Ag, in which the third signal controls the fate of either tolerance or activation [87]. Based on this, the incorporation of IL-12 into a T cell based adoptive immunotherapy has a strong potential to provide T cells with costimulation to counteract tumor-induced immunosuppression.

## CBL-B

Protein ubiquitylation of E3 ligases, in general, through the Casitas B lymphoma-b protein (Cbl-b), can negatively regulate T-cell activation. The E3 ubiquitin ligase Cbl-b is critical in regulating T cell signaling, specifically through the CD28/B7 pathway [88, 89]. Cbl-b has a number of key functions such as controlling the need for costimulation, for the reason that *cblb*$^{-/-}$ T cells have been shown a full activation and producing IL-2 even not being present CD28 costimulation [90]. Cbl-b is also able to moderate the threshold of T cell activation during stimulation with weak agonistic peptides [91]. In summary, Cbl-b displays its gatekeeper function through the ubiquitination of its target protein p85, the regulatory subunit of phosphatidylinositol 3-kinase (PI3K) [92]. Non-degradative ubiquitination of p85 suppresses its recruitment to CD28 [88], therefore, prohibits the activation of PI3K, which is the most relevant signaling pathway that is started by the costimulatory CD28 receptor. The suppressive function of E3 ubiquitin ligases is controlled in the event of a productive T cell costimulation, in which Cbl-b becomes ubiquitinated and degraded by proteasome after a CD28-mediated costimulation [93] through a PKC-θ regulated, CD28-induced inactivation of Cbl-b [94]. Of note, Cbl-b$^{-/-}$ mice had T cell activation being independent to CD28 signaling, T cell hyperactivity, spontaneous autoimmune responses [90, 95], and resistant to Tregs and TGF-β *in vitro* [96, 97], suggest that manipulating Cbl-b in T cells is a promising strategy for cell based cancer therapies.

## TUMOR ESCAPES FROM T CELL SURVEILLANCE

Immunity against tumor and pathogens requires all types of immune cells, such as T cells, B cells, DCs, macrophages, NK cells, granulocytes, and mast cells [96]. T cells perform a critical role in restraining the neoplastic lesion development. However, tumor progresses in immunocompetent hosts, as tumor can handle to escape from the immune surveillance. The escape procedure is diversely attributed to either the incapacity of immune cells to build up an effective anti-tumor response or to break immune surveillance through tumor-derived factors and tumor-induced suppressor cells. Tumor uses multiple mechanisms to escape immune surveillance by interfering with all components of the immune system and affecting the whole immune responses. However, tumor-driven immune suppression is a selective and aggressive suppression of the immune cell functions that particularly responsible for anti-tumor responses, however, not an immunodeficiency. In addition, tumor cells have sophisticated strategies to regulate the development of immune responses, such as the use of inhibitory receptor-ligands, enrollment of major regulatory cells, and production of inhibitory cytokines as well as induction of local inflammation. Although there are multiple mechanisms that tumor use to evade immune surveillance, the following paragraphs will only focus on evasion strategies, which counteract with the T cell recognition: **a**. Tolerance induction to limit tumor-reactive T-cell responses; **b**. Defective recognition of tumors; **c**. Resistance to T-cell-mediated killing; **d**. Induction of anergy in activated T cells; **e**. Induction of immunosuppressive Tregs and myeloid suppressors (myeloid-derived suppressor cell, M2 macrophage and immature dendritic cells) [97-99].

## TOLERANCE INDUCTION

T cell surveillance of tumors primarily depends on the recognition of tumor associated antigen (TAA) peptides loaded on MHC molecules. Most TAAs of solid tumor correspond to self-Ags expressed in tumors and are merely detectable around ordinary cell/tissues. But, to establish a central tolerance, T cells with high affinity TCR for the complex of MHC/self-Ag are removed in the thymus development. As a result, the T cell repertoire associated with self-Ags in the peripheral immune system is limited and most cells usually have a low-affinity TCR against TAA. Under usual circumstances, self-responsive T cells are in an unaware condition termed peripheral tolerance and the self-responsive T cells are re-activated by professional APCs such as DCs, under some circumstances [100]. Although non-primed DCs or immature DCs that have not been primed with hazard signals present self-antigens, they are not able to give a sufficient costimulatory signal for T-cell stimulation. Therefore, T cells that recognize the complexes of MHC/self-Ag with non-primed DCs turn out to be anergy [101]. T cell anergy is a major obstacle for TAA immune responses, which has been observed in a number of tumor tissues in which immature DCs cannot elicit potent T-cell responses [102-104].

## DEFECTIVE RECOGNITION OF TUMORS

It is a common strategy for tumors to escape T cell recognition by modulating antigen presentation machinery (APM) through either down regulation or absolute shutdown of MHC class I molecules, which are also down regulated by point mutations or through sizeable deletions [105, 106]. Another way for tumors to down-modulate MHC class I molecules exists through mutations of *β*2-microglobulin (*β*2m) [107, 108]. Assembly and transportation of MHC class I molecules are critically dependent on the APM that includes transporters related to Ag- processing 1 and 2 (*i.e.*, TAP1, TAP2), the proteasome subunits of low-molecular mass polypeptides 2 and 7 (*i.e.,* LMP2, LMP7), and a number of chaperons (*e.g.*, tapsin) [109]. Some tumor cells have an impaired APM expression, such as TAP1, TAP2, and tapsin, which results in the deficit of surface expression of MHC class I [110, 111].

## RESISTANCE TO CYTOTOXICITY OF T CELLS

Tumors have the ability to avoid T cell killing by interfering with the pathway of perforin/granzyme [112, 113]. The cross linking of death receptors such as CD95 and TRAIL receptor will induce the apoptosis of target tumor cells. However, the signaling of death receptors is inhibited in tumor cells by overexpressing anti-apoptotic protein [114, 115] and down regulating or inactivating of death receptors [116].

## INDUCTION OF T-CELL ANERGY

Costimulatory molecules tightly control T-cell activation and fate. Tumor cells evade T cell attack by preferentially utilizing certain co-inhibitory molecules, such as CTLA4 and PD-1. The possible mechanism is by either expressing these molecules themselves or inducing other cells, such as immature DCs, Tregs and suppressor myeloid cells to express these co-inhibitory molecules. Furthermore, tumor cells induce the production of IL-10, TGF-β, and PGE2, which inhibit activation, proliferation, and differentiation of T-cell homeostasis [117, 118]. The TGF-β causes an insufficient signal transduction in T cells by down regulating the components and signaling molecules of TCR, such as CD3-zeta chain, ZAP70, and ITK (IL2-inducible T-cell kinase) [119]. Furthermore, TGF-β blocks the cytotoxic function of T cells by transcriptional repressing of perforin, granzyme A/B, INF-γ, and FasL [120]. TGF-β also converts effector T cells into Tregs [121]. The inducible cyclooxygenase enzyme COX2 is also overexpressed in a number of tumor forms to induce the production of PGE2 that can further affect tumorigenesis such as angiogenesis, apoptosis and migration [122]. PGE2 changes the immune system from Th1 to Th2 response [123]. PGE2 also augments the induction of Tregs [124]. Tumors could also develop immune evasion through protein-glycan communications engaging galectins. Galectins are natural immunosuppressive proteins which suppress anti-tumor immune responses [125]. It was reported that galectin could interfere with TCR complex assembly in the lipid rafts [126].

## INDUCTION OF IMMUNOSUPPRESSIVE TREGS

Tregs are $CD4^{+}CD25^{high}FOXP3^{+}$ lymphocytes, and professionally suppress effector T cells [127]. Tregs are critical in facilitating peripheral tolerance and avoiding autoimmunity [127]. Treg represents a small portion of entire CD4+ T cells in the periphery (approximately 1–2%) and its frequency is found augmented in the peripheral blood of cancer patients, such as breast, lung, esophageal, gastric, colorectal, and ovarian cancers, lymphomas, as well as melanomas. Also Tregs are found accumulate at tumor sites as well [128-131]. Furthermore, the presence and immunosuppressive activities of Tregs are related to a weak prognosis in those cancer patients [128, 132]. Tregs use several mechanisms to mediate immune evasion of tumor cells. Tumor cells secrete suppressive cytokines such as TGF-β and interleukin-10 (IL-10) and create an immunosuppressive environment that suppresses anti-tumor immunity. Treg also expresses high-affinity CD25, a receptor of IL-2 [133, 134]. Tregs can exhaust IL-2 in the tumor microenvironment. In addition, Tregs occupy more principal homeostatic and antitumor cytokines, including IL-7, IL-15, and IL-12 [135]. Additionally, Tregs express a number of surface proteins, such as CTLA-4, PD-1, and GITR, which bind with B7-1/B7-2, PD-L1, or GITR-L on APCs and T cells. Within tumor tissues, Tregs keep and spread a synchronized, suppressive and tolerogenic environment [130, 131]. Moreover, Tregs can induce the generation of regulatory myeloid cells within the tumor microenvironment [136].

## INDUCTION OF IMMUNOSUPPRESSIVE MYELOID CELLS

Myeloid cells play a pivotal role in tumor initiation, angiogenesis, and metastasis. Myeloid cells contribute to the tumor stroma formation and influence the immune setting during developing tumor masses [137-139]. The subsets of myeloid cells contributing to the immune dysfunction in the tumor stroma consist of DCs, macrophages, and myeloid-derived suppressor cells (MDSC). MDSC are bone marrow (BM)-derived immature myeloid cells that have an increased frequency in tumors, lymphoid organs, and peripheral blood of nearly entire tumor-bearing hosts [140]. Primarily defined as CD11b+/Gr1+ myeloid progenitor cells, which were recruited to the tumor foci by tumor-derived soluble factors, including IL-6, PGE2, VEGF, TGF-β, and IL-10 in tumor-bearing mice. These pro-inflammatory mediators could provoke MDSC tissue accumulations and promote MDSC suppressor activity, thereby helping tumor growth [141, 142]. Because of being short of a Gr-1 homolog, the markers of human MDSCs remain unclear. The initial observations suggested that the phenotypic subset of human MDSCs resided in the population of $Lin^-$ $HLA^-DR^-$ $CD33^+$ cells [143]. MDSC facilitated T-cell suppression is through a direct cell-cell contact by expressing high-level nitric oxide synthase and Arginase 1. Nitric oxide induced T cell apoptosis by suppressing the signaling of STAT5 and the forming of peroxynitrite. Peroxynitrite is an effective oxidant inducing the nitration and nitrosylation of amino acids, which are needed for T-cell function. Arginase 1 can deplete L-arginine in the tumor microenvironment and locally reduce T cell proliferation. Additional suppressive mechanisms of MDSC include the sequestration of cysteine to a limited availability of T cells, the release of suppressive cytokines such as IL-10, and the heavy production of reactive oxygen species [144]. Of note, a latest study similarly suggests that MDSCs can switch the differentiation of $CD4^+$ T cells into Tregs [145]. MDSC induces indoleamine-2, 2-dioxygenase (IDO), which is an amino acid and crucial for T cell differentiation [146, 147]. MDSC is a highly diversified subset of controlling cells, which are able to use varied mechanisms to suppress anti-tumor immunity.

Macrophages are crucial in immune evasion within malignant tumors. In both mice and humans, macrophages are co-opted during the malignancy change to facilitate tumor growth [148-150]. These stromal cells (*i.e.*, mouse $CD11b^+$ $F4/80^+$; human $CD11b^+$ $CD14^+$ $CD33^+$ $CD68^+$) are typically defined as being skewed to a different M2 profile [139, 148, 151]. Of note, in addition of lower levels of proinflammatory cytokines, M2-polarized macrophages can produce higher levels of immunosuppressive mediators, including VEGF, TGF-β, and IL-10 [139, 148, 151].

In the tumor microenvironment, DCs may develop functional impairments and reduce their ability to prime T cells [152]. These functionally impaired DCs frequently have no or low-level expression of costimulatory molecules, but express IDO to suppress anti-tumor immunity [153]. In addition, DCs have defects in the machinery for antigen presentation, such as low-molecular-weight proteins and TAP [152]. As a result, tumors disrupt DC differentiation and function that significantly reduce anti-tumor adaptive immunity.

In summary, tumor cells use multiple ways to escape T cell attack by both decreasing positive T cell stimulation and increasing negative regulation of to T cells, which include: down-regulating co-stimulatory molecules and MHC on APCs and tumors, secreting suppressive cytokines (*e.g.*, TGF-β, IL-10), inducing suppressive cells (*e.g.*, Tregs, MDSCs, immature DCs, and M2 macrophage), and up-regulating PD-1 and CTL-4. A T cell under such strong immunosuppressive environment will eventually end up in the states of anergy, ignorance, AICD, or being induced to become accomplice, such as to become induced Treg, which actually helps tumor escape.

## T CELL COSTIMULATION IN ADOPTIVE T CELL TRANSFER THERAPY

Adoptive immunotherapy using *ex vivo* expanded or genetically modified T cells for the treatment of cancer provides a new venue to fight against tumors. The T cells can be manipulated *ex vivo* with optimized culture systems and genetic modification without the negative influence from the tumor microenvironment for the purpose of rendering them both tumor specificity and costimulatory activation before being infused back into the cancer patients. The commonly targeted costimulatory molecules are listed in Table **1**.

**Table 1:** Targeted costimulatory molecules in cancer adoptive immunotherapy

| Receptor | Ligands | Major function | Utilization |
|---|---|---|---|
| CD28 | CD80 or CD86 | T-cell proliferation<br>T-cell differentiation<br>Anti-apoptosis<br>Decreases TCR signaling threshold | T-cell stimulation/expansion [154]<br>CAR design [155]<br>Receptor switch [156]<br>Direct T-cell modification [157] |
| ICOS | ICOSL | T-cell differentiation<br>B-cell development | T-cell stimulation (Th17 polarization) [25]<br>CAR design [158] |
| CTLA4 | CD80 or CD86 | Blocks T-cell activation/proliferation<br>Cell cycle arrest | Receptor switch [156] |
| PD-1 | PD-L1 or PD-L2 | Blocks T-cell activation/proliferation<br>Cell cycle arrest | Receptor switch [159] |
| OX40 | OX40L | T-cell activation/proliferation<br>Promotes T-cell survival | CAR design [158] |
| 4-1BB | 4-1BBL | Promotes proliferation/cytokine production<br>Promotes T-cell survival<br>Enhances cytotoxic activity | T-cell stimulation/expansion [160]<br>CAR design [158]<br>T-cell modification [157] |
| CD27 | CD70 | T-cell activation and proliferation<br>Promotes T-cell survival<br>Increases memory generation | CAR design [161] |

## ADOPTIVE CELL TRANSFER (ACT)-BASED THERAPY

ACT of tumor-infiltrating T lymphocytes (TIL) mediates a long-term, durable regression of large, vascularized, invasive tumors in patients with advanced metastatic melanoma, which had led to an increase of the objective response rates from 49% to 72% in some pilot clinical trials [162-164]. However, tumor-reactive TIL cannot be obtained from most of other solid tumors. Meanwhile, T lymphocytes can be modified by gene transfer method to express Ag-specific TCR or chimeric Ag receptor (CAR) to enhance their specific anti-tumor activities [165-167]. A series of clinical trials have shown promising outcome when using genetically engineered peripheral blood derived lymphocytes to treat different cancers, including melanoma, synovial sarcoma, neuroblastoma, colorectal carcinoma, renal cell carcinoma, lymphoma and leukemia [168-172]. As these studies demonstrated that adoptive T cell immunotherapy could mediate the regression of established metastatic cancers in human, therefore the T cell-based cancer immunotherapy has drawn the attention from pharmaceutical companies for the commercialization of this technology. Yet to further improve this technology, current efforts are being made to define better procedures for T cell manufacture, to manipulate the tumor microenvironment, and to develop a broad-spectrum pool of tumor-reactive T cells. T cell costimulation as a key element in activation, differentiation, survival, and function, has also been targeted in T cell stimulation/expansion and CAR design. In the studies of adoptive cell therapy for purpose of either directly boosting anti-tumor activities of T cell, or counteracting tumor suppressive microenvironment, the role of costimulatory molecules has been taken into serious consideration.

## GENERATING *EX VIVO* EXPANDED T CELLS WITH HIGH POTENT ANTI-TUMOR ACTIVITIES

To develop a large number of effector T cells for ACT, broad *ex vivo* cell expansion is needed. However, cell expansion usually causes damage to cell differentiation and survival potency. Scientific observations in murine tumor models indicated that ACT efficiency is mostly dependent on the differentiation status of the adoptively transferred T cells, where T cell differentiation is contrariwise connected with *in vivo* anti-tumor effectiveness [173, 174]. Indeed, the use of "young", less-differentiated T cells [174, 175], with longer telomeres [176] and high-level expression of CD27 and CD28 [177], is crucial for the success. Data from clinical trials of TIL ACT has shown that effector-memory $CD8^+$ CTLs are greatly connected to the clinical response, indicating that $CD8^+$ CTLs in the TIL ACT are extremely important in mediating tumor regressions

[174, 178, 179]. Therefore, generating effector-memory T cells expressing both CD28 and CD27 in a short period of time is pursued to establish novel T cell stimulation and expansion systems.

T cell Rapid Expansion Protocol (REP) remains a commonly used method to produce final T cell products for ACT, which is described as taking T cells by means of IL-2 and anti-CD3 antibody in the presence of irradiated PBMC feeder cells to activate them [180]. The PBMC feeder cells can provide Fc receptors for the cross-linking of anti-CD3 antibody as well as co-stimulatory factors and growth factors for T cell expansion [180]. However, the present REP protocol yields T cells that lost the CD28 and CD27 expression [181-183]. These CTLs are prone to apoptosis and hyporesponsive to restimulation with tumor Ags [183]. Signaling *via* 4-1BB in the presence of TCR activation causes T-cell expansion, cytokine induction, upregulation of surviving proteins such as bcl-xL and bcl-2, and prevents activation-induced cell death (AICD). It was reported recently that by adding a fully agonistic human α-4-1BB McAb to the REP culture, it would significantly increase the frequency of CTLs [184]. In the 4-1BB REP, the $CD28^+$ cell frequency in the CTL population remains steady and CD27 expression is also maintained. Interestingly, the supplement of a 4-1BB Ab to the REP culture regulated the CTL phenotype, which was evidenced by the significantly increased perforin and granzyme B expression while there were no changes in Eomesodermin and KLRG-1 expression. This approach could apply to generate TCR/CAR transduced T cells with potentially improved persistence and anti-tumor activity.

Beads immobilized CD3 and CD28 antibodies have been widely employed for T cell stimulation and expansion [154]. The expanded T cells had an improved ability to produce cytokines and to attack target cells without MHC restriction [185]. Subsequently, α-CD3/CD28 magnetic beads are suitable reagents for T cell expansion, which has been utilized to improve T cell immunity in immunosuppressed cancer patients [186, 187] for the enhancement of the anti-tumor effect of both donor-derived lymphocytes [188] and genetically engineered T cells [189-191]. These investigations have confirmed that beads are good to increase functional T cells that could achieve persistence *in vivo* post infusion. Adding CD137 Ab to α-CD3/CD28 beads (α-CD3/CD28/CD137 beads) has a more efficient growth of tumor-reactive $CD8^+$ CTLs over 2 weeks compared with α-CD3/CD28 beads, suggesting that the CD137 conjugation to well-established α-CD3/CD28 beads can progress the expansion ability of tumor-specific $CD8^+$ CTLs. This new artificial APC system is able to be simply created at GMP quality and is likely to be a helpful tool to develop large numbers of tumor-specific CTLs for cell-based therapies [160].

Both beads and antibodies are limiting factors that potentially constitute a hindrance for both cost and supply when large quantities of expanded T cells is required. Cell based artificial APC that has been engineered to express the required stimulatory (CD3) and costimulator (CD28, 4-1BB, and others) molecules provides an alternative option to expand T cells with high quality and quantity [192-195].

## USE CYTOKINES TO BOOST T CELL FUNCTIONS

Human T memory stem cell ($T_{SCM}$) is defined as CD45RO−, CD45RA+, CD28+, CD27+ CCR7+, CD62L+ and IL-7Rα+ T cells with increased levels of IL-2Rβ, LFA-1, CD95, and CXCR3, and exhibited a number of functions that distinctive of memory cells. $T_{SCM}$ showed an increased proliferative capacity, more efficient in reconstituting immunodeficient hosts, and superior anti-tumor activities in animal models as compared with known memory populations. The $T_{SCM}$ identification is directly associated with the vaccine design and T cell-based therapies [196]. $T_{SCM}$ cells can induce an effective tumor regression when a limited cell number is used [196, 197]. Tumor eradication possibly involves various components of the immune system; thus that the transferring T cells keep a constant immunological attack against tumor masses is reasonable. As a result, strategies that generate and expand $T_{SCM}$-like cells is useful to the development of successful T cell-based therapies [198]. It has been shown the success to *in vitro* differentiate, expand, and genetically modify CD8+ $T_{SCM}$ lymphocytes starting from naive precursors in clinically compliant conditions [199]. Human $T_{SCM}$ can be generated by α-CD3/CD28 stimulation with IL-7 and IL-15. Such $T_{SCM}$ displays an improved proliferative ability after ACT into immunodeficient mice and are the only T-cell subsets capable of expanding and mediating a GVHD on serial transplantation. These results represent the most convincing evidence that $T_{SCM}$ specially maintains stem cell–like characters among all human T cells, which would direct researchers in the field to properly investigate the $T_{SCM}$ "pluripotency" in clinical trials.

IL-12 is capable of provoking powerful anti-tumor immune responses [200]. The anti-tumor effects of IL-12 include anti-angiogenesis, improved lytic abilities of immune cells to destroy tumors and augmented production of IFN-γ [200]. However, the mechanisms of IL-12-mediated the anti-tumor immunity are still not clear. In B16 murine melanoma models, IL-12 engineered T cells obviate the demand for vaccine and exogenous IL-2, as well as reduce the cell number for the treatment [201, 202]. In addition, IL-12 delivered by T cells can activate a setting of change in DCs, MDSCs, and macrophages in tumors, which allows the detection of cross-presented TAA [203]. Moreover, the recognition between T cells and professional APCs activated by IL-12 in the tumor microenvironment is crucial in mediating the tumor regression [204]. These conclusions have shaped the basis for clinical trials to treat metastatic melanoma patients with IL-12–engineered TILs (ClinicalTrials.gov ID NCT01236573).

## INTEGRATE COSTIMULATORY IN CAR DESIGNS

ACT can be dramatically enhanced by using peripheral lymphocytes expressing antigen receptors that specifically recognize TAAs. T cells can be re-directed to specifically recognize TAA by two types of receptors: TCR and CAR. TCR is comprised of alpha and beta chains that recognize the MHC/peptide complex; CAR is a fusion protein that links the variable heavy and light chains of a scFv to the intracellular signaling domains of a TCR to recognize TAA on the surface of tumor cells without MHC restriction. CAR is resistant to a number of tumor-evasion mechanisms, including the MHC down-regulation, which would reduce Ag presentation. In addition to a wide application to treat patients with all MHC haplotypes due to unrestricted MHC matching property, the other advantage of CAR over TCR is that costimulatory signaling could be easily incorporated into the CAR structure by simply adding and stacking the intracellular signaling moiety of interested costimulatory molecules. Based on the costimulatroy signaling that incorporated, CAR is categorized into three different generations with increased costimulatory activity. The 1$^{st}$ generation CAR is the CAR utilized constructs made of an scFv linked to the transmembrane and intracellular signaling domains of either CD3ζ or FcRγ lacking the intracellular signaling domains of costimulatory molecules [165]. Early clinical trials by using the first generation CARs caused a temporary cell persistence with no clinical profit as well as no obvious side effects [205-208]. At this point, the "costimless" at least partially accounts for the poor persistence and poor treatment efficacy of the 1$^{st}$ generation CAR.

It is well known that ''Signal 2" (costimulation) is necessary for a complete T-cell activation [5, 6]. The therapeutic success of using CAR highly depends on the introduction of appropriate costimulation. The second generation CARs are incorporated with signaling domains derived from CD28 [155, 208, 209], OX40, 4-1BB, ICOS [158] and CD27 [161, 210]. The third generation CARs that are designed by adding two costimulatory molecules to the CAR together (mostly

CD28 and 4-1BB), have also been generated and tested [211-213]. The inclusion of costimulatory signals in tandem in a CAR would elicit an enhanced Ag-specific cytokine production and an increased target cell killing, as well as prevent apoptosis and facilitate the Ag-specific expansion of the T cells. Second generation CARs with either CD28 or 4-1BB signaling domain have been utilized in numerous clinical studies and interesting preliminary results have been obtained, by using CARs against CD19 to treat B cell leukemia and lymphoma [189-191, 214-216]. A third generation CAR against Her2/neo (ERBB2) [211] has been used in a clinical trial, which treated a colon cancer patient with lungs and liver metastasis, who was refractory to various standard treatments. The patient died five days after the treatment due to cytokine release from large numbers of administering cells, which accumulated in the lung directly following infusion by recognizing low levels of ERBB2 expressed on the epithelial cells of the lung [217]. The therapeutic potential and associated side effect of using the third generation CARs need to be further elucidated, and also, the safety concerns of using costimulation enhanced, new generation CARs are innumberable.

Due to the lack of costimulation, the first generation CAR with only the CD3ζ signaling domain has been proven to be ineffective in treating cancer patients. Adding costimulatory signaling to the CAR constructs increased the CAR-T cell function and survival, as well as the safety concerns of using these CAR targeting TAAs that are mostly self-antigens. Recent data showed that combinatorial Ag recognition with a stable signaling induces the abolition of selective tumors of the CAR-T cells [218]. In a mouse model of prostate tumor, by transducing T cells with both a CAR ($1^{st}$ generation), which gives suboptimal activation upon binding of an Ag with a chimeric costimulatory receptor (CCR, $3^{rd}$ generation without CD3ζ signaling moiety), which recognizes a second Ag, the co-transduced T cells could abolish tumors expressing both Ags, however, did not influence tumors expressing either Ag alone. This 'tumor-sensing' strategy is likely to extend the application and improve the potential therapies of CAR-T cells.

## CO-INHIBITION TO CO-STIMULATION SWITCH

The major challenge of treating cancer patients with any immunotherapies is the suppressive environments that tumor established to evade immune surveillance. Up-regulation of co-inhibitor molecules, including CTLA-4 and PD-1, is a common strategy that tumor uses. Antibodies that used to block these co-inhibitor signals have been widely tested in clinical trials to treat different cancer patients with very promising outcomes [219-222]. Systemic blockade of co-inhibitory signals by using blocking antibodies leads to an enhanced antitumor immunity at the expense of significant autoimmunity. Therefore, selective blockade of co-inhibitory signaling in tumor-specific T cells would be an ideal way to enhance antitumor immunity without causing systemic side effects of autoimmunity. The straightforward way of blocking the co-inhibitory signaling is by silencing the co-inhibitory molecules on the T cells. However, it tends to be a challenge by using current gene silencing technologies to achieve this goal. Making fusing chimeric proteins by exchanging cytoplasmic tail of co-inhibitor molecules with that of CD28, or other co-stimulatory molecules can potentially and selectively inhibit co-inhibitor function in tumor-reactive T cells by genetic modification. The inhibitory function of both PD-1 and CTLA4 were successfully blocked in T cells by transferring such chimeric switch receptors [156, 159]. PD1-CD28 chimeric switch receptor can keep the ability to bind PD-L1 or PD-L2, causing CD28 costimulation, instead of PD1 inhibition, as shown by increased the phosphorylation of ERK, the proliferative capacity, the cytokine secretion, and the expression of granzyme B. This PD1-CD28 chimera likely acts in a dominant-negative manner above endogenous PD-1 through contesting for available PD-L1/PD-L2, and by provoking the PD-1 effects through CD28 signaling [159]. Another group developed a novel CTLA4 mutant named CTLA4-CD28 chimera. This mutant was designed to deliver positive signal instead of the negative signal of CTLA4 and to compete with endogenous CTLA4 for binding to its ligand in a dominant-negative manner. Indeed, retroviral gene transfer of CTLA4-CD28 chimera of murine T cells enhanced cytokine production *in vitro*, and ACT of the tumor-reactive T cells to tumor-bearing mice potentiated therapeutic efficacy of T cells in 2 different syngeneic tumor models. Thus, CTLA4-CD28 chimera modification of T cells provides a novel strategy to facilitate adoptive T-cell therapy by breaking CTLA4-mediated T-cell tolerance [156].

## MODIFICATION OF T CELLS DIRECTLY TO ENHANCE THE COSTIMULATION

Modifying T cells with other molecules, in addition to TCR or CAR, is an attractive way to further enhance T cell functions. Targeting costimulation is always the priority, since, as mentioned above, the major challenge of treating cancer with immunotherapies is to overcome tumor suppressive environments. Tumor cells, by hijacking negative immune suppressive mechanisms, use all possible ways to prevent a full T cell activation through increasing the threshold for T cell activation or decreasing the stimulation signals. Therefore, the ultimate goal of manipulating T cells is to make T cells as sensitive as possible, or as less costimulation-dependent as possible during its tumor antigen-specific recognition and activation. Tumor makes T cell activated in a sub-optimal and thus T cell will undergo either anergy or apoptosis, unless costimulation is provided. Providing costimuation to T cells in tumor environment has been proven challenging, even by using either costimulatory molecule engineered tumor as vaccines [223-225] or systemic antibody administration [226, 227]. TAA-specific T cells constitutively expressing costimulatory ligands could compensate for the costimulatory deficit in the tumor microenvironment. Constitutively expressing costimulatory ligands directly involves with their respective receptors *in cis* (autocostimulation) as well as delivers bystander costimulation to other T cells (transcostimulation) [157]. T cells expressing both B7-1 and 4-1BBL strongly responded to tumor cells, resulting in tumor rejection. Besides costimulation of bystander T cells (transcostimulation), the effect of B7-1 and 4-1BBL binding to their own receptors at the immunological synapse of separated single cells (autocostimulation) is existed [157]. T cells constitutively expressing costimulatory ligands can improve cell-based therapies.

As mentioned above, Cbl-b regulates the essential for CD28 costimulation and the threshold of T- cell activation in response to weak peptide stimulation [91]. Since *cblb*$^{-/-}$ T cells showed a maximum activation and IL-2 production even in the absence of CD28 costimulation [90], ablating Cbl-b could potentially benefit T cells in targeting a tumor. In a clinical relevant setting that needs wide growth of a few tumor-specific CTLs, siRNA are used to knock down Cbl-b expression in two antigen-specific human CD8+/CD28- T cell lines [228]. Cbl-b siRNA-transduced T cells responded to a low-concentration peptide, suggesting that reducing Cbl-b expression in effector cells can improve the functional avidity of these T cells. CD8+/CD28- Cbl-b siRNA-transduced T cells produce IL-2, while unmodified CD8+/CD28- clones fail after antigen stimulation, suggesting Cbl-b siRNA-transduced T cells could be activated and secrete IL 2 bypassing the CD28 costimulation. Therefore, suppressing Cbl-b expression in effector cells with siRNA is likely to improve the therapeutic activity of such T cells, which can be used for cell-based cancer therapies.

Summary, T lymphocytes can be modified by gene transfer to express TCR or CAR to enhance their specific anti-tumor activities, which has been dramatically expanded in the treatment of a broad variety of cancers. T cell costimulation as a key element in activation, differentiation, survival, and effector function, has been extensively applied in T cell manufacture, CAR design and direct T cell modifications for the purpose of either directly boosting T cell antitumor activities or counteracting tumor suppressive microenvironment. Further improvement for T cell based ACT can be achieved by a proper manipulation of both costimulatory and cytokine molecules.

## ACKNOWLEDGEMENTS

This work was supported in part by NIH 2R01CA120409

## CONFLICT OF INTERESTS

The author has financial interests due to intellectual property and patents in the field of cell and gene therapy. Conflicts of interest are managed in accordance with University of Pennsylvania policy and oversight.

## REFERENCES

[1] Quill H, Schwartz RH. Stimulation of normal inducer T cell clones with antigen presented by purified Ia molecules in planar lipid membranes: specific induction of a long-lived state of proliferative nonresponsiveness. J Immunol 1987; 138(11): 3704-12.
[2] Mueller DL, Jenkins MK, Schwartz RH. An accessory cell-derived costimulatory signal acts independently of protein kinase C activation to allow T cell proliferation and prevent the induction of unresponsiveness. J Immunol 1989; 142(8): 2617-28.
[3] Jenkins MK, Chen CA, Jung G, Mueller DL, Schwartz RH. Inhibition of antigen-specific proliferation of type 1 murine T cell clones after stimulation with immobilized anti-CD3 monoclonal antibody. J Immunol 1990; 144(1): 16-22.
[4] Linsley PS, Ledbetter JA. The role of the CD28 receptor during T cell responses to antigen. Annl Rev Immunol 1993; 11: 191-212.
[5] June CH, Ledbetter JA, Gillespie MM, Lindsten T, Thompson CB. T-cell proliferation involving the CD28 pathway is associated with cyclosporine-resistant interleukin 2 gene expression. Mol Cell Biol 1987; 7(12): 4472-81.
[6] Mueller DL, Jenkins MK, Schwartz RH. Clonal expansion *versus* functional clonal inactivation: a costimulatory signalling pathway determines the outcome of T cell antigen receptor occupancy. Annl Rev Immunol 1989; 7: 445-80.
[7] Smith-Garvin JE, Koretzky GA, Jordan MS. T cell activation. Annl Rev Immunol 2009; 27: 591-619.
[8] Gmunder H, Lesslauer W. A 45-kDa human T-cell membrane glycoprotein functions in the regulation of cell proliferative responses. Eur J Biochem 1984; 142(1): 153-60.
[9] Dariavach P, Mattei MG, Golstein P, Lefranc MP. Human Ig superfamily CTLA-4 gene: chromosomal localization and identity of protein sequence between murine and human CTLA-4 cytoplasmic domains. Eur J Immunol 1988; 18(12): 1901-5.
[10] Hutloff A, Dittrich AM, Beier KC, Eljaschewitsch B, Kraft R, Anagnostopoulos I, *et al.* ICOS is an inducible T-cell co-stimulator structurally and functionally related to CD28. Nature 1999; 397(6716): 263-6.
[11] Ishida Y, Agata Y, Shibahara K, Honjo T. Induced expression of PD-1, a novel member of the immunoglobulin gene superfamily, upon programmed cell death. EMBO J 1992; 11(11): 3887-95.
[12] Watanabe N, Gavrieli M, Sedy JR, Yang J, Fallarino F, Loftin SK, *et al.* BTLA is a lymphocyte inhibitory receptor with similarities to CTLA-4 and PD-1. Nat Immunol 2003; 4(7): 670-9
[13] Rudd CE, Taylor A, Schneider H. CD28 and CTLA-4 coreceptor expression and signal transduction. Immunol Rev 2009; 229(1): 12-26.
[14] Shahinian A, Pfeffer K, Lee KP, Kundig TM, Kishihara K, Wakeham A, *et al.* Differential T cell costimulatory requirements in CD28-deficient mice. Science 1993; 261(5121): 609-12.
[15] Bachmann MF, Sebzda E, Kundig TM, Shahinian A, Speiser DE, Mak TW, *et al.* T cell responses are governed by avidity and co-stimulatory thresholds. Eur J Immunol 1996; 26(9): 2017-22.

[16] Bachmann MF, McKall-Faienza K, Schmits R, Bouchard D, Beach J, Speiser DE, *et al.* Distinct roles for LFA-1 and CD28 during activation of naive T cells: adhesion *versus* costimulation. Immunity 1997; 7(4): 549-57.

[17] Lindstein T, June CH, Ledbetter JA, Stella G, Thompson CB. Regulation of lymphokine messenger RNA stability by a surface-mediated T cell activation pathway. Science 1989; 244(4902): 339-43.

[18] Thompson CB, Lindsten T, Ledbetter JA, Kunkel SL, Young HA, Emerson SG, *et al.* CD28 activation pathway regulates the production of multiple T-cell-derived lymphokines/cytokines. Proc Natl Acad Sci USA 1989; 86(4): 1333-7.

[19] Ledbetter JA, Imboden JB, Schieven GL, Grosmaire LS, Rabinovitch PS, Lindsten T, *et al.* CD28 ligation in T-cell activation: evidence for two signal transduction pathways. Blood 1990; 75(7): 1531-9.

[20] Boise LH, Minn AJ, Noel PJ, June CH, Accavitti MA, Lindsten T, *et al.* CD28 costimulation can promote T cell survival by enhancing the expression of Bcl-XL. Immunity 1995; 3(1): 87-98.

[21] Kirchhoff S, Muller WW, Li-Weber M, Krammer PH. Up-regulation of c-FLIPshort and reduction of activation-induced cell death in CD28-costimulated human T cells. Eur J Immunol 2000; 30(10): 2765-74.

[22] Monks CR, Freiberg BA, Kupfer H, Sciaky N, Kupfer A. Three-dimensional segregation of supramolecular activation clusters in T cells. Nature 1998; 395(6697): 82-6.

[23] Huang J, Lo PF, Zal T, Gascoigne NR, Smith BA, Levin SD, *et al.* CD28 plays a critical role in the segregation of PKC theta within the immunologic synapse. Proc Natl Acad Sci USA 2002; 99(14): 9369-73.

[24] Dodson LF, Boomer JS, Deppong CM, Shah DD, Sim J, Bricker TL, *et al.* Targeted knock-in mice expressing mutations of CD28 reveal an essential pathway for costimulation. Mol Cell Biol 2009; 29(13): 3710-21.

[25] Paulos CM, Carpenito C, Plesa G, Suhoski MM, Varela-Rohena A, Golovina TN, *et al.* The inducible costimulator (ICOS) is critical for the development of human T(H)17 cells. Sci Transl Med 2010; 2(55): 55ra78.

[26] Simpson TR, Quezada SA, Allison JP. Regulation of CD4 T cell activation and effector function by inducible costimulator (ICOS). Curr Opin Immunol 2010; 22(3): 326-32.

[27] Kroenke MA, Eto D, Locci M, Cho M, Davidson T, Haddad EK, *et al.* Bcl6 and Maf cooperate to instruct human follicular helper CD4 T cell differentiation. J Immunol 2012; 188(8): 3734-44.

[28] Choi YS, Kageyama R, Eto D, Escobar TC, Johnston RJ, Monticelli L, *et al.* ICOS receptor instructs T follicular helper cell *versus* effector cell differentiation *via* induction of the transcriptional repressor Bcl6. Immunity 2011; 34(6): 932-46.

[29] Yao S, Zhu Y, Zhu G, Augustine M, Zheng L, Goode DJ, *et al.* B7-h2 is a costimulatory ligand for CD28 in human. Immunity 2011; 34(5): 729-40.

[30] Walunas TL, Lenschow DJ, Bakker CY, Linsley PS, Freeman GJ, Green JM, *et al.* CTLA-4 can function as a negative regulator of T cell activation. Immunity 1994; 1(5): 405-13.

[31] Krummel MF, Allison JP. CD28 and CTLA-4 have opposing effects on the response of T cells to stimulation. J Exp Med 1995; 182(2): 459-65.

[32] Driessens G, Kline J, Gajewski TF. Costimulatory and coinhibitory receptors in anti-tumor immunity. Immunol Rev 2009; 229(1): 126-44.

[33] Tivol EA, Borriello F, Schweitzer AN, Lynch WP, Bluestone JA, Sharpe AH. Loss of CTLA-4 leads to massive lymphoproliferation and fatal multiorgan tissue destruction, revealing a critical negative regulatory role of CTLA-4. Immunity 1995; 3(5): 541-7.

[34] Waterhouse P, Penninger JM, Timms E, Wakeham A, Shahinian A, Lee KP, *et al.* Lymphoproliferative disorders with early lethality in mice deficient in Ctla-4. Science 1995; 270(5238): 985-8.

[35] Salomon B, Bluestone JA. Complexities of CD28/B7: CTLA-4 costimulatory pathways in autoimmunity and transplantation. Annl Rev Immunol 2001; 19: 225-52.

[36] Chambers CA, Kuhns MS, Egen JG, Allison JP. CTLA-4-mediated inhibition in regulation of T cell responses: mechanisms and manipulation in tumor immunotherapy. Annl Rev Immunol 2001; 19: 565-94.

[37] Salomon B, Lenschow DJ, Rhee L, Ashourian N, Singh B, Sharpe A, *et al.* B7/CD28 costimulation is essential for the homeostasis of the CD4+CD25+ immunoregulatory T cells that control autoimmune diabetes. Immunity 2000; 12(4): 431-40.

[38] Takahashi T, Tagami T, Yamazaki S, Uede T, Shimizu J, Sakaguchi N, *et al.* Immunologic self-tolerance maintained by CD25(+)CD4(+) regulatory T cells constitutively expressing cytotoxic T lymphocyte-associated antigen 4. J Exp Med 2000; 192(2): 303-10.

[39] Freeman GJ, Wherry EJ, Ahmed R, Sharpe AH. Reinvigorating exhausted HIV-specific T cells *via* PD-1-PD-1 ligand blockade. J Exp Med 2006; 203(10): 2223-7.
[40] Francisco LM, Sage PT, Sharpe AH. The PD-1 pathway in tolerance and autoimmunity. Immunol Rev 2010; 236: 219-42.
[41] Sharpe AH, Wherry EJ, Ahmed R, Freeman GJ. The function of programmed cell death 1 and its ligands in regulating autoimmunity and infection. Nat Immunol 2007; 8(3): 239-45.
[42] Nurieva RI, Liu X, Dong C. Yin-Yang of costimulation: crucial controls of immune tolerance and function. Immunol Rev 2009; 229(1): 88-100.
[43] Chemnitz JM, Parry RV, Nichols KE, June CH, Riley JL. SHP-1 and SHP-2 associate with immunoreceptor tyrosine-based switch motif of programmed death 1 upon primary human T cell stimulation, but only receptor ligation prevents T cell activation. J Immunol 2004; 173(2): 945-54
[44] Riley JL. PD-1 signaling in primary T cells. Immunol Rev 2009; 229(1): 114-25.
[45] Freeman GJ, Long AJ, Iwai Y, Bourque K, Chernova T, Nishimura H, *et al.* Engagement of the PD-1 immunoinhibitory receptor by a novel B7 family member leads to negative regulation of lymphocyte activation. J Exp Med 2000; 192(7): 1027-34.
[46] Carter L, Fouser LA, Jussif J, Fitz L, Deng B, Wood CR, *et al.* PD-1: PD-L inhibitory pathway affects both CD4(+) and CD8(+) T cells and is overcome by IL-2. Eur J Immunol 2002; 32(3): 634-43.
[47] Nurieva R, Thomas S, Nguyen T, Martin-Orozco N, Wang Y, Kaja MK, *et al.* T-cell tolerance or function is determined by combinatorial costimulatory signals. EMBO J 2006; 25(11): 2623-33.
[48] Parry RV, Chemnitz JM, Frauwirth KA, Lanfranco AR, Braunstein I, Kobayashi SV, *et al.* CTLA-4 and PD-1 receptors inhibit T-cell activation by distinct mechanisms. Mol Cell Biol 2005; 25(21): 9543-53.
[49] Bennett F, Luxenberg D, Ling V, Wang IM, Marquette K, Lowe D, *et al.* Program death-1 engagement upon TCR activation has distinct effects on costimulation and cytokine-driven proliferation: attenuation of ICOS, IL-4, and IL-21, but not CD28, IL-7, and IL-15 responses. J Immunol 2003; 170(2): 711-8.
[50] Taylor PA, Lees CJ, Fournier S, Allison JP, Sharpe AH, Blazar BR. B7 expression on T cells down-regulates immune responses through CTLA-4 ligation *via* T-T interactions [corrections]. J Immunol 2004; 172(1): 34-9.
[51] Paust S, Lu L, McCarty N, Cantor H. Engagement of B7 on effector T cells by regulatory T cells prevents autoimmune disease. Proc Natl Acad Sci USA 2004; 101(28): 10398-403.
[52] Butte MJ, Keir ME, Phamduy TB, Sharpe AH, Freeman GJ. Programmed death-1 ligand 1 interacts specifically with the B7-1 costimulatory molecule to inhibit T cell responses. Immunity 2007; 27(1): 111-22.
[53] Park JJ, Omiya R, Matsumura Y, Sakoda Y, Kuramasu A, Augustine MM, *et al.* B7-H1/CD80 interaction is required for the induction and maintenance of peripheral T-cell tolerance. Blood 2010; 116(8): 1291-8.
[54] Croft M, Duan W, Choi H, Eun SY, Madireddi S, Mehta A. TNF superfamily in inflammatory disease: translating basic insights. Trends in immunology 2012; 33(3): 144-52.
[55] Paterson DJ, Jefferies WA, Green JR, Brandon MR, Corthesy P, Puklavec M, *et al.* Antigens of activated rat T lymphocytes including a molecule of 50,000 Mr detected only on CD4 positive T blasts. Mol Immunol 1987; 24(12): 1281-90.
[56] Stuber E, Neurath M, Calderhead D, Fell HP, Strober W. Cross-linking of OX40 ligand, a member of the TNF/NGF cytokine family, induces proliferation and differentiation in murine splenic B cells. Immunity 1995; 2(5): 507-21.
[57] Ohshima Y, Tanaka Y, Tozawa H, Takahashi Y, Maliszewski C, Delespesse G. Expression and function of OX40 ligand on human dendritic cells. J Immunol 1997; 159(8): 3838-48.
[58] Murata K, Ishii N, Takano H, Miura S, Ndhlovu LC, Nose M, *et al.* Impairment of antigen-presenting cell function in mice lacking expression of OX40 ligand. J Exp Med 2000; 191(2): 365-74.
[59] Rogers PR, Song J, Gramaglia I, Killeen N, Croft M. OX40 promotes Bcl-xL and Bcl-2 expression and is essential for long-term survival of CD4 T cells. Immunity 2001; 15(3): 445-55.
[60] Walker LS, Gulbranson-Judge A, Flynn S, Brocker T, Raykundalia C, Goodall M, *et al.* Compromised OX40 function in CD28-deficient mice is linked with failure to develop CXC chemokine receptor 5-positive CD4 cells and germinal centers. J Exp Med 1999; 190(8): 1115-22.
[61] Croft M. Costimulation of T cells by OX40, 4-1BB, and CD27. Cytokine & growth factor reviews 2003; 14(3-4): 265-73.
[62] Vu MD, Xiao X, Gao W, Degauque N, Chen M, Kroemer A, *et al.* OX40 costimulation turns off Foxp3+ Tregs. Blood 2007; 110(7): 2501-10.

[63] So T, Croft M. Cutting edge: OX40 inhibits TGF-beta- and antigen-driven conversion of naive CD4 T cells into CD25+Foxp3+ T cells. J Immunol 2007; 179(3): 1427-30.
[64] Salek-Ardakani S, Song J, Halteman BS, Jember AG, Akiba H, Yagita H, *et al.* OX40 (CD134) controls memory T helper 2 cells that drive lung inflammation. J Exp Med 2003; 198(2): 315-24.
[65] Song A, Tang X, Harms KM, Croft M. OX40 and Bcl-xL promote the persistence of CD8 T cells to recall tumor-associated antigen. J Immunol 2005; 175(6): 3534-41.
[66] Song J, Salek-Ardakani S, Rogers PR, Cheng M, Van Parijs L, Croft M. The costimulation-regulated duration of PKB activation controls T cell longevity. Nat Immunol 2004; 5(2): 150-8.
[67] Song J, So T, Cheng M, Tang X, Croft M. Sustained survivin expression from OX40 costimulatory signals drives T cell clonal expansion. Immunity 2005; 22(5): 621-31.
[68] Song J, Salek-Ardakani S, So T, Croft M. The kinases aurora B and mTOR regulate the G1-S cell cycle progression of T lymphocytes. Nat Immunol 2007; 8(1): 64-73.
[69] Kwon BS, Weissman SM. cDNA sequences of two inducible T-cell genes. Proc Natl Acad Sci USA 1989; 86(6): 1963-7.
[70] Vinay DS, Kwon BS. 4-1BB signaling beyond T cells. Cellular & Mol Immunol 2011; 8(4): 281-4.
[71] Vinay DS, Kwon BS. Role of 4-1BB in immune responses. Seminars in Immunology 1998; 10(6): 481-9.
[72] Croft M. Co-stimulatory members of the TNFR family: keys to effective T-cell immunity? Nat Rev Immunol 2003; 3(8): 609-20.
[73] Watts TH. TNF/TNFR family members in costimulation of T cell responses. Annl Rev Immunol 2005; 23: 23-68.
[74] Goodwin RG, Din WS, Davis-Smith T, Anderson DM, Gimpel SD, Sato TA, *et al.* Molecular cloning of a ligand for the inducible T cell gene 4-1BB: a member of an emerging family of cytokines with homology to tumor necrosis factor. Eur J Immunol 1993; 23(10): 2631-41.
[75] Gramaglia I, Cooper D, Miner KT, Kwon BS, Croft M. Co-stimulation of antigen-specific CD4 T cells by 4-1BB ligand. Eur J Immunol 2000; 30(2): 392-402.
[76] Cannons JL, Lau P, Ghumman B, DeBenedette MA, Yagita H, Okumura K, *et al.* 4-1BB ligand induces cell division, sustains survival, and enhances effector function of CD4 and CD8 T cells with similar efficacy. J Immunol 2001; 167(3): 1313-24.
[77] Zhu Y, Zhu G, Luo L, Flies AS, Chen L. CD137 stimulation delivers an antigen-independent growth signal for T lymphocytes with memory phenotype. Blood 2007; 109(11): 4882-9.
[78] Wilcox RA, Chapoval AI, Gorski KS, Otsuji M, Shin T, Flies DB, *et al.* Cutting edge: Expression of functional CD137 receptor by dendritic cells. J Immunol 2002; 168(9): 4262-7.
[79] van Lier RA, Borst J, Vroom TM, Klein H, Van Mourik P, Zeijlemaker WP, *et al.* Tissue distribution and biochemical and functional properties of Tp55 (CD27), a novel T cell differentiation antigen. J Immunol 1987; 139(5): 1589-96.
[80] Hendriks J, Xiao Y, Borst J. CD27 promotes survival of activated T cells and complements CD28 in generation and establishment of the effector T cell pool. J Exp Med 2003; 198(9): 1369-80.
[81] Hendriks J, Gravestein LA, Tesselaar K, van Lier RA, Schumacher TN, Borst J. CD27 is required for generation and long-term maintenance of T cell immunity. Nat Immunol 2000; 1(5): 433-40.
[82] Keller AM, Xiao Y, Peperzak V, Naik SH, Borst J. Costimulatory ligand CD70 allows induction of CD8+ T-cell immunity by immature dendritic cells in a vaccination setting. Blood 2009; 113(21): 5167-75.
[83] Sharpe AH. Mechanisms of costimulation. Immunol Rev 2009; 229(1): 5-11.
[84] Curtsinger JM, Schmidt CS, Mondino A, Lins DC, Kedl RM, Jenkins MK, *et al.* Inflammatory cytokines provide a third signal for activation of naive CD4+ and CD8+ T cells. J Immunol 1999; 162(6): 3256-62.
[85] Curtsinger JM, Mescher MF. Inflammatory cytokines as a third signal for T cell activation. Curr Opin Immunol 2010; 22(3): 333-40.
[86] Pape KA, Khoruts A, Mondino A, Jenkins MK. Inflammatory cytokines enhance the *in vivo* clonal expansion and differentiation of antigen-activated CD4+ T cells. J Immunol 1997; 159(2): 591-8
[87] Schmidt CS, Mescher MF. Peptide antigen priming of naive, but not memory, CD8 T cells requires a third signal that can be provided by IL-12. J Immunol 2002; 168(11): 5521-9.
[88] Fang D, Liu YC. Proteolysis-independent regulation of PI3K by Cbl-b-mediated ubiquitination in T cells. Nat Immunol 2001; 2(9): 870-5.
[89] Li D, Gal I, Vermes C, Alegre ML, Chong AS, Chen L, *et al.* Cutting edge: Cbl-b: one of the key molecules tuning CD28- and CTLA-4-mediated T cell costimulation. J Immunol 2004; 173(12): 7135-9.

[90] Chiang YJ, Kole HK, Brown K, Naramura M, Fukuhara S, Hu RJ, *et al.* Cbl-b regulates the CD28 dependence of T-cell activation. Nature 2000; 403(6766): 216-20.

[91] Gronski MA, Boulter JM, Moskophidis D, Nguyen LT, Holmberg K, Elford AR, *et al.* TCR affinity and negative regulation limit autoimmunity. Nat Med 2004; 10(11): 1234-9.

[92] Fang D, Wang HY, Fang N, Altman Y, Elly C, Liu YC. Cbl-b, a RING-type E3 ubiquitin ligase, targets phosphatidylinositol 3-kinase for ubiquitination in T cells. J Biol Chem 2001; 276(7): 4872-8.

[93] Zhang J, Bardos T, Li D, Gal I, Vermes C, Xu J, *et al.* Cutting edge: regulation of T cell activation threshold by CD28 costimulation through targeting Cbl-b for ubiquitination. J Immunol 2002; 169(5): 2236-40.

[94] Gruber T, Hermann-Kleiter N, Hinterleitner R, Fresser F, Schneider R, Gastl G, *et al.* PKC-theta modulates the strength of T cell responses by targeting Cbl-b for ubiquitination and degradation. Science Signaling 2009; 2(76): ra30.

[95] Bachmaier K, Krawczyk C, Kozieradzki I, Kong YY, Sasaki T, Oliveira-dos-Santos A, *et al.* Negative regulation of lymphocyte activation and autoimmunity by the molecular adaptor Cbl-b. Nature 2000; 403(6766): 211-6.

[96] Mantovani A, Allavena P, Sica A, Balkwill F. Cancer-related inflammation. Nature 2008; 454(7203): 436-44.

[97] Khong HT, Restifo NP. Natural selection of tumor variants in the generation of "tumor escape" phenotypes. Nat Immunol 2002; 3(11): 999-1005.

[98] Topfer K, Kempe S, Muller N, Schmitz M, Bachmann M, Cartellieri M, *et al.* Tumor evasion from T cell surveillance. J Biomedicine & Biotechnol 2011; 2011: 918471.

[99] Kerkar SP, Restifo NP. Cellular constituents of immune escape within the tumor microenvironment. Cancer Res 2012; 72(13): 3125-30.

[100] Kurts C, Robinson BW, Knolle PA. Cross-priming in health and disease. Nat Rev Immunol 2010; 10(6): 403-14.

[101] Kurts C, Kosaka H, Carbone FR, Miller JF, Heath WR. Class I-restricted cross-presentation of exogenous self-antigens leads to deletion of autoreactive CD8(+) T cells. J Exp Med 1997; 186(2): 239-45.

[102] Troy AJ, Summers KL, Davidson PJ, Atkinson CH, Hart DN. Minimal recruitment and activation of dendritic cells within renal cell carcinoma. Clin Cancer Res 1998; 4(3): 585-93.

[103] Enk AH, Jonuleit H, Saloga J, Knop J. Dendritic cells as mediators of tumor-induced tolerance in metastatic melanoma. International journal of cancer Journal international du cancer 1997; 73(3): 309-16.

[104] Gabrilovich DI, Corak J, Ciernik IF, Kavanaugh D, Carbone DP. Decreased antigen presentation by dendritic cells in patients with breast cancer. Clin Cancer Res 1997; 3(3): 483-90.

[105] Maleno I, Cabrera CM, Cabrera T, Paco L, Lopez-Nevot MA, Collado A, *et al.* Distribution of HLA class I altered phenotypes in colorectal carcinomas: high frequency of HLA haplotype loss associated with loss of heterozygosity in chromosome region 6p21. Immunogenetics 2004; 56(4): 244-53.

[106] Maleno I, Romero JM, Cabrera T, Paco L, Aptsiauri N, Cozar JM, *et al.* LOH at 6p21.3 region and HLA class I altered phenotypes in bladder carcinomas. Immunogenetics 2006; 58(7): 503-10.

[107] Bicknell DC, Rowan A, Bodmer WF. Beta 2-microglobulin gene mutations: a study of established colorectal cell lines and fresh tumors. Proc Natl Acad Sci USA 1994; 91(11): 4751-5.

[108] Hicklin DJ, Wang Z, Arienti F, Rivoltini L, Parmiani G, Ferrone S. beta2-Microglobulin mutations, HLA class I antigen loss, and tumor progression in melanoma. J Clin Invest 1998; 101(12): 2720-9.

[109] Koch J, Tampe R. The macromolecular peptide-loading complex in MHC class I-dependent antigen presentation. Cell Mol Life Sci 2006; 63(6): 653-62.

[110] Manning J, Indrova M, Lubyova B, Pribylova H, Bieblova J, Hejnar J, *et al.* Induction of MHC class I molecule cell surface expression and epigenetic activation of antigen-processing machinery components in a murine model for human papilloma virus 16-associated tumours. Immunology 2008; 123(2): 218-27.

[111] Seliger B. Molecular mechanisms of MHC class I abnormalities and APM components in human tumors. Cancer Immunol Immunother 2008; 57(11): 1719-26.

[112] Medema JP, de Jong J, Peltenburg LT, Verdegaal EM, Gorter A, Bres SA, *et al.* Blockade of the granzyme B/perforin pathway through overexpression of the serine protease inhibitor PI-9/SPI-6 constitutes a mechanism for immune escape by tumors. Proc Natl Acad Sci USA 2001; 98(20): 11515-20.

[113] van Houdt IS, Oudejans JJ, van den Eertwegh AJ, Baars A, Vos W, Bladergroen BA, *et al.* Expression of the apoptosis inhibitor protease inhibitor 9 predicts clinical outcome in vaccinated patients with stage III and IV melanoma. Clin Cancer Res 2005; 11(17): 6400-7.

[114] Griffith TS, Chin WA, Jackson GC, Lynch DH, Kubin MZ. Intracellular regulation of TRAIL-induced apoptosis in human melanoma cells. J Immunol 1998; 161(6): 2833-40.
[115] Zhang X, Jin TG, Yang H, DeWolf WC, Khosravi-Far R, Olumi AF. Persistent c-FLIP(L) expression is necessary and sufficient to maintain resistance to tumor necrosis factor-related apoptosis-inducing ligand-mediated apoptosis in prostate cancer. Cancer Res 2004; 64(19): 7086-91.
[116] Volkmann M, Schiff JH, Hajjar Y, Otto G, Stilgenbauer F, Fiehn W, *et al.* Loss of CD95 expression is linked to most but not all p53 mutants in European hepatocellular carcinoma. J Mol Med (Berl) 2001; 79(10): 594-600.
[117] Kehrl JH, Wakefield LM, Roberts AB, Jakowlew S, Alvarez-Mon M, Derynck R, *et al.* Production of transforming growth factor beta by human T lymphocytes and its potential role in the regulation of T cell growth. J Exp Med 1986; 163(5): 1037-50.
[118] Ranges GE, Figari IS, Espevik T, Palladino MA, Jr. Inhibition of cytotoxic T cell development by transforming growth factor beta and reversal by recombinant tumor necrosis factor alpha. J Exp Med 1987; 166(4): 991-8.
[119] di Bari MG, Lutsiak ME, Takai S, Mostbock S, Farsaci B, Semnani RT, *et al.* TGF-beta modulates the functionality of tumor-infiltrating CD8+ T cells through effects on TCR signaling and Spred1 expression. Cancer Immunol Immunother 2009; 58(11): 1809-18.
[120] Thomas DA, Massague J. TGF-beta directly targets cytotoxic T cell functions during tumor evasion of immune surveillance. Cancer cell 2005; 8(5): 369-80.
[121] Walker MR, Kasprowicz DJ, Gersuk VH, Benard A, Van Landeghen M, Buckner JH, *et al.* Induction of FoxP3 and acquisition of T regulatory activity by stimulated human CD4+CD25- T cells. J Clin Invest 2003; 112(9): 1437-43.
[122] Greenhough A, Smartt HJ, Moore AE, Roberts HR, Williams AC, Paraskeva C, *et al.* The COX-2/PGE2 pathway: key roles in the hallmarks of cancer and adaptation to the tumour microenvironment. Carcinogenesis 2009; 30(3): 377-86.
[123] Pockaj BA, Basu GD, Pathangey LB, Gray RJ, Hernandez JL, Gendler SJ, *et al.* Reduced T-cell and dendritic cell function is related to cyclooxygenase-2 overexpression and prostaglandin E2 secretion in patients with breast cancer. Annals of surgical oncology 2004; 11(3): 328-39.
[124] Baratelli F, Lin Y, Zhu L, Yang SC, Heuze-Vourc'h N, Zeng G, *et al.* Prostaglandin E2 induces FOXP3 gene expression and T regulatory cell function in human CD4+ T cells. J Immunol 2005; 175(3): 1483-90.
[125] Perillo NL, Pace KE, Seilhamer JJ, Baum LG. Apoptosis of T cells mediated by galectin-1. Nature 1995; 378(6558): 736-9.
[126] Chung CD, Patel VP, Moran M, Lewis LA, Miceli MC. Galectin-1 induces partial TCR zeta-chain phosphorylation and antagonizes processive TCR signal transduction. J Immunol 2000; 165(7): 3722-9.
[127] Sakaguchi S, Ono M, Setoguchi R, Yagi H, Hori S, Fehervari Z, *et al.* Foxp3+ CD25+ CD4+ natural regulatory T cells in dominant self-tolerance and autoimmune disease. Immunol Rev 2006; 212: 8-27.
[128] Curiel TJ, Coukos G, Zou L, Alvarez X, Cheng P, Mottram P, *et al.* Specific recruitment of regulatory T cells in ovarian carcinoma fosters immune privilege and predicts reduced survival. Nat Med 2004; 10(9): 942-9.
[129] Priglinger SG, Wolf AH, Kreutzer TC, Kook D, Hofer A, Strauss RW, *et al.* Intravitreal bevacizumab injections for treatment of central retinal vein occlusion: six-month results of a prospective trial. Retina 2007; 27(8): 1004-12.
[130] Shevach EM. Fatal attraction: tumors beckon regulatory T cells. Nat Med 2004; 10(9): 900-1.
[131] Zou W. Regulatory T cells, tumour immunity and immunotherapy. Nat Rev Immunol 2006; 6(4): 295-307.
[132] Siddiqui SA, Frigola X, Bonne-Annee S, Mercader M, Kuntz SM, Krambeck AE, *et al.* Tumor-infiltrating Foxp3-CD4+CD25+ T cells predict poor survival in renal cell carcinoma. Clin Cancer Res 2007; 13(7): 2075-81.
[133] Bluestone JA, Abbas AK. Natural *versus* adaptive regulatory T cells. Nat Rev Immunol 2003; 3(3): 253-7.
[134] Fehervari Z, Sakaguchi S. CD4+ Tregs and immune control. J Clin Invest 2004; 114(9): 1209-17.
[135] Gattinoni L, Finkelstein SE, Klebanoff CA, Antony PA, Palmer DC, Spiess PJ, *et al.* Removal of homeostatic cytokine sinks by lymphodepletion enhances the efficacy of adoptively transferred tumor-specific CD8+ T cells. J Exp Med 2005; 202(7): 907-12.
[136] Tiemessen MM, Jagger AL, Evans HG, van Herwijnen MJ, John S, Taams LS. CD4+CD25+Foxp3+ regulatory T cells induce alternative activation of human monocytes/macrophages. Proc Natl Acad Sci USA 2007; 104(49): 19446-51.

[137] Murdoch C, Muthana M, Coffelt SB, Lewis CE. The role of myeloid cells in the promotion of tumour angiogenesis. Nat Rev Cancer 2008; 8(8): 618-31.

[138] Ostrand-Rosenberg S, Sinha P. Myeloid-derived suppressor cells: linking inflammation and cancer. J Immunol 2009; 182(8): 4499-506.

[139] Sica A, Bronte V. Altered macrophage differentiation and immune dysfunction in tumor development. J Clin Invest 2007; 117(5): 1155-66.

[140] Marigo I, Dolcetti L, Serafini P, Zanovello P, Bronte V. Tumor-induced tolerance and immune suppression by myeloid derived suppressor cells. Immunol Rev 2008; 222: 162-79.

[141] Sinha P, Clements VK, Fulton AM, Ostrand-Rosenberg S. Prostaglandin E2 promotes tumor progression by inducing myeloid-derived suppressor cells. Cancer Res 2007; 67(9): 4507-13.

[142] Bunt SK, Sinha P, Clements VK, Leips J, Ostrand-Rosenberg S. Inflammation induces myeloid-derived suppressor cells that facilitate tumor progression. J Immunol 2006; 176(1): 284-90.

[143] Gabrilovich DI, Nagaraj S. Myeloid-derived suppressor cells as regulators of the immune system. Nat Rev Immunol 2009; 9(3): 162-74.

[144] Srivastava MK, Sinha P, Clements VK, Rodriguez P, Ostrand-Rosenberg S. Myeloid-derived suppressor cells inhibit T-cell activation by depleting cystine and cysteine. Cancer Res 2010; 70(1): 68-77.

[145] Huang B, Pan PY, Li Q, Sato AI, Levy DE, Bromberg J, *et al.* Gr-1+CD115+ immature myeloid suppressor cells mediate the development of tumor-induced T regulatory cells and T-cell anergy in tumor-bearing host. Cancer Res 2006; 66(2): 1123-31.

[146] Viola A, Bronte V. Metabolic mechanisms of cancer-induced inhibition of immune responses. Seminars in cancer biology 2007; 17(4): 309-16.

[147] Munn DH, Mellor AL. Indoleamine 2,3-dioxygenase and tumor-induced tolerance. J Clin Invest 2007; 117(5): 1147-54.

[148] Qian BZ, Pollard JW. Macrophage diversity enhances tumor progression and metastasis. Cell 2010; 141(1): 39-51.

[149] Biswas SK, Mantovani A. Macrophage plasticity and interaction with lymphocyte subsets: cancer as a paradigm. Nat Immunol 2010; 11(10): 889-96.

[150] Gabrilovich DI, Ostrand-Rosenberg S, Bronte V. Coordinated regulation of myeloid cells by tumours. Nat Rev Immunol 2012; 12(4): 253-68.

[151] Mantovani A, Sica A. Macrophages, innate immunity and cancer: balance, tolerance, and diversity. Curr Opin Immunol 2010; 22(2): 231-7.

[152] Gabrilovich D. Mechanisms and functional significance of tumour-induced dendritic-cell defects. Nat Rev Immunol 2004; 4(12): 941-52.

[153] Munn DH, Sharma MD, Lee JR, Jhaver KG, Johnson TS, Keskin DB, *et al.* Potential regulatory function of human dendritic cells expressing indoleamine 2,3-dioxygenase. Science 2002; 297(5588): 1867-70.

[154] Levine BL, Bernstein WB, Connors M, Craighead N, Lindsten T, Thompson CB, *et al.* Effects of CD28 costimulation on long-term proliferation of CD4+ T cells in the absence of exogenous feeder cells. J Immunol 1997; 159(12): 5921-30.

[155] Maher J, Brentjens RJ, Gunset G, Riviere I, Sadelain M. Human T-lymphocyte cytotoxicity and proliferation directed by a single chimeric TCRzeta/CD28 receptor. Nat Biotechnol 2002; 20(1): 70-5.

[156] Shin JH, Park HB, Oh YM, Lim DP, Lee JE, Seo HH, *et al.* Positive conversion of negative signaling of CTLA4 potentiates antitumor efficacy of adoptive T-cell therapy in murine tumor models. Blood 2012; 119(24): 5678-87.

[157] Stephan MT, Ponomarev V, Brentjens RJ, Chang AH, Dobrenkov KV, Heller G, *et al.* T cell-encoded CD80 and 4-1BBL induce auto- and transcostimulation, resulting in potent tumor rejection. Nat Med 2007; 13(12): 1440-9.

[158] Finney HM, Akbar AN, Lawson AD. Activation of resting human primary T cells with chimeric receptors: costimulation from CD28, inducible costimulator, CD134, and CD137 in series with signals from the TCR zeta chain. J Immunol 2004; 172(1): 104-13.

[159] Prosser ME, Brown CE, Shami AF, Forman SJ, Jensen MC. Tumor PD-L1 co-stimulates primary human CD8(+) cytotoxic T cells modified to express a PD1: CD28 chimeric receptor. Mol Immunol 2012; 51(3-4): 263-72.

[160] Teschner D, Wenzel G, Distler E, Schnurer E, Theobald M, Neurauter AA, *et al.* *In vitro* stimulation and expansion of human tumour-reactive CD8+ cytotoxic T lymphocytes by anti-CD3/CD28/CD137 magnetic beads. Scandinavian journal of immunology 2011; 74(2): 155-64.

[161] Shaffer DR, Savoldo B, Yi Z, Chow KK, Kakarla S, Spencer DM, *et al.* T cells redirected against CD70 for the immunotherapy of CD70-positive malignancies. Blood 2011; 117(16): 4304-14.

[162] Dudley ME, Wunderlich JR, Robbins PF, Yang JC, Hwu P, Schwartzentruber DJ, *et al.* Cancer regression and autoimmunity in patients after clonal repopulation with antitumor lymphocytes. Science 2002; 298(5594): 850-4.

[163] Rosenberg SA, Restifo NP, Yang JC, Morgan RA, Dudley ME. Adoptive cell transfer: a clinical path to effective cancer immunotherapy. Nat Rev Cancer 2008; 8(4): 299-308.

[164] Hunder NN, Wallen H, Cao J, Hendricks DW, Reilly JZ, Rodmyre R, *et al.* Treatment of metastatic melanoma with autologous CD4+ T cells against NY-ESO-1. New Eng J Med 2008; 358(25): 2698-703.

[165] Eshhar Z, Waks T, Gross G, Schindler DG. Specific activation and targeting of cytotoxic lymphocytes through chimeric single chains consisting of antibody-binding domains and the gamma or zeta subunits of the immunoglobulin and T-cell receptors. Proc Natl Acad Sci USA 1993; 90(2): 720-4.

[166] Zhao Y, Zheng Z, Robbins PF, Khong HT, Rosenberg SA, Morgan RA. Primary human lymphocytes transduced with NY-ESO-1 antigen-specific TCR genes recognize and kill diverse human tumor cell lines. J Immunol 2005; 174(7): 4415-23.

[167] Zhao Y, Zheng Z, Cohen CJ, Gattinoni L, Palmer DC, Restifo NP, *et al.* High-efficiency transfection of primary human and mouse T lymphocytes using RNA electroporation. Mol Ther 2006; 13(1): 151-9.

[168] Morgan RA, Dudley ME, Wunderlich JR, Hughes MS, Yang JC, Sherry RM, *et al.* Cancer regression in patients after transfer of genetically engineered lymphocytes. Science 2006; 314(5796): 126-9.

[169] Robbins PF, Morgan RA, Feldman SA, Yang JC, Sherry RM, Dudley ME, *et al.* Tumor regression in patients with metastatic synovial cell sarcoma and melanoma using genetically engineered lymphocytes reactive with NY-ESO-1. J Clin Oncol 2011; 29(7): 917-24.

[170] June CH. Adoptive T cell therapy for cancer in the clinic. J Clin Invest 2007; 117(6): 1466-76.

[171] Louis CU, Savoldo B, Dotti G, Pule M, Yvon E, Myers GD, *et al.* Antitumor activity and long-term fate of chimeric antigen receptor-positive T cells in patients with neuroblastoma. Blood 2011; 118(23): 6050-6.

[172] Restifo NP, Dudley ME, Rosenberg SA. Adoptive immunotherapy for cancer: harnessing the T cell response. Nat Rev Immunol 2012; 12(4): 269-81.

[173] Gattinoni L, Klebanoff CA, Palmer DC, Wrzesinski C, Kerstann K, Yu Z, *et al.* Acquisition of full effector function *in vitro* paradoxically impairs the *in vivo* antitumor efficacy of adoptively transferred CD8+ T cells. J Clin Invest 2005; 115(6): 1616-26.

[174] Besser MJ, Shapira-Frommer R, Treves AJ, Zippel D, Itzhaki O, Hershkovitz L, *et al.* Clinical responses in a phase II study using adoptive transfer of short-term cultured tumor infiltration lymphocytes in metastatic melanoma patients. Clin Cancer Res 2010; 16(9): 2646-55.

[175] Dudley ME, Gross CA, Somerville RP, Hong Y, Schaub NP, Rosati SF, *et al.* Randomized Selection Design Trial Evaluating CD8+-Enriched *Versus* Unselected Tumor-Infiltrating Lymphocytes for Adoptive Cell Therapy for Patients With Melanoma. J Clin Oncol. 2013.

[176] Zhou J, Shen X, Huang J, Hodes RJ, Rosenberg SA, Robbins PF. Telomere length of transferred lymphocytes correlates with *in vivo* persistence and tumor regression in melanoma patients receiving cell transfer therapy. J Immunol 2005; 175(10): 7046-52.

[177] Zhou J, Dudley ME, Rosenberg SA, Robbins PF. Persistence of multiple tumor-specific T-cell clones is associated with complete tumor regression in a melanoma patient receiving adoptive cell transfer therapy. J Immunother 2005; 28(1): 53-62.

[178] Radvanyi LG, Bernatchez C, Zhang M, Fox PS, Miller P, Chacon J, *et al.* Specific lymphocyte subsets predict response to adoptive cell therapy using expanded autologous tumor-infiltrating lymphocytes in metastatic melanoma patients. Clin Cancer Res 2012; 18(24): 6758-70.

[179] Besser MJ, Shapira-Frommer R, Treves AJ, Zippel D, Itzhaki O, Schallmach E, *et al.* Minimally cultured or selected autologous tumor-infiltrating lymphocytes after a lympho-depleting chemotherapy regimen in metastatic melanoma patients. J Immunother 2009; 32(4): 415-23

[180] Dudley ME, Wunderlich JR, Shelton TE, Even J, Rosenberg SA. Generation of tumor-infiltrating lymphocyte cultures for use in adoptive transfer therapy for melanoma patients. J Immunother 2003; 26(4): 332-42.

[181] Li Y, Liu S, Hernandez J, Vence L, Hwu P, Radvanyi L. MART-1-specific melanoma tumor-infiltrating lymphocytes maintaining CD28 expression have improved survival and expansion capability following antigenic restimulation *in vitro*. J Immunol 2010; 184(1): 452-65.

[182] Powell DJ, Jr., Dudley ME, Robbins PF, Rosenberg SA. Transition of late-stage effector T cells to CD27+ CD28+ tumor-reactive effector memory T cells in humans after adoptive cell transfer therapy. Blood 2005; 105(1): 241-50.

[183] Hernandez-Chacon JA, Li Y, Wu RC, Bernatchez C, Wang Y, Weber JS, *et al.* Costimulation through the CD137/4-1BB pathway protects human melanoma tumor-infiltrating lymphocytes from activation-induced cell death and enhances antitumor effector function. J Immunother 2011; 34(3): 236-50.

[184] Chacon JA, Wu RC, Sukhumalchandra P, Molldrem JJ, Sarnaik A, Pilon-Thomas S, *et al.* Co-stimulation through 4-1BB/CD137 improves the expansion and function of CD8(+) melanoma tumor-infiltrating lymphocytes for adoptive T-cell therapy. PloS one 2013; 8(4): e60031.

[185] Garlie NK, LeFever AV, Siebenlist RE, Levine BL, June CH, Lum LG. T cells coactivated with immobilized anti-CD3 and anti-CD28 as potential immunotherapy for cancer. J Immunother 1999; 22(4): 336-45.

[186] Rapoport AP, Stadtmauer EA, Aqui N, Badros A, Cotte J, Chrisley L, *et al.* Restoration of immunity in lymphopenic individuals with cancer by vaccination and adoptive T-cell transfer. Nat Med 2005; 11(11): 1230-7.

[187] Laport GG, Levine BL, Stadtmauer EA, Schuster SJ, Luger SM, Grupp S, *et al.* Adoptive transfer of costimulated T cells induces lymphocytosis in patients with relapsed/refractory non-Hodgkin lymphoma following CD34+-selected hematopoietic cell transplantation. Blood 2003; 102(6): 2004-13.

[188] Porter DL, Levine BL, Bunin N, Stadtmauer EA, Luger SM, Goldstein S, *et al.* A phase 1 trial of donor lymphocyte infusions expanded and activated *ex vivo via* CD3/CD28 costimulation. Blood 2006; 107(4): 1325-31.

[189] Porter DL, Levine BL, Kalos M, Bagg A, June CH. Chimeric antigen receptor-modified T cells in chronic lymphoid leukemia. New Eng J Med 2011; 365(8): 725-33.

[190] Kalos M, Levine BL, Porter DL, Katz S, Grupp SA, Bagg A, *et al.* T cells with chimeric antigen receptors have potent antitumor effects and can establish memory in patients with advanced leukemia. Sci Transl Med 2011; 3(95): 95ra73.

[191] Grupp SA, Kalos M, Barrett D, Aplenc R, Porter DL, Rheingold SR, *et al.* Chimeric antigen receptor-modified T cells for acute lymphoid leukemia. New Eng J Med 2013; 368(16): 1509-18.

[192] Suhoski MM, Golovina TN, Aqui NA, Tai VC, Varela-Rohena A, Milone MC, *et al.* Engineering artificial antigen-presenting cells to express a diverse array of co-stimulatory molecules. Mol Ther 2007; 15(5): 981-8.

[193] Maus MV, Thomas AK, Leonard DG, Allman D, Addya K, Schlienger K, *et al. Ex vivo* expansion of polyclonal and antigen-specific cytotoxic T lymphocytes by artificial APCs expressing ligands for the T-cell receptor, CD28 and 4-1BB. Nat Biotechnol 2002; 20(2): 143-8.

[194] Papanicolaou GA, Latouche JB, Tan C, Dupont J, Stiles J, Pamer EG, *et al.* Rapid expansion of cytomegalovirus-specific cytotoxic T lymphocytes by artificial antigen-presenting cells expressing a single HLA allele. Blood 2003; 102(7): 2498-505.

[195] Butler MO, Imataki O, Yamashita Y, Tanaka M, Ansen S, Berezovskaya A, *et al. Ex vivo* expansion of human CD8+ T cells using autologous CD4+ T cell help. PloS one 2012; 7(1): e30229.

[196] Gattinoni L, Lugli E, Ji Y, Pos Z, Paulos CM, Quigley MF, *et al.* A human memory T cell subset with stem cell-like properties. Nat Med 2011; 17(10): 1290-7.

[197] Gattinoni L, Zhong XS, Palmer DC, Ji Y, Hinrichs CS, Yu Z, *et al.* Wnt signaling arrests effector T cell differentiation and generates CD8+ memory stem cells. Nat Med 2009; 15(7): 808-13.

[198] Gattinoni L, Klebanoff CA, Restifo NP. Paths to stemness: building the ultimate antitumour T cell. Nat Rev Cancer 2012; 12(10): 671-84.

[199] Gattinoni L, Restifo NP. Moving T memory stem cells to the clinic. Blood 2013; 121(4): 567-8.

[200] Weiss JM, Subleski JJ, Wigginton JM, Wiltrout RH. Immunotherapy of cancer by IL-12-based cytokine combinations. Expert opinion on biological therapy 2007; 7(11): 1705-21.

[201] Kerkar SP, Muranski P, Kaiser A, Boni A, Sanchez-Perez L, Yu Z, *et al.* Tumor-specific CD8+ T cells expressing interleukin-12 eradicate established cancers in lymphodepleted hosts. Cancer Res 2010; 70(17): 6725-34.

[202] Zhang L, Kerkar SP, Yu Z, Zheng Z, Yang S, Restifo NP, *et al.* Improving adoptive T cell therapy by targeting and controlling IL-12 expression to the tumor environment. Mol Ther 2011; 19(4): 751-9.

[203] Kerkar SP, Goldszmid RS, Muranski P, Chinnasamy D, Yu Z, Reger RN, *et al.* IL-12 triggers a programmatic change in dysfunctional myeloid-derived cells within mouse tumors. J Clin Invest 2011; 121(12): 4746-57.

[204] Kerkar SP, Leonardi AJ, van Panhuys N, Zhang L, Yu Z, Crompton JG, *et al.* Collapse of the Tumor Stroma is Triggered by IL-12 Induction of Fas. Mol Ther. 2013.

[205] Kershaw MH, Westwood JA, Parker LL, Wang G, Eshhar Z, Mavroukakis SA, *et al.* A phase I study on adoptive immunotherapy using gene-modified T cells for ovarian cancer. Clin Cancer Res 2006; 12(20 Pt 1): 6106-15.

[206] Till BG, Jensen MC, Wang J, Chen EY, Wood BL, Greisman HA, *et al.* Adoptive immunotherapy for indolent non-Hodgkin lymphoma and mantle cell lymphoma using genetically modified autologous CD20-specific T cells. Blood 2008; 112(6): 2261-71.

[207] Park JR, Digiusto DL, Slovak M, Wright C, Naranjo A, Wagner J, *et al.* Adoptive transfer of chimeric antigen receptor re-directed cytolytic T lymphocyte clones in patients with neuroblastoma. Mol Ther 2007; 15(4): 825-33.

[208] Lamers CH, Sleijfer S, Vulto AG, Kruit WH, Kliffen M, Debets R, *et al.* Treatment of metastatic renal cell carcinoma with autologous T-lymphocytes genetically retargeted against carbonic anhydrase IX: first clinical experience. J Clin Oncol 2006; 24(13): e20-2.

[209] Hombach A, Wieczarkowiecz A, Marquardt T, Heuser C, Usai L, Pohl C, *et al.* Tumor-specific T cell activation by recombinant immunoreceptors: CD3 zeta signaling and CD28 costimulation are simultaneously required for efficient IL-2 secretion and can be integrated into one combined CD28/CD3 zeta signaling receptor molecule. J Immunol 2001; 167(11): 6123-31.

[210] Song DG, Ye Q, Poussin M, Harms GM, Figini M, Powell DJ, Jr. CD27 costimulation augments the survival and antitumor activity of redirected human T cells *in vivo.* Blood 2012; 119(3): 696-706.

[211] Zhao Y, Wang QJ, Yang S, Kochenderfer JN, Zheng Z, Zhong X, *et al.* A herceptin-based chimeric antigen receptor with modified signaling domains leads to enhanced survival of transduced T lymphocytes and antitumor activity. J Immunol 2009; 183(9): 5563-74.

[212] Zhong XS, Matsushita M, Plotkin J, Riviere I, Sadelain M. Chimeric antigen receptors combining 4-1BB and CD28 signaling domains augment PI3kinase/AKT/Bcl-XL activation and CD8+ T cell-mediated tumor eradication. Mol Ther 2010; 18(2): 413-20.

[213] Carpenito C, Milone MC, Hassan R, Simonet JC, Lakhal M, Suhoski MM, *et al.* Control of large, established tumor xenografts with genetically retargeted human T cells containing CD28 and CD137 domains. Proc Natl Acad Sci USA 2009; 106(9): 3360-5.

[214] Kochenderfer JN, Yu Z, Frasheri D, Restifo NP, Rosenberg SA. Adoptive transfer of syngeneic T cells transduced with a chimeric antigen receptor that recognizes murine CD19 can eradicate lymphoma and normal B cells. Blood 2010; 116(19): 3875-86.

[215] Brentjens RJ, Riviere I, Park JH, Davila ML, Wang X, Stefanski J, *et al.* Safety and persistence of adoptively transferred autologous CD19-targeted T cells in patients with relapsed or chemotherapy refractory B-cell leukemias. Blood 2011; 118(18): 4817-28.

[216] Brentjens RJ, Davila ML, Riviere I, Park J, Wang X, Cowell LG, *et al.* CD19-targeted T cells rapidly induce molecular remissions in adults with chemotherapy-refractory acute lymphoblastic leukemia. Sci Transl Med 2013; 5(177): 177ra38.

[217] Morgan RA, Yang JC, Kitano M, Dudley ME, Laurencot CM, Rosenberg SA. Case report of a serious adverse event following the administration of T cells transduced with a chimeric antigen receptor recognizing ERBB2. Mol Ther 2010; 18(4): 843-51.

[218] Kloss CC, Condomines M, Cartellieri M, Bachmann M, Sadelain M. Combinatorial antigen recognition with balanced signaling promotes selective tumor eradication by engineered T cells. Nat Biotechnol 2013; 31(1): 71-5.

[219] Phan GQ, Yang JC, Sherry RM, Hwu P, Topalian SL, Schwartzentruber DJ, *et al.* Cancer regression and autoimmunity induced by cytotoxic T lymphocyte-associated antigen 4 blockade in patients with metastatic melanoma. Proc Natl Acad Sci USA 2003; 100(14): 8372-7.

[220] Ribas A, Camacho LH, Lopez-Berestein G, Pavlov D, Bulanhagui CA, Millham R, *et al.* Antitumor activity in melanoma and anti-self responses in a phase I trial with the anti-cytotoxic T lymphocyte-associated antigen 4 monoclonal antibody CP-675,206. J Clin Oncol 2005; 23(35): 8968-77.

[221] Topalian SL, Hodi FS, Brahmer JR, Gettinger SN, Smith DC, McDermott DF, *et al.* Safety, activity, and immune correlates of anti-PD-1 antibody in cancer. New Eng J Med 2012; 366(26): 2443-54.

[222] Brahmer JR, Tykodi SS, Chow LQ, Hwu WJ, Topalian SL, Hwu P, *et al.* Safety and activity of anti-PD-L1 antibody in patients with advanced cancer. New Eng J Med 2012; 366(26): 2455-65.

[223] Townsend SE, Allison JP. Tumor rejection after direct costimulation of CD8+ T cells by B7-transfected melanoma cells. Science 1993; 259(5093): 368-70.
[224] Yu P, Lee Y, Liu W, Chin RK, Wang J, Wang Y, *et al.* Priming of naive T cells inside tumors leads to eradication of established tumors. Nat Immunol 2004; 5(2): 141-9.
[225] Andarini S, Kikuchi T, Nukiwa M, Pradono P, Suzuki T, Ohkouchi S, *et al.* Adenovirus vector-mediated *in vivo* gene transfer of OX40 ligand to tumor cells enhances antitumor immunity of tumor-bearing hosts. Cancer Res 2004; 64(9): 3281-7.
[226] Suntharalingam G, Perry MR, Ward S, Brett SJ, Castello-Cortes A, Brunner MD, *et al.* Cytokine storm in a phase 1 trial of the anti-CD28 monoclonal antibody TGN1412. New Eng J Med 2006; 355(10): 1018-28.
[227] Blansfield JA, Beck KE, Tran K, Yang JC, Hughes MS, Kammula US, *et al.* Cytotoxic T-lymphocyte-associated antigen-4 blockage can induce autoimmune hypophysitis in patients with metastatic melanoma and renal cancer. J Immunother 2005; 28(6): 593-8.
[228] Stromnes IM, Blattman JN, Tan X, Jeevanjee S, Gu H, Greenberg PD. Abrogating Cbl-b in effector CD8(+) T cells improves the efficacy of adoptive therapy of leukemia in mice. J Clin Invest 2010; 120(10): 3722-34.

# CHAPTER 10

# Regeneration of Tumor Antigen-Specific T Cells Using iPSC Technology

**Hiroshi Kawamoto***

*Department of Immunology, Institute for Frontier Medical Sciences, Kyoto University, Kyoto 606-8507, Japan*

**Abstract:** In cancer patients, a certain number of cytotoxic T lymphocytes (CTLs) specific for cancer antigen are formed; however, most of these CTLs remain inactive due to various suppressive mechanisms such as improper DC activation (anergy induction) or suppression by regulatory T cells. The conventional strategies have been directed to expand the remaining CTLs *in vitro* or *in vivo*, to diverge the anergic T cells to an activated status, or to inhibit regulatory T cells. Although the resulting activated CTLs exhibit certain activity in killing tumor cells, in most cases the activity of CTLs is not sufficient enough to result in cure of the patient. One of the major limiting factors in this type of approach is the short life span of activated CTLs. Currently we are trying to overcome this problem by utilizing the iPSC (induced pluripotent stem cell) technology. The concept of our strategy is that it is possible to obtain *de novo* generated tumor antigen specific CTLs almost unlimitedly when one firstly produces iPSCs from tumor antigen specific CTLs and subsequently regenerate CTLs from such iPSCs. In line with this concept, we have succeeded in establishing iPSCs from mature CTLs specific for the melanoma antigen MART-1, and in regenerating MART-1 specific T cells from such iPSCs. This approach may provide a breakthrough in the future in the tumor immunotherapy.

**Keywords:** Cloning, cytotoxic T lymphocytes (CTLs), induced pluripotent stem cells (iPSCs), MART-1, melanoma, reprogramming.

## INTRODUCTION

CTLs have long been used in clinical trials of adoptive cell therapy (ACT). The Rosenberg's group has been mainly using CTLs that were collected from tumor lesions (tumor-infiltrating lymphocytes: TILs) for the ACT therapy. In the early trials of their group, only around 5% of patients showed complete response [1]. The low frequency of response was attributed to the rapid decrease of transferred TILs (0.1% of transferred cells remained after 1 week).

***Corresponding author Hiroshi Kawamoto:** Department of Immunology, Institute for Frontier Medical Sciences, Kyoto University Kyoto 606-8507, Japan; Tel: +81(75) 751-3815;
E-mail: kawamoto@frontier.kyoto-u.ac.jp

**Jianxun Song (Ed)**

Subsequent strategies have tried to overcome this rapid decrease of transferred T cells. The Rosenberg's group has recently employed a protocol to intensively deplete patients' lymphocytes by pretreatments [2]. In concrete terms, the patients with metastatic melanoma received massive chemotherapy and whole body irradiation of a lethal dose followed by autologous hematopoietic stem cell transplantation as pretreatment, and transfer of activated TILs. By this protocol, the ratio of patients to achieve a long-term survival (more than 5 years) attained almost 40%. This result strongly suggested that CTLs existing in cancer patients have potential to cure the patients.

## APPROACHES TO UTILIZE YOUNG T CELLS IN ACT

Another possible approach to overcome the rapid decrease of transferred CTLs may be to use "younger" CTLs in ACT. It is known that naïve T cells are the youngest among peripheral T cells (Fig. **1**). When naïve T cells are activated, they undergo proliferation and differentiation to finally become effector T cells. During this process, three different grades of memory T cells are segregated [2]. These are, in order from the young to old, memory stem T cells ($T_{SCM}$), central memory T cells ($T_{CM}$), and effector memory T cells ($T_{EM}$). This order is thought to represent the number of cell divisions that have taken place before their segregation.

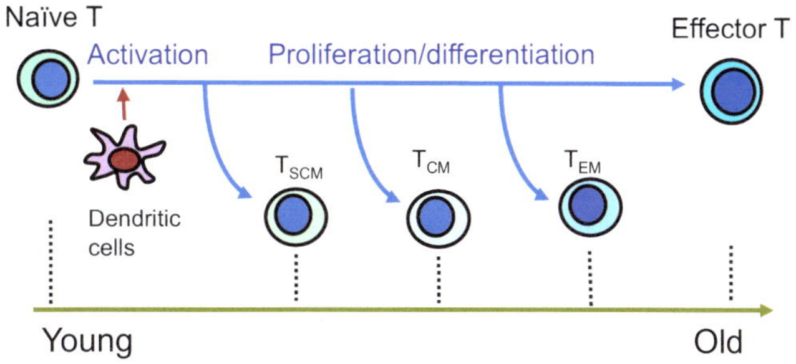


**Figure 1: Differentiation of peripheral T cells.** After activation by antigen presenting dendritic cells, naïve T cells undergo proliferation and differentiation to eventually become effector T cells. During this process, memory stem T cells ($T_{SCM}$), central memory T cells ($T_{CM}$), and effector memory T cells ($T_{EM}$) are segregated.

In conventional methods, during the process of expanding TILs, proliferation is continued by successive stimulation *via* TCR and cytokines, resulting in the generation of effector T cells, which represent the terminal stage and thus have a short life span. Therefore, it is preferable to obtain younger cells that are closer to the starting naïve T cells.

One of such methods may be to modify the culture conditions so that the proportion of the memory T cells can be increased. For example, it was reported that the proportion of memory T cells is increased by using IL-7 and IL-15 in the culture for expansion of CTLs [3]. Another method to make younger T cells may be to genetically transfer specific TCR gene into naïve T cells [4]. In this method, TCR-transfected cells may remain relatively young, because the culture can be initiated with naïve T cells and the culture period can be shortened.

In line with these trials, we propose that the iPSC technology can be applied to make younger T cells, which is very different from other approaches. We think that our method may provide a major breakthrough in cancer immunotherapy.

## ESCs AND iPSCs

Firstly, I will explain the difference in the usage of embryonic stem cells (ESCs) and iPSCs. A fertilized egg develops into a blastocyst, and an inside part of the blastocyst that subsequently develops into the embryo is called the inner cell mass. ESCs can be produced by collecting this part and culturing it. ESCs are plurtipotent in that they can give rise to any kind of tissue. Therefore, ESCs are expected to be used as a cell source in regenerative medicine. However, several problems exist; (i) it is difficult for the patient to obtain HLA-matched ESCs, which are required to ensure long-lasting graft survival, and (ii) the usage of fertilized eggs, which could become an individual human being, raises serious ethical issues.

To avoid graft rejection issues as well as ethical problems, it is desirable to develop a technology to produce ESC-like pluripotent stem cells from a patient's somatic cells. The "nuclear transfer" method realized the idea, in which a nucleus of a somatic cell is transferred to an unfertilized egg. Such a nuclear-transferred egg is endowed to complete the full course of embryogenesis (Fig. **2**, upper lane). In this system, the status of the nucleus of the differentiated somatic cell is changed to obtain pluripotency. Such a phenomenon to change the developmental potential of cells from the original to the remodeled status is generally referred to as "reprogramming". The first success of reprogramming by nuclear transfer was reported in 1962 in amphibia, while a successful nuclear transfer in mammals was reported in 1997 [5].

The nuclear transfer technology has not only made it possible to reproduce a so called "clone animal" but also to establish "ESCs" from somatic cells (Fig. **2**, upper lane). However, this technology has been stagnant in applying to human, since (i) it remains an ethical issue in utilizing fertilized human eggs and (ii) the technology required to do this reprogramming procedure was difficult to learn. As a solution the iPSC technology became available, in 2006, as an in principal easy method of reprogramming, *i.e.,* by transducing somatic cells with a retrovirus containing only four factors (Fig. **2**, lower lane). The first iPSCs reported in 2006 were of murine origin [6], and it took only one year to succeed in making establishing human iPSCs [7].

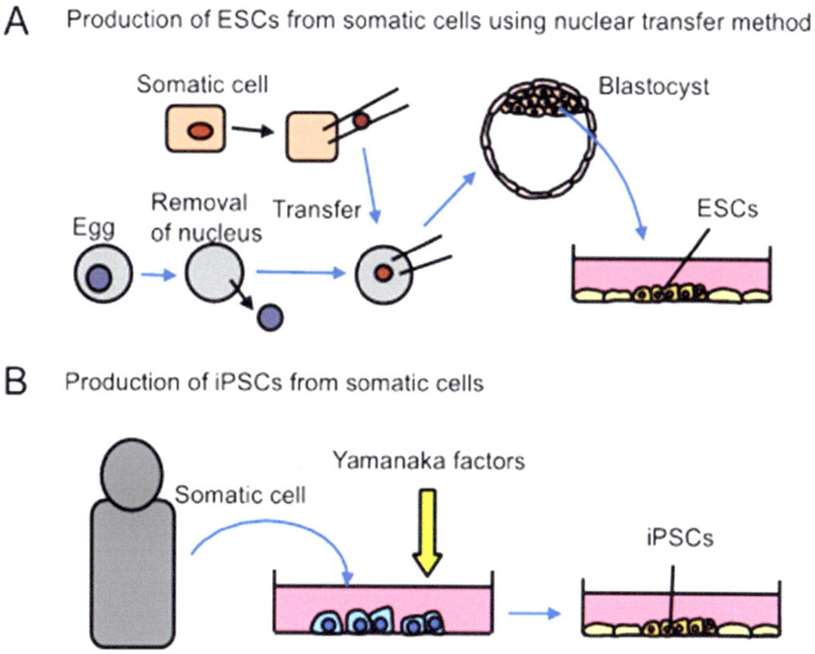


**Figure 2: Two methods for reprogramming somatic cells into pluripotent stem cells.** A) Nuclear transfer method. Remove the nucleus of a somatic cell and transplant it into an unfertilized egg from which a nucleus has been removed. The egg then develops into a blastocyst, and ESCs can be produced by culturing the inner cell mass of the blastocyst. B) iPSC method. Transform somatic cells by enforced expression of Yamanaka factors (Oct3/4、Klf4、Sox2、c-Myc).

## THE IDEA TO CLONE A LYMPHOCYTE BY REPROGRAMMING

Antigen specificity of T cells is defined by T cell receptors (TCR) expressed on individual T cells. Each T cell expresses a TCR with different specificity, and the T cell population as a whole has a broadly diversified repertoire. Such a diversified repertoire is formed by rearrangement of TCR genes, in which the final TCR gene is formed by combining randomly selected gene segments. The resulting repertoire is very broad, thus the frequency of T cells specific to a certain antigen is very low (less than 1 in 100,000).

The method to select a T cell of certain specificity and to expand it is termed "cloning". Note that the reprogramming of a T cell into ESC/iPSCs serves not only as a strategy for rejuvenation of T cells but also as a cloning method (Fig. **3**). When a T cell with certain specificity is reprogrammed into ESC/iPSCs, the rearranged genomic combination of TCR genes of the original T cell is inherited to ESC/iPSCs. When T cells are regenerated from such ESC/iPSCs, all regenerated T cells are expected to express the same TCR as that of the original T cell.

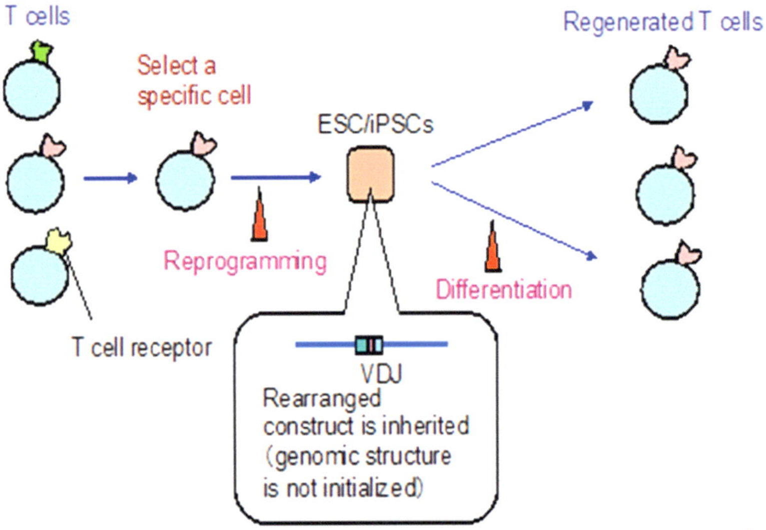


**Figure 3: Reprogramming of a T cell with a certain antigen specificity into ESC/iPSCs serves as a method of cloning.** ESC/iPSCs produced by reprogramming a T cell having a defined antigen specificity inherit rearranged genomic constructs of TCR genes of the original T cell. All T cells regenerated from such ESC/iPSCs are expected to express the same TCR as the original T cell.

## REPROGRAMMING OF NKT CELLS

We initially tried to apply the nuclear transfer technology to reprogram T cells. We actually used NKT cells as a source of T cells. NKT cells do not recognize cancer antigens, but do recognize glycolipid antigens presented on the CD1d molecule expressed on antigen presenting cells. By administering a stimulating antigen to cancer patients, NKT cells may be activated and consequently enhance anti-tumor immune response.

Several years ago, we produced a murine NKT cell clone by transferring the nucleus from a NKT cell to an unfertilized egg [8]. Subsequently, we established ESCs and then it was shown that T cells regenerated *in vitro* from such ESCs were almost exclusively NKT cells [9]. After the invention of the iPSC method by S. Yamanaka, we applied the iPSC technology to clone NKT cells. Thus, iPSCs were produced from murine NKT cells and functional NKT cells were regenerated *in vitro* from such iPSCs [10].

These results demonstrated that the idea to use the reprogramming technology to clone a T cell is a feasible approach. However, as mentioned earlier, NKT cells do not possess specificity for a tumor antigen. We therefore decided to focus on CTLs, which have been used as the main effector cells in antigen specific cancer immunotherapy.

## PRODUCTION OF iPSCS FROM TUMOR ANTIGEN-SPECIFIC CTLS

The ideas of our strategy are (i) to produce iPSCs from a tumor antigen specific CTL, and (ii) to regenerate CTLs with the same antigen-specificity as the original T cell from such iPSCs (Fig. **4**) with the purpose to generate an unlimited supply.

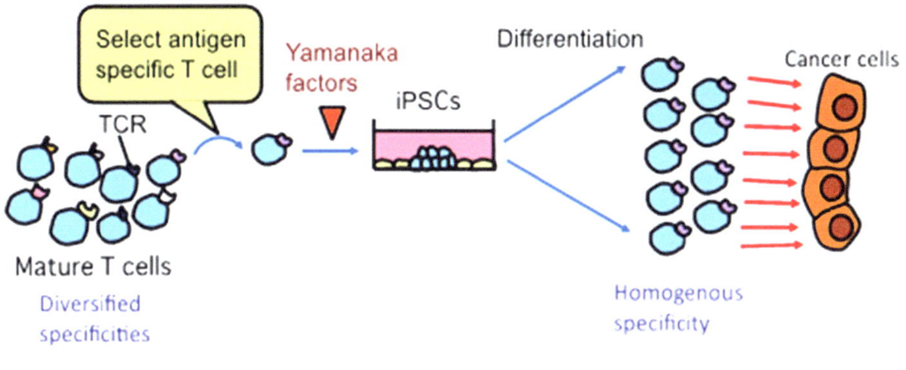


**Figure 4: The concept of our strategy: regeneration of tumor-antigen specific T cells using the iPSC technology.** A tumor antigen-specific T cell is isolated from a heterogeneous mature T cell population, and iPSCs are made from the cell. Then, T cells are regenerated from such iPSCs. All of these regenerated T cells are expected to express the same TCR as the original T cells.

As a cell source we decided to use a CTL clone specific for the melanoma antigen MART-1 (Fig. **5**) [11]. We obtained such CTLs (JKF6 cells) as kind donation from the Surgery Branch of the National Cancer Institute. JKF6 cells are long-term cultured TILs that were originally derived from a melanoma patient [12]. Some previous studies reported that iPSCs can be produced from human peripheral T cells by using Yamanaka factors [13, 14], which was reproducible by our group, but the same procedure was inefficient to establish iPSCs from antigen-specific T cells. We therefore employed SV40 [15] to be used with the Yamanaka factors to increase efficiency of reprogramming. For transduction, we used the Sendai virus system [16]. This way, we succeeded in establishing human iPSCs from MART-1 specific CTLs (MAR1-T-iPSCs).

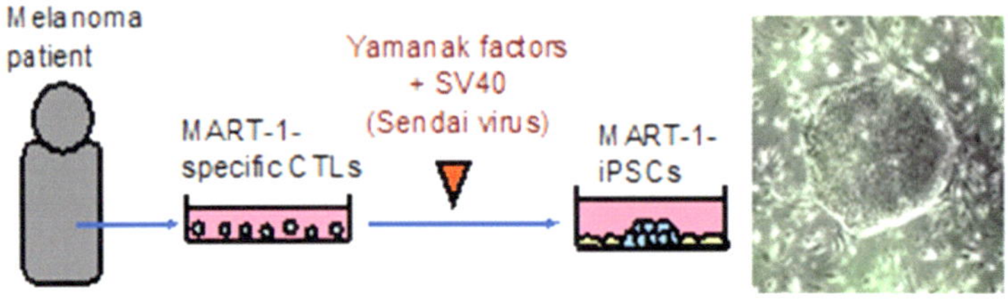


**Figure 5: Generation of iPSCs from MART-1 specific CTLs.** Long-term cultured MART-1 specific CTLs (JKF6 cells) were transduced with Yamanaka factors and SV40, and iPSCs were established.

## REGENERATION OF TUMOR ANTIGEN-SPECIFIC CTLS FROM iPSCS

We then induced differentiation of T cells from the MART1-T-iPSCs (Fig. **6A**) by using a modified method from one previously published [17]. On the 35th day of cultivation, $CD4^{+}CD8^{+}$ double positive (DP) cells were generated. The majority of the DP cells generated from MART1-T-iPSCs expressed a TCR specific to MART-1 antigen, although about 30% of $CD3^{+}$ DP cells were negative or only weakly positive after MART-1-tetramer staining (Fig. **6B**). To induce further differentiation, we added anti-CD3 monoclonal antibody (mAb) to the culture on day 35. The proportion of $CD8^{+}$ T cells clearly increased during 6 days following TCR stimulation (Fig. **6C**, left panel), and these cells expanded by 300 fold during 6 days. Importantly, the resulting $CD8^{+}$ T cells were almost exclusively specific for the MART-1 antigen (Fig. **6C**, right panel). These regenerated T cells were surface-phenotypically similar to naïve T cells (Fig. **6D**).

We next examined whether the generated CD8+ cells are functionally mature. MART-$1^{+}CD3^{+}CD8^{+}$ T cells were stimulated with beads coated with a mixture of anti-CD3 mAb and anti-CD28 mAb. IFNγ production by the $CD8^{+}$ T cells was detected following this CD3/CD28 stimulation, and the production of IFNγ was synergistically enhanced by the addition of hIL-2 (Fig. **6E**). To examine whether the $CD8^{+}$ T cells can be activated in an antigen-specific manner, they were co-cultured with target cells (human EBV-lymphoblastoid cell line) with or without MART-1 peptide. The $CD8^{+}$ T cells produced a substantial amount of IFNγ only in the presence of specific peptide (Fig. **6F**). Thus, this iPSC-based approach appears to be effective in regenerating functional antigen-specific CTLs.

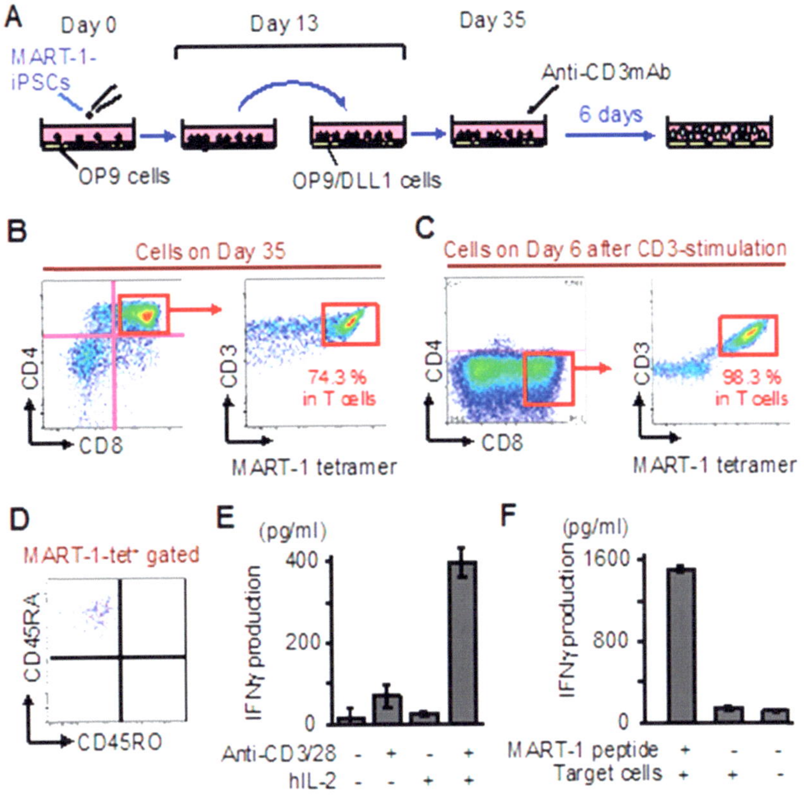


**Figure 6: Regeneration of MART-1 specific CTLs from MART1-T-iPSCs.** A) MART1-T-iPSCs were sequentially cultured with two types of feeder cells, OP9 and OP9/DLL1 cells. On day 35 of cultivation, anti-CD3 mAb was added to induce the generation of mature T cells. B) CD4/CD8 DP cells were generated on day 35 of cultivation, 70% of them expressed a TCR specific for the MART-1 antigen. C) A large number of CD8 + cells were generated 6 days after the stimulation with anti-CD3 mAb. Virtually all of them expressed a TCR specific for the MART-1 antigen. D) Flowcytometric profile of cells generated 6 days after CD3 stimulation. Expression profile for CD45RA *vs* CD45RO on $CD3^{+}$MART-1-$tetramer^{+}$ cells is shown. E) Production of IFNγ by regenerated $CD8^{+}$ T cells upon TCR stimulation. $CD8^{+}$ T cells were stimulated by adding human T-Activator CD3/CD28 Dynabeads, in the absence or presence of hIL-2. After 16 hours, the concentration of IFNγ in medium was measured by ELISA. Mean ±SE of triplicates is shown. F) Production of IFNγ by regenerated $CD8^{+}$ T cells upon antigen specific stimulation. IFNγ secretion by $CD8^{+}$ T cells was measured by ELISA from the supernatant after co-culturing $1x10^{5}$ regenerated $CD8^{+}$ T cells for 24 hours with $1x10^{4}$ HLA-A*02:01-positive EBV-lymphoblastoid cells (CIRA0201) pulsed or not with MART-1 peptide (EAAGIGILTV). Mean ±SE of triplicates is shown.

## A NOVEL METHOD FOR CLONING OF T CELLS

The method for T cell cloning using the iPSC method presented here can be regarded as a technological innovation comparable to the method to clone B cells for the production of mAbs.

B cells can be immortalized by using the hybridoma method of Kohler and Millstein in which a B cell producing mAb to a desired antigen is fused with an immortalized cell. Infinite amounts of mAb can be obtained from the culture supernatant of the hybridoma; Several mAbs are already used in the clinical setting (Fig. 7).

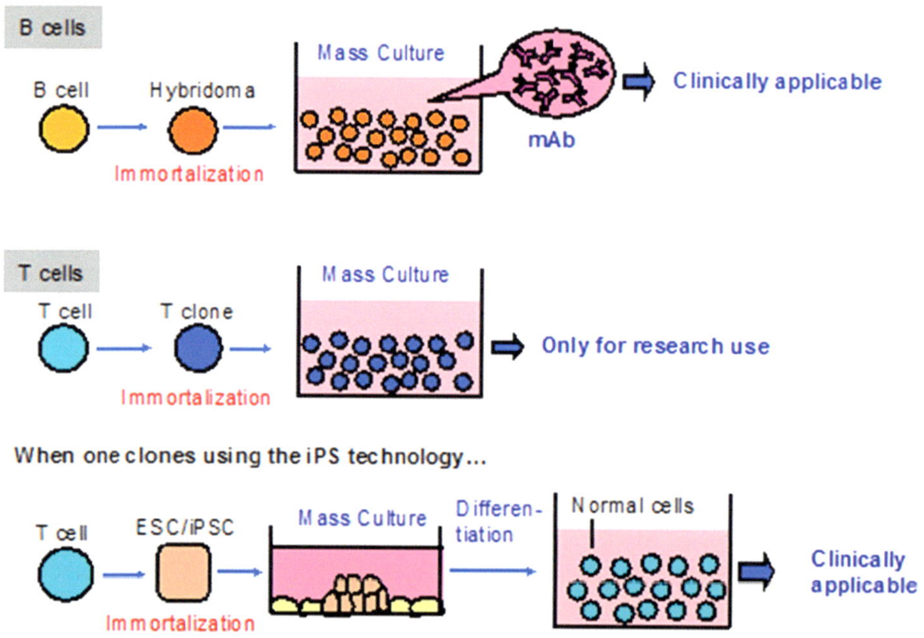


**Figure 7: The reprogramming method provides a novel tool for T cell cloning.** B cells can be cloned by immortalizing primary B cells using the hybridoma method. mAb obtained from the culture supernatant can be used in the clinical setting. T cells can also be cloned by using a similar hybridoma method or after long-term culture, clones may ultimately appear. These cloned T cells have been mostly used in experimental settings, because they may develop into leukemic cells upon transfer into the patients. By cloning T cells as iPSCs, it is possible to infinitely expand them, and the regenerated cells from these iPSCs could be directly applied for clinical use.

T cells can also be cloned by immortalization with a similar hybridoma method or just by long-term culture in certain conditions. However, it is very difficult to use such immortalized cells in clinical setting.

In this context, the method presented here may represent a novel tool for the cloning of T cells. By cloning T cells as iPSCs, it is possible to infinitely expand at the stage of iPSCs, and the regenerated cells from these iPSCs will be normal and thus should be directly applicable in clinical use.

## TARGET PATIENTS OF REGENERATIVE MEDICINE CAN BE BROADENED

In this article I have introduced the strategy to regenerate CTLs using iPSC technology as a novel method in cancer immunotherapy. However, this strategy can also be categorized as one of the therapeutic approaches in regenerative medicine. In our method, "clonal expansion" of antigen specific T cells, which is a key phenomenon in acquired immunity, is artificially reproduced *in vitro*. It can thus be said that this approach represents the reconstruction of the immune system.

Whereas the possible applications of the iPSC technology may include the use for screening of drugs or for testing toxicity of drugs, the primary application has been directed to cases in which compensation of lost organs is required. However, the number of target patients so far seems still small. For example, some trials to use iPSC-derived tissues are in the planning phase to be clinically tested within several years, and these include Parkinson's disease, spinal injury, retinal disease, arthrosis, diabetes mellitus, cardiac infarction, *etc*. Most of these diseases have alternative therapeutic methods in place, albeit not optimal. Furthermore, although the incidence of diabetes mellitus is high, the number of patients who require the cell transfer therapy is only limited. The same is true for cardiac infarction.

Cancer patients with metastatic lesions are incurable and will die. Virtually no effective alternative strategies exist at present. Now, our approach could make it possible to put cancer patients as targets of regenerative medicine. We have shown the case of malignant melanoma, but a large variety of peptide antigens recognized by CTLs have been identified for various types of solid tumors, including gastric cancer, colon cancer, lung cancer, breast cancer, and so on. This means that the CTL-iPSC strategy has a potential to target a broad range of cancer cases.

Furthermore, this strategy can also be applied for infectious diseases. For example, H. Nakauchi, S. Kaneko and their colleagues have shown that, using a very similar approach to ours, successful regeneration of CTLs against human immunodeficiency virus [18]. One of the possible applications may be to use the regenerated CTLs specific for viral antigens to prevent or cure opportunistic viral infections by CMV or EBV occurring after bone marrow transplantation.

## PERSPECTIVE

In this article we have introduced our strategy as one of the possible approaches for the use of young CTLs that can survive for longer period in recipients after ACT. This strategy is advantageous in that it is possible to almost unlimitedly produce CTLs for ACT once one establishes iPSCs from antigen specific CTLs. As mentioned earlier, the TCR gene transfer method may also result in the production of relatively young CTLs with a fixed specificity [4]. However, any "gene therapy" may have a risk of hitting some oncogene by retroviral integration into the genome. Another concern of the TCR gene transfer method is that it may be difficult to perfectly suppress the expression of endogenous TCR genes, which could make TCR exhibiting unexpected reactivity.

In T-iPSC strategy, the genome is not damaged during reprogramming process as long as the Sendai virus vector is used. On the other hand, as to the reproducibility of antigen specificity, there exists some risk of generation of harmful TCR. The TCR$\alpha$ chain gene formed after rearrangement still retains remaining V and J segments upstream and downstream of the rearranged V-J construct, leaving the possibility to yield further rearrangement replacing the original V-J construct. Such possibility should be carefully tested in *in vivo* experiments using animal models before clinical application, although in our experiment virtually all TCR expressed in the regenerated mature T cells were found to express the same TCR as original one (Fig. **6C**).

One of the possible approaches to avoid the side effect by autoreactive T cells is to use T cell progenitors induced from antigen-specific iPSCs as cell source to be trasferred to patients. It is highly probable that the transferred T cell progenitors migrate into the thymus and produce a large number of naïve CTLs that are specific for the tumor antigen in thymus. In such a case, even if a portion of regenerated T cells comes to express autoreactive TCR, they may be negatively selected in the thymus.

Undesired immune reaction could occur even when original TCR is faithfully recapitulated in the regenerated CTLs. Since most of the tumor antigens are endogenous molecules, they could be expressed in some other normal tissue. For example, it has been reported that some melanoma patients receiving CTLs genetically engineered to express a TCR specific for MART-1 exhibited patchy vitiligo, uvetitis or hearing loss, since normal melanocytes exist in skin, eye and ear do more or less express MART-1 [19]. However, this apparent side effect is true evidence that this line of immune therapy does work. Even if the tumor antigen is exclusively expressed in cancer cells, the side effect caused by cross reactivity should be considered. Therefore, it is important to select those tumor antigens that will not lead to serious side effects. However, such information can only be really obtained during carefully monitored clinical trials.

Before these approaches go into clinical trials, it is required to develop more efficient culture systems to induce the differentiation of T cells from T-iPSCs. We have developed various culture systems that support T cell generation from both mouse and human stem cells [20, 21]. By improving these culture systems, we are now developing a feeder free culture system to induce human T cells starting from iPSCs. We are also testing whether the regeneration of antigen-specific CTLs is also possible for other tumor antigens or the origin of T cells.

## ACKNOWLEDGEMENT

The author is grateful to Y. Katsura and W. T. V. Germeraad for critical reading of the manuscript.

## CONFLICT OF INTEREST

The authors confirm that this chapter contents have no conflict of interest.

## REFERENCES

[1] Rosenberg SA, Packard BS, Aebersold PM, Solomon D, Topalian SL, Toy ST, Simon P, Lotze MT, Yang JC, Seipp CA, Simpson C, Carter C, Bock S, Schwartzentruber D, Wei JP, White DE. Use of tumor infiltrating lymphocytes and interleukin-2 in the immunotherapy of patients with metastatic melanoma. A preliminary report. N Engl J Med 1988; 319(25): 1676-1680.

[2] Rosenberg SA. Cell transfer immunotherapy for metastatic solid cancer--what clinicians need to know. Nat Rev Clin Oncol. 2011; 8: 577-585.

[3] Cieri N, Camisa B, Cocchiarella F, *et al.* IL-7 and IL-15 instruct the generation of human memory stem T cells from naive precursors. Blood 2013; 121: 573-584.

[4] Morgan RA, Dudley ME, Wunderlich JR, *et al.* Cancer regression in patients after transfer of genetically engineered lymphocytes. Science 2006; 314: 126-129.

[5] Wilmut I, Schnieke AE, McWhir J, *et al.* Viable offspring derived from fetal and adult mammalian cells. Nature 1997; 385: 810-813.

[6] Takahashi K, Yamanaka S. Induction of pluripotent stem cells from mouse embryonic and adult fibroblast cultures by defined factors. Cell 2006; 126: 663-676.

[7] Takahashi K, Tanabe K, Ohnuki M, *et al.* Induction of pluripotent stem cells from adult human fibroblasts by defined factors. Cell 2007, 131, 861-872.

[8] Wakao H, Kawamoto H, Sakata S, *et al.* A novel mouse model for invariant NKT cell study. J Immunol. 2007; 179: 3888-3895.

[9] Watarai H, Rybouchkin A, Hongo N, *et al.* Generation of functional NKT cells *in vitro* from embryonic stem cells bearing rearranged invariant Valpha14-Jalpha18 TCRalpha gene. Blood 2010; 115: 230-237.

[10] Watarai H, Fujii S, Yamada D, *et al.* Murine induced pluripotent stem cells can be derived from and differentiate into natural killer T cells. J Clin Invest. 2010; 120: 2610-2618.

[11] Vizcardo R, Masuda K, Yamada D, *et al.* Regeneration of human tumor antigen-specific T cells from iPSCs derived from mature $CD8^+$ T cells. Cell Stem Cell 2013; 12: 31-36.

[12] Yang S, Liu F, Wang QJ, *et al.* The shedding of CD62L (L-selectin) regulates the acquisition of lytic activity in human tumor reactive T lymphocytes. PLoS One 2011; 6: e22560.

[13] Seki T, Yuasa S, Oda M, *et al.* Generation of induced pluripotent stem cells from human terminally differentiated circulating T cells. Cell Stem Cell 2010; 7: 11-14.

[14] Loh YH, Hartung O, Li H, *et al.* Reprogramming of T cells from human peripheral blood. Cell Stem Cell 2010; 7: 15-19.

[15] Park IH, Zhao R, West JA, Y *et al.* Reprogramming of human somatic cells to pluripotency with defined factors. Nature 2008; 451: 141-146.

[16] Fusaki N, Han H, Nishiyama A, *et al.* Efficient induction of transgene-free human pluripotent stem cells using a vector based on Sendai virus, an RNA virus that does not integrate into the host genome. Proc Jpn Acad Ser B, Phys Biol Sci. 2009; 85: 348-362.

[17] Timmermans F, Velghe I, Vanwalleghem L, *et al.* Generation of T cells from human embryonic stem cell-derived hematopoietic zones. J Immunol. 2009; 182: 6879-6888.

[18] Nishimura T, Kaneko S, Kawana-Tachikawa A, *et al.* Generation of rejuvenated antigen-specific T cells by reprogramming to pluripotency and redifferentiation. Cell Stem Cell 2013; 12: 114-126.

[19] Johnson LA, Morgan RA, Dudley ME, *et al.* Gene therapy with human and mouse T-cell receptors mediates cancer regression and targets normal tissues expressing cognate antigen. Blood 2009; 114: 535-546.

[20] Ikawa T, Hirose S, Masuda K, *et al.* An essential developmental checkpoint for production of the T cell lineage. Science 2010; 329: 93-96.

[21] Meek B, Cloosen S, Borsotti C, *et al.* *In vitro*-differentiated T/natural killer-cell progenitors derived from human $CD34^+$ cells mature in the thymus. Blood 2010; 115: 261-264.

**CHAPTER 11**

# Neutralizing Regulatory T Cells

**Ivan Shevchenko and Viktor Umansky***

*Skin Cancer Unit, German Cancer Research Center, Heidelberg and Department of Dermatology, Venereology and Allergology, University Medical Center Mannheim, Ruprecht-Karl University of Heidelberg, Mannheim, Heidelberg, Germany*

**Abstract:** The maintenance of peripheral tolerance against self and environmental antigens needs regulatory T cells (Treg) that deploy a variety of suppressive mechanisms to control potentially harmful inflammatory and autoimmune reactions. These mechanisms include production of suppressive cytokines and small molecules, expression of inhibitory receptors as well as direct cytolysis and intracellular transfer of second messengers. However, the tumors may hijack Treg immunosuppressive function to escape the anti-cancer immune responses. Expression of self- or altered-self antigens on tumor cells may drive Treg expansion and enhance their suppressive activity. Therefore, Treg-mediated immunosuppression represents one of the main hurdles to the anti-tumor immunity accounting for the failure of anti-tumor therapies including the vaccination and adoptive cell transfer. It has been shown that inhibition of Treg development, survival, and function can alleviate tumor-induced immunosuppression and improve the efficacy of anticancer immunotherapy. Here we discuss current strategies of targeting Treg development and function, including Treg depletion, inhibition of extracellular adenosine production and modulation of signaling pathways in Treg through cell surface receptors.

**Keywords:** CD25, CD73, costimulatory molecules, CTLA-4, FoxP3, GITR, IL-2, immunotoxins, OX40, regulatory T cells, suppression, vaccination.

## INTRODUCTION

The major role of the immune system in defending the host from malignancies has been progressively recognized over the last decades. Multiple investigations in humans and animal systems have confirmed vigorous activation of innate and adaptive immunity in response to tumors [1]. This is highlighted by the correlation between tumor infiltration and prognosis [1-4]. The outcome of tumorigenesis is thus largely determined by the balance between the anti-tumor

***Corresponding author Viktor Umansky:** Skin Cancer Unit, German Cancer Research Center, Heidelberg and Department of Dermatology, Venereology and Allergology, University Medical Center Mannheim, Ruprecht-Karl University of Heidelberg, Mannheim, Heidelberg, Germany; Tel: +49 (621) 383-3773; E-mail: V.Umansky@dkfz-heidelberg.de

**Jianxun Song (Ed)**

immunity and numerous mechanisms of immune escape and suppression developed by the tumor [1]. One of the main factors of tumor-associated immune suppression is activation and recruitment of inhibitory immune cells [1, 5].

Under physiological conditions, regulatory CD4 T cells (Tregs), characterized by the expression of the transcription factor forkhead box P3 (FoxP3), and CD25, the interleukin-2 (IL-2) receptor α-chain. Tregs serve to prevent adverse immune reactions against self, food and environmental antigens (6). Mice with a loss-of-function mutation in FoxP3 lack functional Tregs and die of multi-organ autoimmune and lymphoproliferative reactions early in life [6]. In humans, hypomorphic mutations in FoxP3 cause a similar pathology termed IPEX (immune dysregulation, polyendocrinopathy, enteropathy, and X-linked) syndrome [7].

Numerous studies have linked Treg accumulation in tumors and peripheral blood of cancer patients to poor prognosis, making Tregs an attractive target for cancer immunotherapy [8, 9]. Studies in animal models demonstrate that the depletion of Treg or inhibition of Treg suppressive mechanisms can restore anti-tumor immunity, eventually leading to decreased tumor growth or even tumor regression [4, 10].

However, many recent publications have challenged this simplistic view of Tregs as a major pro-tumorigenic cell population in the tumor microenvironment. First, a variety of other cells have been concerned in the negative regulation of the antitumor immune response [5, 11]. Second, it has been established that in certain malignancies, Treg accumulation can diminish tumorigenic inflammation and serve as a positive prognostic factor [12-14]. Third, Tregs exhibit significant phenotypical and functional heterogeneity with different subsets showing distinct suppressive efficacy and exploiting distinct suppressive mechanisms [15]. Moreover, Treg phenotype and function strongly differs between tumors, underlining the necessity to investigate the specific role of Tregs in particular malignancies [16].

In the current review, the role of Tregs in the suppression of anti-tumor immunity is discussed, focusing on therapeutic targeting of Treg-mediated immunosuppressive mechanisms.

## TREG DEVELOPMENT: NATURALLY OCCURRING AND INDUCED TREGS

During thymic differentiation, the intermediate-strength signals of T cell receptor (TCR) (together with IL-2 signaling) enable a number of CD4 single-positive thymocytes to escape deletion [6]. This population is enriched for cells instructed to differentiate into naturally occurring FoxP3$^+$ Treg cells (nTregs) [6]. The development of nTreg cells in the thymus is promoted by increased affinity interactions with self-peptide-MHC complexes. Meanwhile, in the periphery, conventional CD4$^+$CD25$^-$FoxP3$^-$ T cells (Tcons) are switched into induced Tregs (iTregs), as a result of high-affinity TCR signaling together with suboptimal costimulation in the presence of cytokines such as transforming growth factor (TGF)-β and IL-2 [6, 17]. These cells can arise in response to stimulation with foreign as well as tumor-associated self- or altered self-antigens under tolerogenic conditions [6, 17]. The TCR repertoire of iTregs largely differs from that of nTregs [6]. In particular, it has been suggested that iTregs often descend from Tcons recognizing antigens from the environment or commensal microbiota [18-21]. This implies that iTregs have a critical role in the post-thymic education of the immune system and adaptive tolerance [21].

TGF-β signaling is usually essential for FoxP3 induction in CD4$^+$ T cells from the peripheral blood [6]. IL-2 is also needed for TGF-β-mediated FoxP3 induction in peripheral T cells *in vitro* [6, 17, 22]. In the presence of TGF-β, IL-2 activates the FoxP3 locus through STAT5 and enhances the viability and proliferation rate of target cells [23]. IL-2 also inhibits the development of T helper 17 (Th17) cells [24]. Moreover, IL-2 is indispensable for the homeostasis of fully differentiated Treg cells [25].

Type 1 regulatory T cells (Tr1), characterized by the IL-10 production, can be induced by suboptimal activation and TGF-β signaling [26, 27]. However, Tr1 differentiation requires high IL-10 levels and they might be FoxP3$^-$ [26, 28]. In addition, although retinoic acid promotes the induction of FoxP3, it can supress the expression of IL-10 [29]. Altogether, these data indicate that iTregs and Tr1 likely stand for competing and alternative cell lineages. It has been suggested that tumor-reactive nTregs and iTregs both independently give to the pool of tumor-infiltrating Tregs [30]. Moreover, the stimulation of Tregs with tumor antigens possibly trigger strong proliferation of both nTregs and iTregs, substantially increasing their numbers in the tumor [31]. Rudensky's group newly generated mice with a deleted CNS1-element, an intronic FoxP3 enhancer which is essential for the differentiation of iTreg but not nTreg cells [32]. This model has already been applied to determine the role of iTregs in mucosal Th2 inflammation [33] and maternal-foetal conflict [34]. It might also significantly facilitate further elucidation of iTreg function in cancer.

## TREG PHENOTYPE AND IDENTIFICATION

In mice, FoxP3 seems to be an essential and adequate marker for the identification of *bona fide* Tregs [6], although it has been detected in a minor fraction of recently activated Tcons [35]. However, in humans, FoxP3 is expressed in a significant proportion of activated Tcons [7], which means additional markers are needed for accurate analysis of human Tregs. Regulatory T cells are routinely defined and isolated based on the surface expression of CD25, although it can also be expressed on activated Tcons [26]. Therefore, much attention has been focused on finding further markers that would allow robust detection and sorting of Tregs. For instance, several studies suggested that the IL-7 receptor CD127 is mainly expressed on conventional but not on Tregs [36]. Unfortunately, it was shown later that CD127 is not an ideal biomarker for the identification of Tregs, because some early activated Tcon also downregulate CD127 expression [37] and some activated Tregs can be $CD127^{+}$ [38]. Another study [39] showed that the integrin CD49d is present on most pro-inflammatory $CD25^{high}$ cells, but virtually absent in the Treg compartment; it can be used in conjunction with CD127 to improve the purity of sorted Treg preparations. Indeed, sorting of $CD25^{high}CD127^{low/-}CD49d^{-}$ Tregs, with subsequent analysis of FoxP3 expression, is now becoming a standard method for human Treg isolation [40].

## MECHANISMS OF SUPPRESSION

Tregs inhibit the activity of various immune cell types, *e.g.* CD4 and CD8 T cells, dendritic cells (DC), B cells, natural killer (NK), and NKT cells both *in vitro* and *in vivo* [6, 41]. *In vitro*, Tregs show hyporesponsiveness, *i.e.,* low proliferation rate in response to stimulation [7, 28]. However, a significant proportion of Tregs exhibit vigorous homeostatic proliferation *in vivo,* probably reflecting a high turnover rate or representing a consequence of recurrent interactions with cognate antigens [16]. Tregs inhibit immune responses in an antigen-unspecific manner, but their suppressive function is activated upon antigen-specific stimulation [42].

The suppressive effects of Tregs are mediated by a wide variety of mechanisms. These include surface expression of inhibitory or cell-death-inducing molecules, secretion of immunosuppressive cytokines, production of inhibitory molecules, and direct cytolysis. Tregs express high-level CD25 (*i.e.*, IL-2 receptor α-chain) and consequently can compete with effector T cells (Teff) for IL-2 as well as hamper their proliferation [43]. CTLA-4, an inhibitory co-receptor cytotoxic T lymphocyte antigen, is constitutively expressed on Tregs at high levels and has an imperative role in Treg suppressive activity [44]. CTLA-4 interaction with costimulatory molecules B7-1 (CD80) and B7-2 (CD86) on DC leads to upregulation of the suppressive enzyme indoleamine 2, 3-dioxygenase (IDO) in antigen-presenting cells (APC), and following T cell suppression [45]. Moreover, IDO itself is a strong inducer of Treg differentiation [46].

There are several other surface molecules that Tregs use to inhibit the APC activity. For instance, LAG-3, a CD4 homolog and a high-affinity ligand of MHC class II, contributes to the suppressive activity of both nTregs and iTregs [47]. Ligation of MHC II by LAG-3 leads to the inhibition of DC maturation and function [48]. Another recently discovered protein, TIGIT, is highly expressed on Tregs and activated Tcons, representing another example of Treg-mediated control of DC activity. During Treg-DC interactions, TIGIT induces IL-10 and TGF-β production by DC [49]. Besides contact-dependent immune suppression, Tregs can also secrete suppressive cytokines, most notably TGFβ and IL-10, which have proved to be essential for the Treg homeostasis and function *in vivo* [50-52].

Several mechanisms of Treg-mediated immune suppression involve production of molecules disrupting metabolic pathways and signaling in target cells. For instance, Tregs can transfer the second messenger cyclic AMP (cAMP) into target cells through gap junctions, which dampens the proliferation and activity of target cells [53]. Another mechanism leading to cAMP elevation in effector cells is Treg-mediated adenosine production through the enzymatic activity of cell-surface enzymes CD39 and CD73 [54]. These proteins can convert pro-inflammatory ATP into immunosuppressive adenosine in a two-step process: CD39 hydrolyses ATP or ADP into AMP, and CD73, in turn, cleaves AMP yielding adenosine [55]. However, extracellular enzymes adenylate kinase and NDP kinase can phosphorylate AMP and ADP, respectively, thus antagonizing CD39 activity [56]. In contrast, adenosine can only be phosphorylated inside the cell by adenosine kinase, although it can also be inactivated in the extracellular space by adenosine deaminase. Remarkably, despite the necessity of CD73 for adenosine synthesis under physiological conditions, CD73 deficiency is usually complemented by compensatory overproduction of alkaline phosphatases [56].

Adenosine activates four individual G-protein-coupled receptors: A1, A2A, A2B, and A3 [55]. The A1 and A3 adenosine receptors are attached to the Gi/o subunit, and their activation inhibits adenylate cyclase activity, leading to reduce the production of cAMP and the activation of protein kinase A (PKA). In addition, engagement of these receptors activates the phosphatidylinositol 3-kinase (PI3K) pathway. Activation of A2A and A2B largely accounts for the immunosuppressive effects of adenosine. These receptors are coupled to the Gs subunit that activates adenylate cyclase, thus leading to enhanced cAMP synthesis and subsequent inhibitory effects on target cells [54]. However, in contrast to other adenosine receptors, A2B is a low-affinity receptor and can only be activated by high levels of adenosine generated in response to pathological conditions [55].

A2A receptors (A2AR) are expressed on a variety of immune cells (*i.e.*, monocytes/macrophages, granulocytes, lymphocytes, DC and NK cells) [55, 57]. A2AR-triggered cAMP elevation inhibits effector functions of all these cell populations. In particular, adenosine impedes the phagocytic capacity of macrophages, degranulation of neutrophils and the production of IFN-γ by NK cells [55]. It also drives DC differentiation towards a population producing immune suppressive factors, such as TGF-β, prostaglandin E2, IDO *etc.* [58]. Adenosine-mediated cAMP accumulation and inhibition of the NF-κB pathway [59] in T cells hinders their activation, proliferation, survival and effector functions [60, 61].

Adenosine production also strongly contributes to Treg immunosuppressive activity [56, 62]. Tregs from CD39-deficient mice are constantly activated but fail to suppress effector T cell proliferation [61]. Furthermore, activated CD4 T cells in CD73-deficient animals show enhanced production of pro-inflammatory cytokines, including IFN-γ, IL-2 and TNF-α, and their Tregs completely lack suppressive activities [63]. Therefore, it has been hypothesized that CD73-derived adenosine ensures a tonic inhibition of NF-κB in $CD4^+$ T-cells, restricting thereby the development of effector T cell responses. CD39 and CD73 on Tregs have a vital role in regulating the balance between pro-inflammatory ATP and immunosuppressive adenosine. ATP can accumulate outside the cell both under normal and pathological conditions. In the context of inflammation and cancer, ATP is released by activated leukocytes, dying, injured or stressed cells [56].

The effects of ATP-mediated signaling are concentration-dependent. High ATP concentrations activate the NLRP3 inflammasome through P2X7 receptors, which leads to caspase activation and cell death [64]. Low ATP concentrations can trigger the influx of calcium into the cytoplasm or inhibit the synthesis of immunosuppressive cAMP through various P2Y receptors [65]. Thus, the regulation of the ratio between extracellular ATP and adenosine by CD39 and CD73 on Tregs provides a means of tipping the balance between an immune activation and suppression. However, the role of CD73 in the human immune system appears to differ significantly from that in animal models. Importantly, while murine Tregs stably express CD73 on the cell surface, in human Tregs CD73 can only be detected inside the cell [66]. This challenges the notion that human Tregs can mediate the whole cascade of ATP conversion into adenosine, suggesting thereby that other cell populations might be involved in catalyzing AMP dephosphorylation.

Another means for Treg-mediated immune suppression is direct cytotoxic activity against effector cells of the immune system [28]. Tregs can release cytolytic molecules, including granzyme A/B and perforin, or activate the pathway of the tumor necrosis factor (TNF) related apoptosis inducing ligand (TRAIL)-death receptor (DR)-5.

Thus, Tregs deploy a wide variety of mechanisms to control the effector arm of immunity (Fig. **1**). This paves the way for the development of a number of strategies to alleviate the suppressor function of Tregs in cancer patients aiming to improve anti-tumor immune responses.

## THERAPEUTIC NEUTRALIZATION OF TREGS

Multiple studies implicate Tregs in a variety of pro-tumor activities, such as tumor-associated immunosuppression, tumor growth, invasion, angiogenesis, and metastasis formation. Current strategies to target Tregs in cancer include Treg depletion as well as blockades of Treg immunosuppressive activity and migration. Here we focus on the first two strategies since therapeutic approaches to inhibit Treg migration have recently been extensively reviewed elsewhere [10, 16, 17, 67].

Treg depletion has been widely used to restore antitumor immunity and to develop the efficacy of vaccination and cell-based therapies, in both human and animal hosts [10]. Depletion agents used in clinical and preclinical studies include anti-CD25 antibody (daclizumab), IL-2-diphtheria toxin fusion protein (denileukin diftitox, ONTAK), low-dose chemotherapeutics, and CD25-targeting immunotoxins [16, 68]. Current depletion strategies do not allow specific Treg targeting, since they share CD25 expression with activated Tcons [16]. However, these approaches have proved instrumental when Tregs significantly outnumber activated Tcons in the tumor microenvironment. Therefore, Treg depletion might restore the activation, migration, proliferation and activity of remaining Tcons [10].

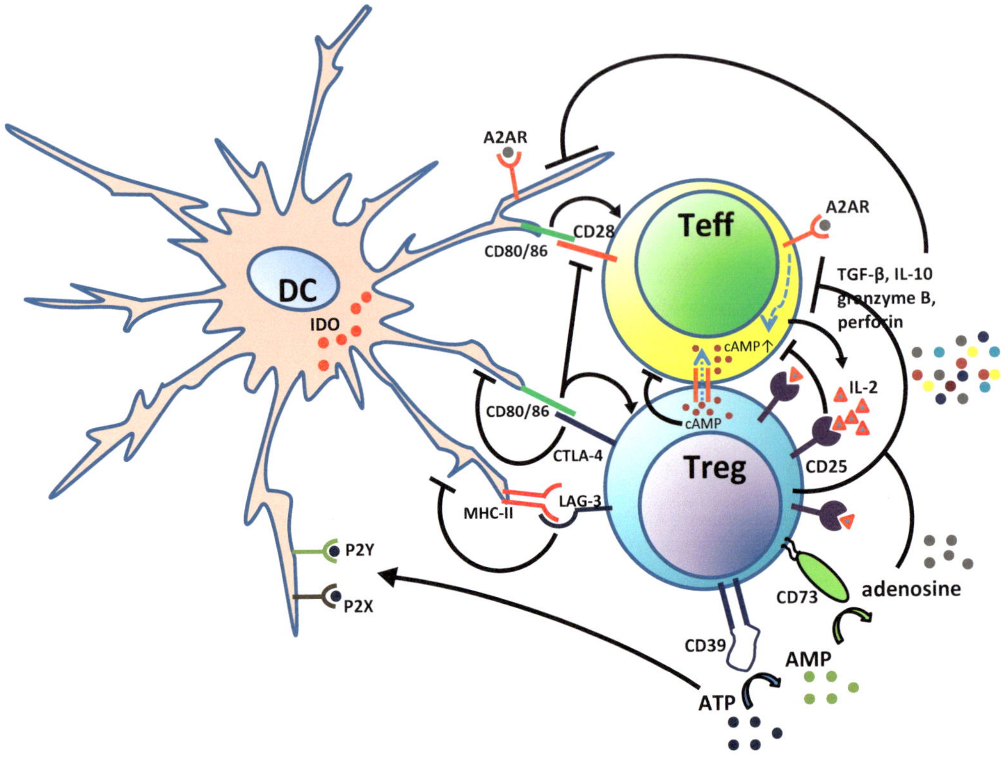


**Figure 1: Mechanisms of Treg-mediated immunosuppression.** Tregs suppress the function of effector T cells (Teff) and dendritic cells (DC) both in a contact-dependent manner and through soluble mediators. High-level IL-2 receptor α-chain (CD25) on Tregs lead to the IL-2 depletion in the microenvironment, hindering Teff proliferation and activity. Conversion of extracellular ATP into adenosine by CD39 and CD73 inhibits Teff function and prevents ATP-mediated DC stimulation through P2 receptors. Extracellular adenosine, activates A2a receptors on DC and Teff, triggering the synthesis of immunosuppressive cAMP. Tregs transfer cAMP into Teff *via* gap-junctions. CTLA-4 on Tregs binds to the costimulatory molecules CD80 and CD86 on DC with high affinity. This prevents the CD28-dependent costimulation of Teff and leads to the downregulation of CD80 and CD86 on DC. The activity of indoleamine 2,3-dioxygenase (IDO) in DC is induced, which mediates tryptophan depletion and triggers thereby Teff apoptosis. Ligation of MHC-II molecules on DC through Treg-derived LAG-3 results in the suppression of DC maturation and function. Upon activation, Tregs kill both responder Teff or DC by releasing granzyme B and perforin. Tregs secrete a number of immunosuppressive cytokines, including TGF-β and IL-10 to inhibit both Teff and DC.

## LOW-DOSE CHEMOTHERAPY

The high proliferation rate of Tregs makes them more sensitive to chemotherapy than effector T cells [16]. Therefore, certain chemotherapeutic regimens might lead to fairly selective Treg depletion. This was confirmed by studies showing that anti-tumor effects of certain chemotherapeutic agents have distinct mechanisms, depending on the dose regimen [69]. Metronomic (low-dose) cyclophosphamide (CTX) administration has been shown to improve anti-tumor immunity and vaccination efficacy through Treg depletion, whereas high-dose regimens exerted direct cytolytic effects on tumor cells but also caused immunosuppression [69].

The results of an early study by Polak and Turk [70] indicated that CTX might reverse immune tolerance by targeting a yet unidentified suppressive T-cell population. Further investigations confirmed this hypothesis. For instance, Machiels *et al.* [71] showed that immune-modulating doses of CTX, doxorubicin, and paclitaxel can boost the anti-tumor effects of HER-2/neu-expressing whole cell vaccines and reduce mammary tumor growth in *neu* transgenic mice. The tolerance to the *neu* transgene observed in these mice recapitulates irresponsiveness to tumor antigens in cancer patients. Administration of CTX at 50-150 mg/kg one day before vaccination was superior to CTX or vaccination alone. The reversed order of treatment proved to be ineffective, and higher doses of CTX were detrimental for vaccine efficacy. Metronomic CTX treatment resulted in an augmented Th1 HER-2/neu-specific T cell response, indicating the reversal of tolerance.

In a rat model of colon carcinoma, Ghiringhelli *et al.* [72] demonstrated that CTX indeed decreases the number of Tregs, resulting in a restoration of peripheral T cell proliferation with innate killing actions. A single administration of CTX at 25 to 30 mg/kg depleted $CD4^+CD25^+$ T cells while sparing other lymphocytes, delayed tumor growth, and led to a complete tumor regression when followed by immunotherapy that had no curative effect when administered alone.

Later, it was shown that metronomic CTX could also selectively deplete $CD4^+CD25^+FoxP3^+$ Treg cells in advanced cancer patients. For instance, in a study reported by Ge *et al.* [73], daily oral administration of 50 mg cyclophosphamide in patients with treatment-refractory metastatic breast cancer initially caused a depletion of more than 40% of Treg in the peripheral blood. However, during the treatment, Treg numbers gradually recovered. Nevertheless, the transient Treg depletion allowed an expansion of tumor antigen-specific T cells that persisted during the whole period of treatment. Notably, numbers of tumor-reactive T effectors, but not Tregs correlated with disease stabilization and increased overall survival.

Preclinical studies showed that low-dose CTX also decreases the functional activity of Treg cells. Lutsiak *et al.* [74] compared Tregs from cyclophosphamide-treated (2 mg intraperitoneally) and control mice 2 and 10 days after treatment. Tregs from CTX-treated animals had a significantly diminished suppressive capacity, which was restored by day 10 upon the treatment. Furthermore, CTX also decreased the homeostatic proliferation of Tregs, enhanced their susceptibility to apoptosis, and downregulated FoxP3 expression.

In the recent phase II trial [75], Treg numbers, phenotype and function were rigorously monitored in the lymph nodes and peripheral blood of stage II-III melanoma patients vaccinated by HLA-A*0201-modified tumor peptides in conjunction with the low-dose CTX and IL-2 administration. CTX slightly reduced the Treg number in the immunized patients. Again, the transient Treg depletion after the first CTX injection was followed by complete recovery of Treg numbers, in spite of the following administration of extra CTX doses. However, the treatment resulted in a substantial reduction in Treg numbers as well as IL-10 and TGFβ production in regional lymph nodes. Interestingly, the Treg frequency in the lymph nodes (LNs) was lower in patients treated with CTX than controls. This study is consistent with the preclinical results indicating that CTX selectively depletes cycling and effector/memory Tregs with enhanced tumor-homing activity. These findings suggest that metronomic CTX depletes iTregs at the tumor site rather than in the peripheral blood.

However, despite certain insights gained in these studies, the elucidation of universal immunological mechanisms of metronomic chemotherapy is substantially hindered by the differences in therapeutic regimens and the methods used to detect and analyze Tregs.

## TREG DEPLETION BY CD25-TARGETING AGENTS

### Anti-CD25

Several groups showed that prophylactic Treg depletion by way of anti-CD25 mAb in animals triggered the rejection of syngeneic tumors [76, 77], although after tumor induction the treatment of anti-CD25 mAb was greatly less efficient. However, tumor rejection was substantially facilitated when anti-CD25 mAb administration was used with the DC vaccination [78, 79], CTLA-4 blockade [80] or GITR stimulation [28, 81]. Since both Tregs and activated $CD4^+$ and $CD8^+$ T cells express CD25, anti-CD25 therapy may entail concomitant deletion of effector T cells. Accordingly, in B16 melanoma model, it was observed that although $CD25^+$ T cell depletion before vaccination enhanced treatment efficacy, the administration of anti-CD25 mAbs prior to a rechallenge in pre-vaccinated animals significantly reduceed the protecting effect of vaccination [78, 80].

In a clinical study, Jacobs *et al.* [82] evaluated the impact of anti-CD25 mAb management on vaccination efficacy. Thirty HLA-$A2.1^+$ patients with metastatic melanoma were immunized with mature DC loaded with tumor peptide plus keyhole limpet hemocyanin (KLH). Fifteen patients were pretreated with the drug of daclizumab that is a humanized anti-CD25 blocking antibody. Daclizumab efficiently depleted all circulating $CD25^{high}$ leukocytes (including $CD4^+FoxP3^+CD25^{high}$ cells) within four days after daclizumab injection. Thirty days following the administration, daclizumab clearance from the blood was manifested by the recovery of entire $CD25^+$ cells. The daclizumab presence for the duration of DC vaccinations prohibited the induction of specific antibodies, however, not the existence of antigen-specific T cells. These $CD25^+$ T cells did not acquire effector functions. As a consequence, notably fewer patients pretreated with daclizumab built up functional and specific effector T cells as well as antibodies than controls. Compared to the control group, the pretreatment of Daclizumab had no important effect on the progression-free survival.

A more recent study published by Rech *et al.* [83] showed that daclizumab does not act through antibody-dependent or complement-mediated cytotoxicity rather than suppresses FoxP3 expression selectively in $CD25^{high}CD45RA^-$ Tregs. Furthermore, daclizumab-treated $CD45RA^-$ Tregs vanished suppressive function and acquired the capacity to produce IFN-γ, indicating their reprogramming towards Th1 lineage. In a clinical trial monitored by the same group [83], in patients with metastatic breast cancer daclizumab was administered in arrangement with a tentative cancer vaccine. The treatment resulted in a substantial and extended reduction of Tregs. Effective $CD8^+$ and $CD4^+$ T cell priming and responsiveness to all vaccine antigens were confirmed, along with an absence of autoimmune reactions.

Thus, studies on anti-CD25 mAb-mediated Treg depletion show conflicting results, underscoring the necessity to investigate the impact of various treatment regimens on the effects of daclizumab.

## IL-2-Difteria Toxin Fusion Protein

Another CD25-targeting agent, denileukin diftitox (ONTAK), was initially approved by FDA as an anti-neoplastic agent for the management of cutaneous T cell lymphoma [68]. Denileukin diftitox consists of a portion of diphtheria toxin that is fused to IL-2. Upon internalization, diphtheria toxin permanently hampers protein synthesis, eventually causing cell death. In patients with renal cell carcinoma, ONTAK significantly reduced circulating Treg numbers and promoted the expansion of $CD4^+$ and $CD8^+$ T cells producing IFN-γ after DC vaccination [84]. However, clinical studies of ONTAK in patients with melanoma showed inconsistent efficacy of Treg depletion and contradictory data on the clinical outcome. For instance, it has been reported that ONTAK administration altered neither FoxP3 mRNA levels in $CD4^+$ T cells nor the suppressive activity of $CD4^+CD25^+$ T cells [85]. None of the patients in this investigation showed an objective clinical response. In contrast, Telang *et al.* [86] showed that ONTAK caused a transient depletion of Tregs, promoting melanoma antigen-specific $CD8^+$ T cells. Moreover, in a phase II clinical trial, ONTAK treatment resulted in a partial response in 16.7% of 60 patients and markedly increased the one-year survival in the cohort of partial responders as compared to patients with the progressive disease.

## CD25-Targeting Immunotoxins

Two clinical trials explored the management of immunotoxins linked to CD25 antibodies: RFT5-SMPT-dgIgA, which is a CD25-specific murine antibody linked to a deglycosylated ricin A chain (dgA) [87], and LMB-2, which is a fusion of a single-chain Fγ fragment of the CD25-specific, anti-Tac monoclonal antibody to a truncated form of *Pseudomonas* exotoxin A [88]. The administration of RFT5-SMPT-dgA in six patients with metastatic melanoma led to a transient but consistent decrease in the number of $CD25^{high}CD4^+$ T cells *in vivo* [87]. However, the reduction in total $FoxP3^+CD4^+$ T cell numbers was not as drastic, since the $CD25^{low/-}FoxP3^+$ subpopulation of $CD4^+$ T cells escaped the depletion and persisted at stable numbers. No objective antitumor responses were observed. In another study, eight patients with metastatic melanoma were given LMB-2 followed by MART-1 and gp100-specific peptide vaccination [88]. LMB-2 administration led to a special, short-lived reduction (up to 79.1%) in circulating $CD25^+CD4^+$ T cell numbers. Again, $FoxP3^+CD4^+$ Tregs that escaped the depletion mediated by LMB-2 were $CD25^{low/-}$. However, despite the decrease in Treg numbers, LMB-2 therapy failed to improve the immune response to vaccination and no patient practiced an objective response or autoimmunity.

Thus, the above-mentioned Treg-depleting strategies transiently reduce the Treg numbers and function in the peripheral blood of some cancer patients. However, the Tregs come back and it becomes again necessary to block their activity.

# FOXP3 VACCINATION

Since FoxP3 is a "master regulator" transcription factor of Treg development and function, the vaccination against FoxP3 might lead to efficient Treg depletion, representing an interesting approach to neutralize the tumor-associated immune suppression. In the B16 melanoma model, it was shown that the vaccination with FoxP3 mRNA leads to a local intratumoral but not systemic depletion of FoxP3$^+$ cells [78]. Nevertheless, the paucity of tumor Treg was associated with the improved anti-tumor reactivity of TRP-2-specific cytotoxic T lymphocytes after an additional vaccination with TRP-2-loaded DC. The mechanisms of this preferential depletion of tumor Treg remain obscure.

# INHIBITING TREG FUNCTION

## CTLA-4

Similar to many other markers, the CTLA-4 expression is shared by regulatory and activated T cells [28]. There have been some conflicting data on the specific role of CTLA-4 expression in either subset. Mice with Treg-specific CTLA-4 knockout succumb to lymphoproliferation and autoimmune diseases, similar to FoxP3 deficiency [89]. Nude mice reconstituted with splenocytes with CTLA-4-deficient Tregs showed an enhanced survival and decreased tumor growth (or even teh tumor rejection) as compared with the recipients of control splenocytes [89]. On the other hand, it has been demonstrated [90] that although antibody-mediated CTLA-4 blockade on T effector cells significantly improved the survival of mice with B16 melanoma, a specific blockade of CTLA-4 expressed on Tregs alone had no antitumor effects. However, the maximal prolongation of survival was achieved by associating blockade of CTLA-4 in both regulatory and effector T cells.

In stage IV melanoma patients, therapy with anti-CTLA-4 antibodies (ipilimumab) reduced Treg numbers and restored TCR-dependent proliferation of effector T cells [72]. Importantly, a randomised trial in a number of patients with formerly treated metastatic melanoma [91] showed a significantly increased overall survival upon ipilimumab treatment. However, such therapy often triggers severe systemic toxicity that outweighs the antitumor effects of the treatment [92].

## GITR

Glucocorticoid-induced TNFR-related protein (GITR) is a co-stimulatory molecule constitutively expressed in Tregs [16]. It is also expressed at lower levels in resting effector T cells and is upregulated upon T cell activation [10]. GITR stimulation by agonistic antibodies or GITR ligands leads to suppression of Treg activity and increased proliferation of effector T cells [16]. Administration of anti-GITR mAbs elicited a concomitant immunity in B16 melanoma-bearing mice, *i.e.,* promoted rejection of B16 at a remote site [77]. Moreover, GITR activation triggered tumor regression in animals with methylcholanthrene-induced fibrosarcoma (93). In contrast to most depletion strategies, anti-GITR mAb therapy has shown higher efficacy in animals with established tumors as compared with in prophylactic settings [93]. In addition, the combination of GITR activation with tumor Ag stimulation promotes tumor-reactive effector T cells [94]. Thus, GITR represents an attractive target for cancer immunotherapy.

## OX40

OX40 (CD134) is a costimulatory receptor expressed on Treg and activated Teff [16]. OX40 ligation promotes T cell proliferation, cytokine production, and survival [95]. Furthermore, it can also inhibit Treg differentiation and suppressive activity [96, 97]. Studies in preclinical models have demonstrated that OX40 activation provides strong protection against immunogenic tumors, although poorly immunogenic tumors are more refractory to the therapy [98]. Interestingly, a recent study showed that, in the context of chemotherapy-induced lymphopenia, OX40 activation induced a novel $CD4^+$ T cell population, expressing the transcription factor eomesodermin and producing Th1 and Th2 cytokines [99]. This subpopulation promoted eradication of advanced B16 tumors in mice, supporting the use of immune modulation in redirecting the polarization of $CD4^+$ T cells. These promising results suggest the need for further research to achieve a better understanding how OX40 plays in antitumor immunity.

## Extracellular Adenosine Metabolism and Signaling

In mice, Tregs coexpress ectoenzymes CD39 and CD73 which turn ATP into immunosuppressive adenosine [54]. Over the last years, multiple studies have observed that adenosine production by Treg is part of their inhibitory activity, and have shown that targeting adenosine synthesis *in vivo* is a promising strategy to diminish tumor-mediated immunosuppression [60, 61, 66, 100-103].

It has been well documented that inhibiting adenosine signaling, either targeting the receptor or the enzyme that produces it, significantly reduces tumor growth by improving the anti-tumor immune response [60, 100-104]. One seminal study showed that A2A receptor deficiency promoted the rejection of established immunogenic tumors, and that the administration of A2AR antagonists reduced tumor growth and metastasis [60]. The antitumor outcomes of A2AR targeting were CTL-dependent. Furthermore, in a transplantable breast cancer model, Stagg *et al.* [101] demonstrated the efficacy of anti-CD73 mAb therapy in reducing tumorigenesis and metastasis. This study, together with several others [60, 103], showed the importance of CD73 expressed on tumor cells in hindering anti-tumor immune reactivity.

More recently, research has centered on the host CD73 in tumor-mediated immunosuppression and on the specific contribution of various cell lineages to adenosine production. Using four different transplantable tumor models, Stagg *et al.* [100] found that CD73-deficiency enhanced anti-tumor immune responses and resistance to experimental metastasis. The anti-tumor effect of CD73 deletion was dependent on CTL and related to an expansion of antigen-specific interferon-γ-producing CTL in the peripheral circulation and the tumor microenvironment. Experiments with bone marrow chimeras indicated that both hematopoietic and non-hematopoietic expression of CD73 non-redundantly contribute to the tumor immune escape. Furthermore, CD73 expression at least partially accounted for the tumor-promoting effects of Tregs. The pro-metastatic effect of host-derived CD73 was not independent of the expression of CD73 on non-hematopoietic cells. Complementary data of Wang *et al.* [102] suggested that the enzymatic activity of CD73 on non-hematopoietic cells hindered leukocyte migration into the tumor site, whereas CD73 on hematopoietic cells suppressed a systemic anti-tumor T cell expansion and their effector functions. Both groups demonstrated the anti-tumor and anti-metastatic effects of CD73 targeting, with a monoclonal antibody or APCP, the selective inhibitor α, β-methylene adenosine diphosphate. Moreover, Wang *et al.* [102] showed that anti-CD73 mAbs could completely restore the efficacy of T cell-based therapy in tumor-bearing mice. The translational significance of these findings is underscored by the fact that various adenosine receptor antagonists are already used in clinical settings for other indications [16].

Thus, targeting adenosine production and signaling represents a promising strategy to restore spontaneous T cell-mediated anti-tumor reactivity and to progress the efficiency of adoptive cellular immunotherapy in cancer patients. Additional investigations are needed to determine the adenosine role in human immune cells and their interactions with tumor cells in the tumor microenvironment and in the periphery.

# CONCLUSION

Tregs are essential in tumor escape from the anti-cancer immune response. Treg-targeting strategies developed over the last years include variations on Treg depletion and inhibition of their suppressive activity and migration. Although many of these strategies showed significant anti-tumor efficacy in animal cancer models, only a few were demonstrated to lead to objective responses and prolongation of survival in clinical trials. The limited success of Treg depletion is largely attributed to the lack of truly specific surface markers of Tregs, which would allow them to target without affecting tumor-specific effector T cells. Moreover, these therapies only cause a transient decrease, as the number of Tregs eventually recovers in all studies. Finally, agents targeting Tregs or important negative checkpoints (*e.g.* CTLA-4) often entail a severe and potentially fatal systemic toxicity. Therefore, less toxic substances inhibiting Tregs and activating effector T cells, such as anti-OX40 mAbs or adenosine receptor antagonists may be hopeful candidates for the development of new schemes of cancer immunotherapy.


# ACKNOWLEDGEMENTS

Declared None.


# CONFLICT OF INTEREST

The authors confirm that this chapter contents have no conflict of interest.

# REFERENCES


[1] Schreiber RD, Old LJ, Smyth MJ. Cancer immunoediting: integrating immunity's roles in cancer suppression and promotion. Science 2011; 331(6024): 1565-70.

[2] Clark WH, Jr., Elder DE, Guerry Dt, Braitman LE, Trock BJ, Schultz D, *et al.* Model predicting survival in stage I melanoma based on tumor progression. J Natl Cancer Inst 1989; 81(24): 1893-904.

[3] Naito Y, Saito K, Shiiba K, Ohuchi A, Saigenji K, Nagura H, *et al.* CD8+ T cells infiltrated within cancer cell nests as a prognostic factor in human colorectal cancer. Cancer Res 1998; 58(16): 3491-4.

[4] Oleinika K, Nibbs RJ, Graham GJ, Fraser AR. Suppression, subversion and escape: the role of regulatory T cells in cancer progression. Clin Exp Immunol 2013; 171(1): 36-45.

[5] Umansky V, Sevko, A. Melanoma-induced immunosuppression and its neutralization. Semin Cancer Biol 2012; 22(4): 319-26.

[6] Josefowicz SZ, Lu LF, Rudensky AY. Regulatory T cells: mechanisms of differentiation and function. Annu Rev Immunol 2012; 30: 531-64.

[7] Sakaguchi S, Miyara M, Costantino CM, Hafler DA. FOXP3+ regulatory T cells in the human immune system. Nat Rev Immunol 2010; 10(7): 490-500.

[8] Badoual C, Hans S, Fridman WH, Brasnu D, Erdman S, Tartour E. Revisiting the prognostic value of regulatory T cells in patients with cancer. J Clin Oncol 2009; 27(19): e5-6; author reply e7.

[9] Fridman WH, Galon J, Pages F, Tartour E, Sautes-Fridman C, Kroemer G. Prognostic and predictive impact of intra- and peritumoral immune infiltrates. Cancer Res 2011; 71(17): 5601-5.
[10] Byrne WL, Mills KH, Lederer JA, O'Sullivan GC. Targeting regulatory T cells in cancer. Cancer Res 2011; 71(22): 6915-20.
[11] Gabrilovich DI, Ostrand-Rosenberg S, Bronte V. Coordinated regulation of myeloid cells by tumours. Nat Rev Immunol 2012; 12(4): 253-68.
[12] Erdman SE, Rao VP, Olipitz W, Taylor CL, Jackson EA, Levkovich T, *et al.* Unifying roles for regulatory T cells and inflammation in cancer. Int J Cancer 2010; 126(7): 1651-65.
[13] Erdman SE, Poutahidis T. Cancer inflammation and regulatory T cells. Int J Cancer 2010; 127(4): 768-79.
[14] Badoual C, Hans S, Rodriguez J, Peyrard S, Klein C, Agueznay Nel H, *et al.* Prognostic value of tumor-infiltrating CD4+ T-cell subpopulations in head and neck cancers. Clin Cancer Res 2006; 12(2): 465-72.
[15] Campbell DJ, Koch MA. Phenotypical and functional specialization of FOXP3+ regulatory T cells. Nat Rev Immunol 2011; 11(2): 119-30.
[16] Pere H, Tanchot C, Bayry J, Terme M, Taieb J, Badoual C, *et al.* Comprehensive analysis of current approaches to inhibit regulatory T cells in cancer. Oncoimmunology 2012; 1(3): 326-33
[17] Tanchot C, Terme M, Pere H, Tran T, Benhamouda N, Strioga M, *et al.* Tumor-Infiltrating Regulatory T Cells: Phenotype, Role, Mechanism of Expansion *In Situ* and Clinical Significance. Cancer Microenviron 2013; 6(2): 147-57.
[18] Kretschmer K, Apostolou I, Hawiger D, Khazaie K, Nussenzweig MC, von Boehmer H. Inducing and expanding regulatory T cell populations by foreign antigen. Nat Immunol 2005; 6(12): 1219-27.
[19] Kretschmer K, Heng TS, von Boehmer H. *De novo* production of antigen-specific suppressor cells *in vivo*. Nat Protoc 2006; 1(2): 653-61.
[20] Verginis P, McLaughlin KA, Wucherpfennig KW, von Boehmer H, Apostolou I. Induction of antigen-specific regulatory T cells in wild-type mice: visualization and targets of suppression. Proc Natl Acad Sci U S A 2008; 105(9): 3479-84.
[21] Lathrop SK, Bloom SM, Rao SM, Nutsch K, Lio CW, Santacruz N, *et al.* Peripheral education of the immune system by colonic commensal microbiota. Nature 2011; 478(7368): 250-4.
[22] Davidson TS, DiPaolo RJ, Andersson J, Shevach EM. Cutting Edge: IL-2 is essential for TGF-beta-mediated induction of Foxp3+ T regulatory cells. J Immunol 2007; 178(7): 4022-6.
[23] Burchill MA, Yang J, Vang KB, Moon JJ, Chu HH, Lio CW, *et al.* Linked T cell receptor and cytokine signaling govern the development of the regulatory T cell repertoire. Immunity 2008; 28(1): 112-21.
[24] Laurence A, Tato CM, Davidson TS, Kanno Y, Chen Z, Yao Z, *et al.* Interleukin-2 signaling *via* STAT5 constrains T helper 17 cell generation. Immunity 2007; 26(3): 371-81.
[25] Fontenot JD, Rasmussen JP, Gavin MA, Rudensky AY. A function for interleukin 2 in Foxp3-expressing regulatory T cells. Nat Immunol 2005; 6(11): 1142-51.
[26] Roncarolo MG, Gregori S, Battaglia M, Bacchetta R, Fleischhauer K, Levings MK. Interleukin-10-secreting type 1 regulatory T cells in rodents and humans. Immunol Rev 2006; 212: 28-50.
[27] Groux H, O'Garra A, Bigler M, Rouleau M, Antonenko S, de Vries JE, *et al.* A CD4+ T-cell subset inhibits antigen-specific T-cell responses and prevents colitis. Nature 1997; 389(6652): 737-42.
[28] Shalev I, Schmelzle M, Robson SC, Levy G. Making sense of regulatory T cell suppressive function. Semin Immunol 2011; 23(4): 282-92.
[29] Maynard CL, Hatton RD, Helms WS, Oliver JR, Stephensen CB, Weaver CT. Contrasting roles for all-trans retinoic acid in TGF-beta-mediated induction of Foxp3 and Il10 genes in developing regulatory T cells. J Exp Med 2009; 206(2): 343-57.
[30] Zhou G, Levitsky HI. Natural regulatory T cells and *de novo*-induced regulatory T cells contribute independently to tumor-specific tolerance. J Immunol 2007; 178(4): 2155-62.
[31] Bilate AM, Lafaille JJ. Induced CD4+Foxp3+ regulatory T cells in immune tolerance. Annu Rev Immunol 2012; 30: 733-58.
[32] Zheng Y, Josefowicz S, Chaudhry A, Peng XP, Forbush K, Rudensky AY. Role of conserved non-coding DNA elements in the Foxp3 gene in regulatory T-cell fate. Nature 2010; 463(7282): 808-12.
[33] Josefowicz SZ, Niec RE, Kim HY, Treuting P, Chinen T, Zheng Y, *et al.* Extrathymically generated regulatory T cells control mucosal TH2 inflammation. Nature 2012; 482(7385): 395-9.

[34] Samstein RM, Josefowicz SZ, Arvey A, Treuting PM, Rudensky AY. Extrathymic generation of regulatory T cells in placental mammals mitigates maternal-fetal conflict. Cell 2012; 150(1): 29-38.

[35] Miyao T, Floess S, Setoguchi R, Luche H, Fehling HJ, Waldmann H, *et al.* Plasticity of Foxp3(+) T cells reflects promiscuous Foxp3 expression in conventional T cells but not reprogramming of regulatory T cells. Immunity 2012; 36(2): 262-75.

[36] Liu W, Putnam AL, Xu-Yu Z, Szot GL, Lee MR, Zhu S, *et al.* CD127 expression inversely correlates with FoxP3 and suppressive function of human CD4+ T reg cells. J Exp Med 2006; 203(7): 1701-11.

[37] Allan SE, Alstad AN, Merindol N, Crellin NK, Amendola M, Bacchetta R, *et al.* Generation of potent and stable human CD4+ T regulatory cells by activation-independent expression of FOXP3. Mol Ther 2008; 16(1): 194-202.

[38] Simonetta F, Chiali A, Cordier C, Urrutia A, Girault I, Bloquet S, *et al.* Increased CD127 expression on activated FOXP3+CD4+ regulatory T cells. Eur J Immunol 2010; 40(9): 2528-38.

[39] Kleinewietfeld M, Starke M, Di Mitri D, Borsellino G, Battistini L, Rotzschke O, *et al.* CD49d provides access to "untouched" human Foxp3+ Treg free of contaminating effector cells. Blood 2009; 113(4): 827-36.

[40] Peters JH, Preijers FW, Woestenenk R, Hilbrands LB, Koenen HJ, Joosten I. Clinical grade Treg: GMP isolation, improvement of purity by CD127 Depletion, Treg expansion, and Treg cryopreservation. PLoS One 2008; 3(9): e3161.

[41] Mougiakakos D, Choudhury A, Lladser A, Kiessling R, Johansson CC. Regulatory T cells in cancer. Adv Cancer Res 2010; 107: 57-117.

[42] Yamaguchi T, Hirota K, Nagahama K, Ohkawa K, Takahashi T, Nomura T, *et al.* Control of immune responses by antigen-specific regulatory T cells expressing the folate receptor. Immunity 2007; 27(1): 145-59.

[43] Pandiyan P, Zheng L, Ishihara S, Reed J, Lenardo MJ. CD4+CD25+Foxp3+ regulatory T cells induce cytokine deprivation-mediated apoptosis of effector CD4+ T cells. Nat Immunol 2007; 8(12): 1353-62.

[44] Bachmann MF, Kohler G, Ecabert B, Mak TW, Kopf M. Cutting edge: lymphoproliferative disease in the absence of CTLA-4 is not T cell autonomous. J Immunol 1999; 163(3): 1128-31.

[45] Miyara M, Sakaguchi S. Natural regulatory T cells: mechanisms of suppression. Trends Mol Med 2007; 13(3): 108-16.

[46] Curti A, Pandolfi S, Valzasina B, Aluigi M, Isidori A, Ferri E, *et al.* Modulation of tryptophan catabolism by human leukemic cells results in the conversion of CD25- into CD25+ T regulatory cells. Blood 2007; 109(7): 2871-7.

[47] Huang CT, Workman CJ, Flies D, Pan X, Marson AL, Zhou G, *et al.* Role of LAG-3 in regulatory T cells. Immunity 2004; 21(4): 503-13.

[48] Liang B, Workman C, Lee J, Chew C, Dale BM, Colonna L, *et al.* Regulatory T cells inhibit dendritic cells by lymphocyte activation gene-3 engagement of MHC class II. J Immunol 2008; 180(9): 5916-26.

[49] Yu X, Harden K, Gonzalez LC, Francesco M, Chiang E, Irving B, *et al.* The surface protein TIGIT suppresses T cell activation by promoting the generation of mature immunoregulatory dendritic cells. Nat Immunol 2009; 10(1): 48-57.

[50] von Boehmer H. Mechanisms of suppression by suppressor T cells. Nat Immunol 2005; 6(4): 338-44.

[51] Rubtsov YP, Rasmussen JP, Chi EY, Fontenot J, Castelli L, Ye X, *et al.* Regulatory T cell-derived interleukin-10 limits inflammation at environmental interfaces. Immunity 2008; 28(4): 546-58.

[52] Marie JC, Liggitt D, Rudensky AY. Cellular mechanisms of fatal early-onset autoimmunity in mice with the T cell-specific targeting of transforming growth factor-beta receptor. Immunity 2006; 25(3): 441-54.

[53] Bopp T, Becker C, Klein M, Klein-Hessling S, Palmetshofer A, Serfling E, *et al.* Cyclic adenosine monophosphate is a key component of regulatory T cell-mediated suppression. J Exp Med 2007; 204(6): 1303-10.

[54] Allard B, Turcotte M, Stagg J. CD73-generated adenosine: orchestrating the tumor-stroma interplay to promote cancer growth. J Biomed Biotechnol 2012; 2012: 485156.

[55] Stagg J, Smyth MJ. Extracellular adenosine triphosphate and adenosine in cancer. Oncogene 2010; 29(39): 5346-58.

[56] Beavis PA, Stagg J, Darcy PK, Smyth MJ. CD73: a potent suppressor of antitumor immune responses. Trends Immunol 2012; 33(5): 231-7.

[57] Fredholm BB, Chern Y, Franco R, Sitkovsky M. Aspects of the general biology of adenosine A2A signaling. Prog Neurobiol 2007; 83(5): 263-76.

[58] Novitskiy SV, Ryzhov S, Zaynagetdinov R, Goldstein AE, Huang Y, Tikhomirov OY, *et al.* Adenosine receptors in regulation of dendritic cell differentiation and function. Blood 2008; 112(5): 1822-31.

[59] Majumdar S, Aggarwal BB. Adenosine suppresses activation of nuclear factor-kappaB selectively induced by tumor necrosis factor in different cell types. Oncogene 2003; 22(8): 1206-18.

[60] Ohta A, Gorelik E, Prasad SJ, Ronchese F, Lukashev D, Wong MK, *et al.* A2A adenosine receptor protects tumors from antitumor T cells. Proc Natl Acad Sci U S A 2006; 103(35): 13132-7.

[61] Deaglio S, Dwyer KM, Gao W, Friedman D, Usheva A, Erat A, *et al.* Adenosine generation catalyzed by CD39 and CD73 expressed on regulatory T cells mediates immune suppression. J Exp Med 2007; 204(6): 1257-65.

[62] Whiteside TL, Mandapathil M, Schuler P. The role of the adenosinergic pathway in immunosuppression mediated by human regulatory T cells (Treg). Curr Med Chem 2011; 18(34): 5217-23.

[63] Romio M, Reinbeck B, Bongardt S, Huls S, Burghoff S, Schrader J. Extracellular purine metabolism and signaling of CD73-derived adenosine in murine Treg and Teff cells. Am J Physiol Cell Physiol 2011; 301(2): C530-9.

[64] Kanneganti TD, Lamkanfi M, Kim YG, Chen G, Park JH, Franchi L, *et al.* Pannexin-1-mediated recognition of bacterial molecules activates the cryopyrin inflammasome independent of Toll-like receptor signaling. Immunity 2007; 26(4): 433-43.

[65] Abbracchio MP, Burnstock G, Verkhratsky A, Zimmermann H. Purinergic signalling in the nervous system: an overview. Trends Neurosci 2009; 32(1): 19-29.

[66] Mandapathil M, Hilldorfer B, Szczepanski MJ, Czystowska M, Szajnik M, Ren J, *et al.* Generation and accumulation of immunosuppressive adenosine by human CD4+CD25highFOXP3+ regulatory T cells. J Biol Chem 2010; 285(10): 7176-86.

[67] Mailloux AW, Young MR. Regulatory T-cell trafficking: from thymic development to tumor-induced immune suppression. Crit Rev Immunol 2010; 30(5): 435-47.

[68] Jacobs JF, Nierkens S, Figdor CG, de Vries IJ, Adema GJ. Regulatory T cells in melanoma: the final hurdle towards effective immunotherapy? Lancet Oncol 2012; 13(1): e32-42.

[69] Le DT, Jaffee EM. Regulatory T-cell modulation using cyclophosphamide in vaccine approaches: a current perspective. Cancer Res 2012; 72(14): 3439-44.

[70] Polak L, Turk JL. Reversal of immunological tolerance by cyclophosphamide through inhibition of suppressor cell activity. Nature 1974; 249(458): 654-6.

[71] Machiels JP, Reilly RT, Emens LA, Ercolini AM, Lei RY, Weintraub D, *et al.* Cyclophosphamide, doxorubicin, and paclitaxel enhance the antitumor immune response of granulocyte/macrophage-colony stimulating factor-secreting whole-cell vaccines in HER-2/neu tolerized mice. Cancer Res 2001; 61(9): 3689-97.

[72] Ghiringhelli F, Larmonier N, Schmitt E, Parcellier A, Cathelin D, Garrido C, *et al.* CD4+CD25+ regulatory T cells suppress tumor immunity but are sensitive to cyclophosphamide which allows immunotherapy of established tumors to be curative. Eur J Immunol 2004; 34(2): 336-44.

[73] Ge Y, Domschke C, Stoiber N, Schott S, Heil J, Rom J, *et al.* Metronomic cyclophosphamide treatment in metastasized breast cancer patients: immunological effects and clinical outcome. Cancer Immunol Immunother 2012; 61(3): 353-62.

[74] Lutsiak ME, Semnani RT, De Pascalis R, Kashmiri SV, Schlom J, Sabzevari H. Inhibition of CD4(+)25+ T regulatory cell function implicated in enhanced immune response by low-dose cyclophosphamide. Blood 2005; 105(7): 2862-8.

[75] Camisaschi C, Filipazzi P, Tazzari M, Casati C, Beretta V, Pilla L, *et al.* Effects of cyclophosphamide and IL-2 on regulatory CD4(+) T cell frequency and function in melanoma patients vaccinated with HLA-class I peptides: impact on the antigen-specific T cell response. Cancer Immunol Immunother 2013; 62(5): 897-908.

[76] Onizuka S, Tawara I, Shimizu J, Sakaguchi S, Fujita T, Nakayama E. Tumor rejection by *in vivo* administration of anti-CD25 (interleukin-2 receptor alpha) monoclonal antibody. Cancer Res 1999; 59(13): 3128-33.

[77] Turk MJ, Guevara-Patino JA, Rizzuto GA, Engelhorn ME, Sakaguchi S, Houghton AN. Concomitant tumor immunity to a poorly immunogenic melanoma is prevented by regulatory T cells. J Exp Med 2004; 200(6): 771-82.

[78] Nair S, Boczkowski D, Fassnacht M, Pisetsky D, Gilboa E. Vaccination against the forkhead family transcription factor Foxp3 enhances tumor immunity. Cancer Res 2007; 67(1): 371-80.

[79] Matsushita N, Pilon-Thomas SA, Martin LM, Riker AI. Comparative methodologies of regulatory T cell depletion in a murine melanoma model. J Immunol Method 2008; 333(1-2): 167-79.

[80] Sutmuller RP, van Duivenvoorde LM, van Elsas A, Schumacher TN, Wildenberg ME, Allison JP, *et al.* Synergism of cytotoxic T lymphocyte-associated antigen 4 blockade and depletion of CD25(+) regulatory T cells in antitumor therapy reveals alternative pathways for suppression of autoreactive cytotoxic T lymphocyte responses. J Exp Med 2001; 194(6): 823-32.

[81] Ramirez-Montagut T, Chow A, Hirschhorn-Cymerman D, Terwey TH, Kochman AA, Lu S, *et al.* Glucocorticoid-induced TNF receptor family related gene activation overcomes tolerance/ignorance to melanoma differentiation antigens and enhances antitumor immunity. J Immunol 2006; 176(11): 6434-42.

[82] Jacobs JF, Punt CJ, Lesterhuis WJ, Sutmuller RP, Brouwer HM, Scharenborg NM, *et al.* Dendritic cell vaccination in combination with anti-CD25 monoclonal antibody treatment: a phase I/II study in metastatic melanoma patients. Clin Cancer Res 2010; 16(20): 5067-78.

[83] Rech AJ, Mick R, Martin S, Recio A, Aqui NA, Powell DJ, Jr., *et al.* CD25 blockade depletes and selectively reprograms regulatory T cells in concert with immunotherapy in cancer patients. Sci Transl Med 2012; 4(134): 134ra62.

[84] Dannull J, Su Z, Rizzieri D, Yang BK, Coleman D, Yancey D, *et al.* Enhancement of vaccine-mediated antitumor immunity in cancer patients after depletion of regulatory T cells. J Clin Invest 2005; 115(12): 3623-33.

[85] Attia P, Maker AV, Haworth LR, Rogers-Freezer L, Rosenberg SA. Inability of a fusion protein of IL-2 and diphtheria toxin (Denileukin Diftitox, DAB389IL-2, ONTAK) to eliminate regulatory T lymphocytes in patients with melanoma. J Immunother 2005; 28(6): 582-92.

[86] Telang S, Rasku MA, Clem AL, Carter K, Klarer AC, Badger WR, *et al.* Phase II trial of the regulatory T cell-depleting agent, denileukin diftitox, in patients with unresectable stage IV melanoma. BMC Cancer 2011; 11: 515.

[87] Powell DJ, Jr., Attia P, Ghetie V, Schindler J, Vitetta ES, Rosenberg SA. Partial reduction of human FOXP3+ CD4 T cells *in vivo* after CD25-directed recombinant immunotoxin administration. J Immunother 2008; 31(2): 189-98.

[88] Powell DJ, Jr., Felipe-Silva A, Merino MJ, Ahmadzadeh M, Allen T, Levy C, *et al.* Administration of a CD25-directed immunotoxin, LMB-2, to patients with metastatic melanoma induces a selective partial reduction in regulatory T cells *in vivo*. J Immunol 2007; 179(7): 4919-28.

[89] Wing K, Onishi Y, Prieto-Martin P, Yamaguchi T, Miyara M, Fehervari Z, *et al.* CTLA-4 control over Foxp3+ regulatory T cell function. Science 2008; 322(5899): 271-5.

[90] Peggs KS, Quezada SA, Chambers CA, Korman AJ, Allison JP. Blockade of CTLA-4 on both effector and regulatory T cell compartments contributes to the antitumor activity of anti-CTLA-4 antibodies. J Exp Med 2009; 206(8): 1717-25.

[91] Hodi FS, O'Day SJ, McDermott DF, Weber RW, Sosman JA, Haanen JB, *et al.* Improved survival with ipilimumab in patients with metastatic melanoma. N Engl J Med 2010; 363(8): 711-23.

[92] Pardoll DM. The blockade of immune checkpoints in cancer immunotherapy. Nat Rev. Cancer 2012; 12(4): 252-64.

[93] Ko K, Yamazaki S, Nakamura K, Nishioka T, Hirota K, Yamaguchi T, *et al.* Treatment of advanced tumors with agonistic anti-GITR mAb and its effects on tumor-infiltrating Foxp3+CD25+CD4+ regulatory T cells. J Exp Med 2005; 202(7): 885-91.

[94] Nishikawa H, Kato T, Hirayama M, Orito Y, Sato E, Harada N, *et al.* Regulatory T cell-resistant CD8+ T cells induced by glucocorticoid-induced tumor necrosis factor receptor signaling. Cancer Res 2008; 68(14): 5948-54.

[95] Jensen SM, Maston LD, Gough MJ, Ruby CE, Redmond WL, Crittenden M, *et al.* Signaling through OX40 enhances antitumor immunity. Semin Oncol 2010; 37(5): 524-32.

[96] Valzasina B, Guiducci C, Dislich H, Killeen N, Weinberg AD, Colombo MP. Triggering of OX40 (CD134) on CD4(+)CD25+ T cells blocks their inhibitory activity: a novel regulatory role for OX40 and its comparison with GITR. Blood 2005; 105(7): 2845-51.

[97] Piconese S, Valzasina B, Colombo MP. OX40 triggering blocks suppression by regulatory T cells and facilitates tumor rejection. J Exp Med 2008; 205(4): 825-39.

[98] Kjaergaard J, Tanaka J, Kim JA, Rothchild K, Weinberg A, Shu S. Therapeutic efficacy of OX-40 receptor antibody depends on tumor immunogenicity and anatomic site of tumor growth. Cancer Res 2000; 60(19): 5514-21.

[99] Hirschhorn-Cymerman D, Budhu S, Kitano S, Liu C, Zhao F, Zhong H, *et al.* Induction of tumoricidal function in CD4+ T cells is associated with concomitant memory and terminally differentiated phenotype. J Exp Med 2012; 209(11): 2113-26.

[100] Stagg J, Divisekera U, Duret H, Sparwasser T, Teng MW, Darcy PK, *et al.* CD73-deficient mice have increased antitumor immunity and are resistant to experimental metastasis. Cancer Res 2011; 71(8): 2892-900.

[101] Stagg J, Divisekera U, McLaughlin N, Sharkey J, Pommey S, Denoyer D, *et al.* Anti-CD73 antibody therapy inhibits breast tumor growth and metastasis. Proc Natl Acad Sci U S A 2010; 107(4): 1547-52.

[102] Wang L, Fan J, Thompson LF, Zhang Y, Shin T, Curiel TJ, *et al.* CD73 has distinct roles in nonhematopoietic and hematopoietic cells to promote tumor growth in mice. J Clin Invest 2011; 121(6): 2371-82.

[103] Jin D, Fan J, Wang L, Thompson LF, Liu A, Daniel BJ, *et al.* CD73 on tumor cells impairs antitumor T-cell responses: a novel mechanism of tumor-induced immune suppression. Cancer Res 2010; 70(6): 2245-55.

[104] Stagg J, Beavis PA, Divisekera U, Liu MC, Moller A, Darcy PK, *et al.* CD73-deficient mice are resistant to carcinogenesis. Cancer Res 2012; 72(9): 2190-6.

CHAPTER 12

# Cancer Vaccines: Current Status and Future Perspectives

**Yu Sawada, Toshiaki Yoshikawa, Kazuya Ofuji, Mayuko Sakai, Tetsuya Nakatsura***

*Division of Cancer Immunotherapy, Exploratory Oncology Research and Clinical Trial Center, National Cancer Center, Japan*

**Abstract:** This chapter will review the current status and future perspectives in the field of cancer vaccine development, and also introduce the glypican-3 (GPC3) peptide-based vaccine for hepatocellular carcinoma (HCC).

Cancer vaccine is administered to promote the induction of immune cells that respond to such antigens. Tumor-associated antigens (TAAs) are the principal targets of cancer vaccine therapy, which include peptide or protein vaccines, dendritic cell (DC) vaccines, tumor lysate vaccines, and genetic vaccines. TAA-specific immunotherapy is considered as an advantageous treatment, because it is likely that adverse effects could be reduced due to the high specificity. Several phase II/III clinical trials of vaccine-based immunotherapy to augment antitumor immunity in a number of cancer patients have been conducted and it is shown that immunotherapy could decrease the possibility of recurrence after therapeutic treatment in adjuvant settings. In 2010, for the first time, the US FDA approved a curative cancer vaccine, Provenge (sipuleucel-T), which is used for prostate cancer patients. However, vaccines as sole therapy do not substantially impact on patients with advanced solid tumors.

Therefore, a thorough understanding of tumor immunity would facilitate an improved application of potential vaccine-based therapy. The future perspectives of cancer vaccine application will likely focus on the combinatorial therapies, such as with vaccines and other immunomodulators.

Recently, we showed that a GPC3-derived peptide vaccination is considerably tolerated, and anti-tumor immunity are significant in a phase I trial in HCC patients. Based on these observations, we anticipate that the outcome of the current work will provide insights into a greater randomized clinical trial of the GPC3 peptide-based vaccine.

**Keywords:** Adjuvant, antigen-presenting cell (APC), cancer vaccine, cancer/testis (CT) antigen, clinical trial, cytotoxic T-cell (CTL), dendritic cell (DC) vaccine,

***Corresponding author Tetsuya Nakatsura:** Division of Cancer Immunotherapy, Exploratory Oncology Research and Clinical Trial Center, National Cancer Center, Japan; Tel: +81(4) 7131-5490; E-mail: tnakatsu@east.ncc.go.jp

**Jianxun Song (Ed)**

differentiation antigen, genetic vaccine, glypican-3 (GPC3), immune checkpoint, intratumoral peptide injection, ipilimumab, major histocompatibility complex (MHC), peptide vaccine, regulatory T cell (Treg), sipuleucel-T, tumor lysate, tumor-associated antigen (TAA), virus vaccine.

## INTRODUCTION

Immunotherapy has long been proposed as a method to treat cancer. Generally, immunotherapeutic strategies include cytokine therapy, monoclonal antibody therapy, gene transfer therapy, adoptive T cell therapy, and vaccine therapy (further subgrouped as peptide or protein vaccine, dendritic cell (DC) vaccine, tumor lysate vaccine, or genetic vaccine). Recently, a number of studies have suggested immunotherapy as an innovative and alternative cancer treatment, for instance, the US FDA approved ipilimumab that is an engineered antibody against cytotoxic T-lymphocyte antigen 4 (CTLA-4) for the metastatic melanoma immunotherapy. Thus, some immunotherapeutic strategies have shown sufficient efficacies for clinical uses.

Identification of tumor antigens has made it possible to develop tumor-specific immunotherapy. As cancer vaccines, such antigens could be administered directly to the cancer patient, to promote *in vivo* activation of immune cells in response to these antigens. First, a large number of animal studies worldwide have shown cancer vaccination achieved certain efficacy and they are clinically safe of which prepared them for the stage of human use. Second, several phase II/III clinical trials of vaccine-based immunotherapy have been performed for patients with advanced cancer, or after receiving a curative treatment in adjuvant settings. In the early 2010, the US FDA granted the earliest curative vaccine, Provenge (sipuleucel-T) for metastatic hormone-refractory prostate cancer. Most cancer vaccine trials are conducted in patients with advanced cancer, which makes it difficult to show adequate clinical outcomes, because patients with advanced cancer are immunocompromised after receiving previous treatments and/or due to the immune evasion mechanisms of the tumor. Therefore, only a better understanding of tumor immunity would facilitate the improved application of a potent vaccine-based therapy. In contrast, therapeutic vaccines may be applied preventively to lower the cancer incidences. Vaccine therapy, in the preventive settings, can reduce the risk of cancer occurrence, for example, as chronic human papillomavirus (HPV) and hepatitis B virus (HBV) are two most common viral causes to hepatocellular carcinoma (HCC) and vulvar and vaginal cancers respectively. In order to reduce cancer incidences in the context of eliminating viral infections, to date, two types of cancer-preventive vaccines - against HBV and against HPV types 16 and 18 respectively have been approved by the FDA.

In this chapter, we will review vaccine therapies for cancer, and also introduce our clinical investigation of the GPC3 peptide vaccine against HCC.

## VACCINE STRATEGY

Tumor-associated antigens (TAAs) are the principal targets of cancer vaccine therapy. TAA-specific immunotherapy is considered attractive as a treatment, because adverse effects would, theoretically, occur at a lower frequency than with traditional treatments due to its specificity. Vaccine strategies, including peptide or protein vaccine, DC vaccine, genetic vaccine, and tumor lysate are described in this section (Fig. **1**).

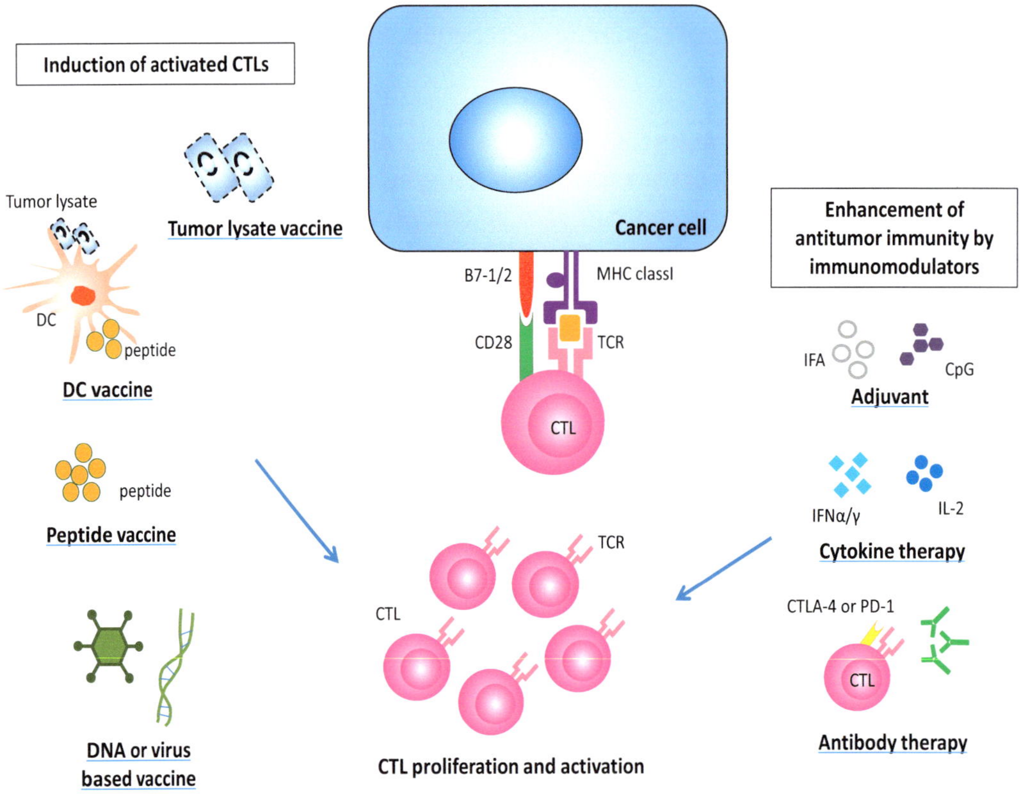


**Figure 1:** Tumor-reactive CTLs stimulated by various cancer vaccines have the ability of distinguishing and destroying cancer cells. Various immunomodulators, including adjuvants, cytokines, and immune checkpoint blockade are expected to enhance antitumor immunity.

## TUMOR-ASSOCIATED ANTIGENS

Identification of appropriate TAAs is the first and most significant step in the development of cancer vaccine therapy. Boon *et al.* initially identified MAGE-A as a human TAA from a melanoma patient [1]. Tumor-specific cytotoxic T lymphocytes (CTLs) can distinguish MHC-I/peptides (8-11 aa) complexes. Therefore, it is not necessary that the antigenic protein itself be expressed on the cell surface. Proteins present in cytoplasm or nucleus, when broken down into peptides and properly coupled to major MHC-I molecules are recognized by CTLs *via* their TCR recognition. This drastically expands the number of molecules that could act as TAAs, and following this a number of both them and their CTL epitopes have been identified and further investigated.

**Table. Classification of tumor associated antigens (TAAs)**

| TAA | | characteristics |
|---|---|---|
| **Cancer / testis antigens** | **MAGE**<br>**NY-ESO-1** | An antigen group expressed only in testis, ovary, placenta, and tumor tissue. These antigens are the principal targets of cancer-specific therapy, because MHC molecules are not expressed, or are expressed at lower levels, on germ-line cells. |
| **Differentiation antigens** | **tyrosinase**<br>**gp100**<br>**Melan-A(MART-1)**<br>**PSA** | An antigen group expressed specifically in cancer cells and in normal tissues from which the cancer cells arose. |
| **Antigens derived from genetic abnormality** | | |
| **point mutation** | **p53** | An antigen group associated with a gene product with single- or multiple-nucleotide mutations. |
| **overexpression** | **HER2**<br>**hTERT** | An antigen group in which a gene is amplified or its product is otherwise over-expressed. |
| **splicing variant** | **survivin-2B** | An antigen group associated with molecules derived from aberrant splicing. |
| **fusion protein** | **bcr/abl** | An antigen group associated with a fusion gene product. |
| **Virus antigens** | **HPV E6,7** | An antigen group associated with virus-related sequences. |

TAAs are separated into cancer/testis (CT) antigens, differentiation antigens, genetic abnormality antigens (point mutation, overexpression, splicing variant, or fusion protein), and viral antigens [2-5] (Table). CT antigens are expressed only in testis, ovary, placenta, and tumor tissues, as their name implies. More than 100 molecules have been identified as CT antigens, and a database project has been established to fully describe them (CT antigen data base, http://www.cta.lncc.br/index.php). Differentiation antigens are expressed specifically in ordinary tissues and in tumors may be recognized as antigenic by the immune systems of cancer patients. For example, CTLs recognizing Melan-A (MART-1), tyrosinase, and gp100, which is also expressed in regular melanocytes, have been isolated from melanoma patients [2]. Many studies have aimed to determine whether the immune system in cancer patients responds to the products of mutated genes. Tumor antigens attributable to genetic abnormalities have been identified and are recognized by CTLs [3]. Some of the epitopes derived from the mutant genes have been identified [4], and a database of these has been created for documentation (http://cancerimmunity.org/peptide/mutations/).

Clinical trials of cancer vaccines target TAAs, including randomized controlled trials, have been conducted. The National Cancer Institute (NCI) evaluates the usefulness of tumor Ags by introducing these nine criteria: (1) curative function, (2) immunogenicity, (3) role in oncogenicity, (4) specificity, (5) expression level in cancer and percentage of $Ag^+$ cancers, (6) stem cell expression, (7) number of $Ag^+$ patients, (8) number of antigenic epitopes, and (9) cellular location [5]. For 46 of 75 antigens, clinical immunogenicity was evaluated in the NCI project, and 20 showed possible clinical efficacy. Clinical trials using novel TAAs are now being conducted, and further analysis will be followed.

## PEPTIDE OR PROTEIN VACCINES

Ags for use in vaccines could be DNA, mRNA, protein, or peptides of 8-15 amino acids. Peptides represent short segments of tumor proteins, which might be synthesized following the present cGMP (good manufacturing practices) circumstances which permit for the use as pharmaceutical agents. These agents can be easily manufactured and are generally safe. Large numbers of vaccines, including peptides and proteins that target various cancer types, are currently being verified.

The MHC-I/tumor epitope complexes on the tumor cells could stimulate and activate CTLs. The MHC-II/tumor epitope complexes on Ag-presenting cells (APCs) and occasionally on tumor cells are recognized by helper T cells (Th). Every peptide binds with a distinct MHC molecule, which is applicable only to patients, who express the specific MHC molecule.

A variety of tumor Ags and their CTL epitope peptides have been defined previously. The MHC-I/peptide complexes on the tumor surface drive the development of tumor-reactive CTLs, and is essential for antigen-associated T cell immunotherapy. The epitope peptides are capable to be adapted to augment the binding ability of MHC-I molecules, resulting in improved CTL responses. Because of the poor immunogenicity of tumor self-proteins due to immune tolerance [6], the modified peptides which contain single-amino-acid substitutions that improve the peptide affinity for the HLA peptide-binding site and increase immunogenicity have been designed [7-11]. However, the peptide analogues frequently activate and induce peptide-reactive, however, not tumor-specific CTLs that cannot progress tumor regression [12, 13].

Early creations of peptide vaccines had one or several CTL-epitope peptides. At present, a variety of types of new peptide vaccines are under development. Immunization with multiple epitopes vaccines is more effective than with single-epitope ones [14] which reduces the risk of antigen loss caused by tumor immune selection [6, 15]. Because $CD4^+$ T cells are critical in developing the persistence of memory $CD8^+$ T cells that target tumor cells [16, 17], numerous MHC II-restricted helper epitopes have been known among the target molecules of MHC I-restricted CTL-epitope vaccines, and both of them are also used as cancer vaccines. Of note, the same tumor epitopes induce both $CD4^+$ Th cells and Tregs that have capable of suppressing the CTL effectors [18]. Therefore, other strategies to specially advance the expansion of tumor-reactive Th cells are required. The classical types of peptide vaccines have one to several epitope peptides of CTLs or Th cells. Conversely, the original protein of the peptide vaccines typically contains a number of HLA-type-restricted epitopes of both $CD8^+$ CTLs and $CD4^+$ Th cells. A major weakness of protein-based vaccines is their inefficient stimulation of effector T cells; particularly, protein vaccines are likely to bring out incomplete responses, because they have the ability to stimulate tumor-reactive $CD4^+$ T cells, however, they weakly stimulate tumor-reactive $CD8^+$ T cells [19, 20].

The significance of Th cells in the CTL induction has been known, and protein vaccines can induce the activation of both CTLs and Th cells, however, the protein vaccines have a number of disadvantages concerning manufacturing processes and safety restraints. To overcome the problems, long-peptide vaccines have been used. Such vaccines are taken up primarily by APCs, within which they are processed for Ag presentation with MHC molecules. Synthetic long peptides possibly contain a number of MHC T-cell epitopes that permits the use of this peptide vaccine in MHC-nonresistricted manner.

Peptides and proteins administered lonely as vaccines induce poor immune responses. The use of immunological adjuvants, which slow Ag release and increase Ag presentation, leads to a generation of more efficient immune responses.

A number of researchers have tried to generate more operational cancer vaccines. The role of immune checkpoint molecules, such as CTLA-4 and programmed cell death-1 (PD-1), in antitumor immunity has been identified, and promising outcomes have been shown from clinical trials of combining peptide vaccines with immune checkpoint blockade [21-23]. Additional randomized phase III trials are needed to demonstrate the clinical advantages of these vaccine therapies such as the immune checkpoint blockade combination therapies.

## DENDRITIC CELL VACCINES

Dendritic cells (DCs) are professional APCs, comprising a number of subsets, including conventional and plasmacytoid DCs [24]. DCs play a central role in the generation of both antitumor immune response and tolerance. DC vaccines, usually pulsed with tumor-reactive Ags, induce specific T-cell response. DCs present MHC-I/tumor-derived peptides to naive $CD8^+$ T cells and initial their CTL differentiation.

Various signals such as costimulatory and cytokine signals drive the following $CD8^+$ T cell expansion and differentiation. $CD4^+$ T cells further regulate $CD8^+$ T cell differentiation, as they manipulate the differentiation and expansion of tumor-reactive CTLs and the generation of durable CTL memory. Meanwhile, $CD4^+$ T cells activate macrophages at tumor sites and actively kill tumor cells.

The research and development approach to develop DCs *ex vivo* have avoided several problems associating with the dysfunction of endogenous DCs in cancer patients. Several methods to load DCs with Ag have been introduced, such as peptide-pulsing, whole protein-loading, and genetic engineering. DC-based immunotherapy remains tremendously difficult and involves a number of strategic choices, including the preference of DC subset, the process of Ag pulsing, and the method of management, such as subcutaneous injections. Figdor *et al.* decribed an overall schedule for the standardization and quality control in order to systemically describe these DC-based vaccines [25].

The therapeutic cancer vaccine needs overcome the suppression of the tumor environment generated by the established tumors and the dysfunctional immune system, including the suppressive regulatory T (Treg) cells and myeloid-derived suppressor cells (MDSCs) [26-29]. To reach this goal, the *in vitro* generation of mature DCs that obtain important resistance to suppressive factors for *in vivo* re-infusion is an optimal approach [30-32]. To bypass the limitation of immature or partially matured DCs in the vaccines, a number of approaches to the induction of fully matured DCs for clinical use have been used. Originally, two modalities implicating prostaglandin E2 (PGE2) have been tested to achieve induced DC maturation: (1) macrophage-conditioned medium [33, 34], and (2) a cytokine cocktail, containing IL-1$\alpha$, IL-6, TNF-$\alpha$ and PGE2 [35]. These methods sought to induce mature DCs, which express costimulatory molecules and surface CCR7 at high levels, and the chemokines CCL19 and CCL21 [36, 37]. The negative impact of PGE2 is it results in the production of IL-12p70 [38], which induces Th1 differentiation [39], and is capable of mediating the interaction between Treg cells and DCs presented in cancer patients are potential limitations. Maturation processes for DCs used in cancer treatment are selected based on its ability to stimulate maturation which defines the direction of its immune response.

## TUMOR LYSATE VACCINES

Tumor lysate vaccines have the advantage of transporting and presenting tumor antigens to both $CD8^+$ and $CD4^+$ T cells. Both autologous and allogeneic tumor cells can be used to prepare for this type of vaccine. Tumor lysate vaccines from autologous tumor cells may contain unique TAAs that could be ideal targets for immunotherapy, since these TAAs could generate antitumor immune responses. Although such vaccines are promising, the challenge is to acquire enough tumor cells. Thus, allogeneic tumor cells are valuable alternatives. Allogeneic tumor cells can be utilized as a resource of TAAs, because tumors have an overlapping antigen expression profile, and also the cross-priming to match patients' the HLA haplotype drives antitumor immunity.

Mitchell *et al.* performed a phase I trial using melanoma lysate as cancer vaccine [40]. They administered the lysate without adjuvant to patients with stage IV melanoma, and assessed toxicity and immunological activity. No toxicity of the tumor lysate vaccine has been found and improved immunological reactivity to melanoma cells has been reported. In their study, eight of fifteen patients showed an increased number of cytotoxic T cell precursors. Based on this finding, the investigators expect this treatment approach could be approved for clinical use, with the addition of appropriate adjuvant materials. Based on this, Melacine is an allogeneic melanoma cell lysate along with an immunologic adjuvant, DETOX has been developed. Sondak *et al.* performed phase I and II studies in patients with stage-IV melanoma to test Melacine which showed a low-level antitumor activity. However, this vaccine showed it's a greater promise in combining with adjuvant. They also held a phase III trial, which showed a survival benefit in the subset of melanoma patients who expressed the HLA class I antigens A2 and/or HLA-C3 [41].

Clinically, tumor lysate may also be used as a source of TAAs for DC vaccines. DCs are the most effective APCs, which mediate T cell immunity. Tumor lysate would provide a potent source of Ag to increase the efficiency of the DC-based immunotherapy. El Ansary *et al.* reported that DC-based vaccine was safe and well tolerated in patients with advanced HCC, who received an inoculation of autologous DCs loaded with cell lysate of liver tumors. Compared with patients received supportive treatment, an overall survival improvement was observed. It is also shown that both $CD8^{+}$T cells and serum interferon gamma levels were elevated after DC injection [42].

Thus, tumor cell lysates have a potential to become the sources of TAAs that could induce a strong antitumor immunity. However, the low immunogenicity of tumor cells must be taken into account. Therefore, new approaches that enhance their immunogenicity are necessary.

## RECOMBINANT VIRUS VACCINES

Therapeutic cancer vaccines must overcome the unfavorable mechanisms of tolerance and immune suppression to induce antitumor immune responses. This may be favored if vaccines present TAAs in the context of hazard signals. Genetic engineered immunogenic virus particle, by using recombinant viral vectors expressing tumor antigens and/or cytokines falls on this approach. Virus expressing TAAs with costimulatory molecules is able to infect APCs or other cell types to induce the expression of costimulatory signals that are needed to fully activate TAA-specific T cells. Genetic engineering has facilitated the development of techniques that use vectors based on effectively immunogenic pathogens aimed at delivery and expression of exogenous proteins to achieve a desired immune response. Thus, it is an exciting area of cancer vaccine development. In this section, we will review some viral vectors, which have been utilized for inducing antitumor immunity. Around 40 clinical trials are under investigation, in which the treatment regimen is designed as the utilization of recombinant virus containing Ag, cytokine, or costimulatory receptor/ligand.

TG4010 is a modified vaccinia Ankara (MVA) vector that encodes TAAs called MUC-1, which is considered as an interesting target for tumor immunotherapy. A randomized phase II trial using TG4010 with conventional chemotherapy in patients with the non-small cell lung cancer (NSCLC) has shown an increased progression-free survival rate [43]. A PANVAC vaccine containing two TAAs (CEA and MUC1) along the TRICOM has also been tested in pancreatic cancer. Although a phase II study presented an enhanced median survival, a phase III trial failed to achieve such survival benefit [44-45]. Of note, new observations in patients who had various malignancies demonstrated to induce TAA-specific immune responses as well as achieve a survival advantage [45]. Odunsi *et al.* performed a phase II study of vaccination using the recombinant vaccine and fowlpox vectors expressing NY-ESO-1 Ag, in patients who had advanced tumors. NY-ESO-1-specific antitumor immunity was confirmed in the vaccinated patients. This study provided the groundwork support of clinical advantages of recombinant poxvirus-based cancer vaccines [46].

## CLINICAL TRIALS

Several phase II/III clinical trials of vaccine-based immunotherapy in patients who had advanced cancer were conducted to augment antitumor immunity, or to decrease the recurrence possibility. We will briefly review vaccine-based phase II/III clinical trials for solid tumors, which will be focused on melanoma, prostate cancer, lung cancer, renal cell carcinoma, pancreatic cancer, and hepatocellular carcinoma.

## MELANOMA

The development of long-term, tumor-specific reactions without autoimmunity is the goal for an optimal immunotherapy. Tumor antigens identified in melanoma are among the best targets for cancer immunotherapy. For example, gp100 is a well-studied tumor antigen in melanoma. A phase III study using the gp100 peptide vaccine followed by IL-2, against HLA-A*0201-positive melanoma in advanced stage III or stage IV, showed a significant progress in the general clinical responses and the longer progression-free survival. The median overall survival was also longer in the vaccine group than in the control group (IL-2 only) [47].

CTLA-4 is a coinhibitory receptor expressing on T cells. Ligand with B7-1 and B7-2, CTLA-4-mediated inhibitory signals result in the reduction of T-cell proliferation and IL-2 secretion. Ipilimumab, a McAb which blocks CTLA-4, has been approved by the FDA for treating metastatic melanoma since 2011. In a randomized phase III study against metastatic melanoma, a combination of ipilimumab and gp100 peptide vaccine was tested, however, failed to show any superior activity compared to ipilimumab alone. The median overall survival was 10.0 or 10.1 months using ipilimumab + gp100 or ipilimumab only [21]. This study confirmed that the treatment using ipilimumab with gp100 does not achieve clinical benefit in the overall survival. Nevertheless, the long-term follow-up showed that ipilimumab caused ongoing tumor regression in patients with metastatic melanoma treated with ipilimumab plus either gp100 or IL-2; furthermore, the combination with IL-2 resulted in the whole response rate [48].

MAGE-A3 is another promising tumor antigen that has potential clinical value. A phase III study using a MAGE-A3 Ag-specific vaccine (GSK2132231A) in patients who have the resected stage IIIc melanoma is ongoing (NCT00796445). The rationale of this study is to estimate the advantage of GSK2132231A in preventing disease relapse. Meanwhile, Vitespen is a heat-shock protein (hsp, gp96)-peptide complex isolated from resected autologous tumors, which has been tested in clinical trials as cancer vaccine. In a phase III study using vitespen in patients with stage IV melanoma, one arm of the patients was arbitrarily given the vitespen and the other was allocated as the physician's choice arm. Although, the overall survival between these two arms in this study had no statistically significant difference, in other exploratory landmark analyses, AJCC substages M1a and M1b patients getting at least 10 doses of vaccine had better survival than those in the physician's choice arm [49].

## PROSTATE CANCER

In April 2010, the FDA approved sipuleucel-T as the first cancer treatment vaccine for patients who have metastatic prostate cancer. As a DC-based vaccine, Sipuleucel-T is targeting to the prostatic acid phosphatase (PAP), which is an Ag presented in the majority of prostate cancer cells. In a phase III study, sipuleucel-T showed a virtual decrease of 22% in the death risk and a progress in median survival [50].

Prostvac is considered a promising treatment for prostate cancer. Prostvac is made up of recombinant vaccinia and fowlpox viral vectors, encoding prostate-specific antigen (PSA) and three costimulatory molecules, including B7.1, ICAM-1 and LFA-3. Compared with a control group, a randomized phase II trial showed a prolonged overall survival in the Prostvac group, (median survival time 25.1 *vs.* 16.6 months, hazard ratio 0.56, $P$=0.061) [51]. A randomized phase III trial using the combination of Prostvac and GM-CSF against metastatic prostate cancer is in progress (NCT01322490).

Combination approaches of cancer vaccine with chemotherapy are considered as promising treatment strategies. A personalized peptide vaccine strategy by using no more than four peptides that was chosen underlying the host immunity before vaccination has been determined. In a phase II study in Japan of such a personalized peptide vaccine in the combination with chemotherapy for prostate cancer, two-group patients were randomly assigned: peptide vaccine + low-dose estramustine phosphate (EMP) group and a standard-dose EMP group. This study showed a better progression-free survival (PFS) in the peptide vaccine + low-dose EMP group compared with the group with the standard EMP [52].

## NON-SMALL CELL LUNG CANCER (NSCLC)

Several vaccine-based phase III studies for NSCLC have been conducted. The expression of MAGE-A3 in the early stage of NSCLC has been demonstrated in 35% of cases which could serve as a good target for vaccine development [53]. In a phase II study, patients who had MAGE-A3$^+$ NSCLC were randomly, allocated into a MAGE-A3 vaccine treatment group for adjuvant therapy or into a placebo group. In this study, there was a tendency toward improved PFS in the MAGE-A3 vaccine treatment group compared to the placebo group [53, 54].

The glycoprotein Mucin-1 (MUC1) is over-expressed and aberrantly glycosylated in various human cancers, making it an excellent target for cancer immunotherapy [55]. L-BLP 25 is a liposomal vaccine consisting by BLP25 lipopeptide and immunoadjuvant monophosphoryl lipid A, which targets the uncovered core peptide of the MUC1 Ag. A randomized phase IIb study using L-BLP25 in NSCLC patients was conducted to investigate its clinical value. Although this trial did not show a significant survival advantage, in some stage IIIb locoregional patients, a tendency to improve survival was observed [56]. An updated analysis showed that with an additional 2 years of follow up, the median overall survival in the L-BLP25 or the BSC group was 17.2 or 13 months (hazard ratio 0.745), and the three-year survival rate was 31% *vs.* 17% ($P$=0.035) [57]. Based on these observations, a phase III study or the START trial was performed to further evaluate L-BLP25. The START trial is a randomized, placebo-controlled trial for the efficiency and safety of L-BLP25 as a maintenance therapy of the NSCLC patients from North America, South America, Europe, and Australia (NCT00409188). Recently, Merck Serono declared that "the Phase III START study of L-BLP25 in NSCLC patients did not achieve its primary endpoint to show a statistically considerable advance in the overall survival. In spite of not reaching the primary endpoint, prominent treatment effects were found using L-BLP25 in particular subgroups". The results of further analyses are awaited. The

INSPIRE study of the treatment effect of L-BLP25, as compared with placebo, on overall survival time in East-Asian NSCLC patients is ongoing (NCT01015443).

The TG4010 (MVA-MUC1-IL2) is also a vaccine designed to target the MUC1 antigen. This vaccine is underlying a recombinant vaccinia virus expressing both the MUC1 Ag and IL-2. In a phase IIb study using TG4010, total 148 $MUC1^{+}$ NSCLC patients were allocated to the combination therapy group (cisplatin and gemcitabine plus TG4010), or to the control group (same chemotherapy without TG4010). The primary PFS at endpoint was 43.2% (32 of 74) in the TG4010 plus chemotherapy group and 35.1% (26 of 74) in the control group. Median overall survival in patients with an objective response was longer in the TG4010 group than in the control group. Furthermore, in a subgroup analysis, patients who had normal levels of activated $CD16^{+}$ $CD56^{+}$ $CD69^{+}$ NK cells, had a longer median overall survival than patients with augmented numbers of activated NK cells [43]. A phase III study is underway to determine the efficiency and safety of the first-line chemotherapy plus TG4010 for patients with MUC1-expressing stage IV NSCLC (NCT01383148).

The EGFR pathway is another promising target candidate in the treatment of NSCLC. The CIMAvax EGF vaccine was intended to stimulate the immune response and to provoke the production of anti-EGF antibodies. CIMAvax EGF is composed of human recombinant EGF and the *Neisseria meningitides* P64K recombinant protein, which has been developed and approved in Cuba for clinical use [58]. In a phase II trial, NSCLC patients were assigned after receiving an initial chemotherapy to either EGF vaccine or to BSC. A good anti-EGF antibody response (GAR: an antibody response to a titer > 1:4000) was detected around 51.3% of patients in the group of EGF vaccine. The vaccinated group developed a longer survival than the control group (median overall survival, 6.47 *vs.* 5.33 months). A strong relationship was found between survival and immune response, and patients with GAR had a longer median overall survival than patients with poor antibody response [59]. Underlying the results of earlier research, a phase III study in patients who have NSCLC at the IIIB/IV stage is ongoing in the UK (NCT01444118).

## RENAL CELL CARCINOMA (RCC)

One of the strategies to advance the effectiveness of peptide vaccines is the utilization of multiple immunogenic epitope peptides. IMA901 consists of ten various TAAs (TUMAPs), which are greatly expressed in RCC. In a phase II trial using IMA901 in patients who had advanced RCC, a significantly longer survival was observed in patients who had a response to multiple TUMAPs [60]. A phase III study is in progress to assess the survival improvement of IMA901 coupled with sunitinib in patients who have metastatic and/or locally advanced RCC (NCT01265901).

In 2008, vitespen was approved in Russia for the RCC treatment in patients at an intermediate risk of recurrence. In a phase III trial in patients who had high risk RCC recurrence after nephrectomy, vitespen did not show any improvement in RFS over the no-treatment group [61], although patients with early stage disease who received vitespen showed a potential improvement in a recurrence-free survival.

## PANCREATIC CANCER

The whole-cell HyperAcute-Pancreas (algenpantucel-L) allovaccine is comprised of two different pancreatic cancer cells that genetically modified to express alpha-Gal. A phase III trial is presently proceeding to assess the overall survival in post-resection pancreatic cancer patients treated with HyperAcute-Pancreas besides chemotherapy and chemoradiotherapy in the adjuvant settings (NCT01072981).

In Japan, a phase III study, COMPETE-PC, for patients with refractory pancreatic cancer to standard therapy is ongoing. It aims to evaluate the survival benefit of the cocktail vaccine OCV-C01, which consists by VEGFR1-, 2- with KIF20A-derived peptides (UMIN-CTR number: 000007279).

## HEPATOCELLULAR CARCINOMA (HCC)

To date, only sorafenib that is a multi-targeted tyrosine kinase inhibitor has been demonstrated to significantly sustain survival in patients who have advanced HCC [62]. And no second-line treatment or standard adjuvant therapy has been launched. Latest treatment regimens are directly needed to sustain survival in patients who have advanced HCC, and help induce the development of an effective protective approach, including vaccination for preventing the HCC occurrence and recurrence.

Previous clinical trials of immunotherapy in patients who had advanced HCC have substantially demonstrated the feasibility and safety [63]. Nevertheless, there is no phase I or II study showing that cancer vaccine has a high response rate in advanced HCC [64]. On the other hand, a number of studies have reported the potential to decrease the HCC occurrence and recurrence [64].

Although alpha-fetoprotein (AFP)-based vaccines have been widely tested in patients who had advanced HCC, no valuable clinical benefits were achieved [65, 66]. In 31 HCC patients who were immunized with DC-based vaccine loaded by autologous tumor lysates, 4 incomplete immune responses with 17 disease stabilizations have been documented [67]. Among 25 patients who were immunized with DC-based vaccine loaded by the HepG2 lysate, there was only one partial response [68]. Autologous DC-based vaccines in HCC patients is safe and clearly accepted by the body, and has shown an objective response in some cases. A randomized controlled trial showed a significantly longer recurrence-free survival after treatment with autologous formalin-fixed tumor vaccine [69] or with cytokine-induced killer cells [70], compared to no treatment. Greten *et al.* showed a result from 40 patients who had advanced HCC by a treatment using low-dose cyclophosphamide combined with telomerase peptide (GV1001) vaccination [71]. Although the use of GV1001 reduced the number of $CD4^{+}CD25^{+}Foxp3^{+}$ regulatory T cells, there were no GV1001-specific immune responses that were detected behind this regimen. Nakamoto *et al.* demonstrated that in 10 patients who had cirrhosis and HCC, a regimen using DC infusion into tumor tissues through transcatheter arteries and transarterial embolization was feasible and safe [72]. A number of patients infused with DCs did not present the HCC occurrence and recurrence. As a result, the infusion of transcatheter arterial is likely to be a feasible approach to induce effective immune responses specifically in the target lesion.

## GPC3 PEPTIDE VACCINE

Glypican-3 (GPC3) may be an excellent TAA for HCC immunotherapy. Our cDNA microarray data have suggested that GPC3 is highly expressed in human HCC [73]. GPC3 can promote the growth of HCC through the canonical Wnt [74] or the Hippo pathway [75]. We have demonstrated that both human and mouse $GPC3_{298\text{-}306}$ (EYILSLEEL) and human $GPC3_{144\text{-}152}$ (FVGEFFTDV) stimulated GPC3-specific CTL responses and did not induce any autoimmune activities [76, 77].

Underlying these data, we performed a phase I study using GPC3-based peptide in patients who had advanced HCC [78-80]. In this trial, 33 patients were intradermally given the GPC3 peptide vaccination. Specifically, HLA-A24 positive patients were given $GPC3_{298\text{-}306}$ (EYILSLEEL); while HLA-A2 positive patients were injected with $GPC3_{144\text{-}152}$ (FVGEFFTDV). First, it is shown that GPC3 peptide vaccination was relatively accepted. One patient presented an incomplete response, and 19 displayed stable disease following the beginning of treatment. Therefore, this trial achieved a 60.6% disease-control rate (partial response + stable disease). In addition, we examined the GPC3-specific CTL frequency using the ELISPOT assay. In most patients' periphery, the numbers of GPC3 peptide-specific CTLs were increased in a dose-dependent manner after the GPC3 peptide vaccination. Of note, in this trial, we established a number of $GPC3_{144-152}$ peptide-specific CTL clones from the vaccinated patients' PBMCs [81]. This study demonstrated that the CTL frequency was correlated with the overall survival in the HCC patients who took the vaccination. The median overall survival was 12.2 or 8.5 months in patients who had high GPC3-specific CTL frequencies or low GPC3-specific CTL frequencies, separately. The frequency of the GPC3 peptide-specific CTLs could be a predictive element for the overall survival of these tests. This trial gave a lot immunological indications, indicating that the GPC3-based peptide vaccine has the possibility to improve the overall survival.

Next, we performed a phase II trial using the GPC3-based peptides in patients who had HCC (UMIN-CTR number: 000002614). Forty HCC patients who had gone through either surgery and/or radiofrequency ablation were included in this phase II study. More than one year, patients received 10 vaccinations after the therapeutic treatment. The recurrence rates of 1 - 2 years were used as the primary endpoints; the immunological responses determined by the IFN-γ ELISPOT assay were set as the secondary endpoints. Presently, we are studying the correlation between the recurrence time and the immunological responses.

We are doing a study of the GPC3-based peptide vaccination in patients who have advanced HCC to evaluate the histopathological results. In this study, we are conducting liver biopsies before and after the GPC3 peptide vaccination. We reported the clinical course and pathological study, including an autopsy of an HCC patient who had remarkable tumor regression following the second inoculation [82]. In that trial, we also visulized the specific CTLs in the liver biopsy specimens by flow cytometric analysis.

## NEW OR COMBINATION STRATEGIES

Cancer vaccine is an attractive treatment regimen, however, vaccine alone cannot attain an impressive benefits for advanced cancer patients. As a result, it is needed to develop an advanced strategy to connect the antitumor immunity and the clinical response to maximize the ability of tumor Ag-reactive cancer immunotherapy.

## OUR PROPOSAL—INTRATUMORAL PEPTIDE INJECTION

In cancer vaccination, the function of tumor Ag-reactive CTLs are in association with their cell-surface MHC class I molecules. One of the potential problems in cancer immunotherapy is the insufficient presentation of tumor Ag-derived peptide on the tumor cell surface. We hypothesized that Ag-specific cancer immunotherapy would be dramatically improved by strengthening the presentation density of an Ag-derived peptide. We found that the peptide administration of the intratumoral injection resulted in an improved peptide presentation that increased tumor cell recognition by the Ag-specific CTLs in mice, which received the peptide vaccine [83, 84]. Furthermore, we confirmed an antigen-spread effect following intratumoral peptide injection in mice inoculated with tumor cells. These clinical studies associated with a number of original immunological methods will bring about the progress of additional new treatment regimens.

## COMBINATORIAL STRATEGIES

Combinatorial strategies include an arrangement of traditional chemo-, radiotherapy or concurrent employment of various immunotherapeutic methods. Blockade of immune checkpoints is a promising strategy. Specifically, a number of agonist or antagonist antibodies can bind to crucial receptors to regulate immune reactions [85]. Combined antibody injection of anti-CTLA-4, PD-1, or others possibly modulate the tumor microenvironment, thus enhancing the potency of a cancer vaccine [86, 87]. Preclinical studies in a murine model showed that the combined treatment of anti-CTLA-4 and vaccine therapy resulted in synergistic antitumor effects [86]. However, a phase III trial showed that the combined ipilimumab, the anti-CTLA-4 antibody, with gp100 peptide vaccine did not improve the overall survival in patients who had metastatic melanoma [21]. These results suggest that the antitumor effect is a result of targeting CTLA-4 alone, as anti-CTLA-4 blockade did not lead to an increase in peptide-specific immune responses in the peripheral blood [88].

Removal or suppression of regulatory T cells (Tregs) using a low-dose cyclophosphamide [87] or anti-CD25 [89] or GITR [90] antibodies appears to be a rational approach. In an early stage clinical trial, daclizumab, a humanized antibody against CD25, did not enhance the efficacy of a dendritic cell vaccine [89]. On the other hand, a phase II study using an RCC-associated peptide vaccine verified that a single dosage of cyclophosphamide decreased the Treg number and prolonged the survival of immune responders [60]. However, no significant difference in survival of non-immune responders was observed between the groups in the use and no use of cyclophosphamide. Consequently, the interactive effects of cyclophosphamide are likely to demand a specific immune reaction.

Promising observations will show cancer vaccines having synergistic effects of combining with other strategies, especially when the mechanisms of tumor immunity have been elucidated fully. The future of cancer vaccine therapies will likely involve the combination therapies, comprised by both vaccines and immunomodulators.

## CONCLUSION

To characterize the clinical efficacy of vaccine therapy, large-scale clinical trials for a variety of tumors are currently in progress. A better understanding of tumor immunity based on the results of clinical trials, which could be applied in additional clinical setting, is desired. The progress and practice of such vaccines, in addition to varying clinical efficiency, has improved our understanding of the particular mechanisms by which tumor cells manage to resist vaccine-induced anti-tumor immunity. The gained knowledge will also be significant for optimizing potential vaccines, giving information essential to improve the individual components required developing and administrating more efficient vaccines/immunotherapy. It is indispensable to develop studies to suitably assess other new cancer vaccine therapies or combined treatment regimens, which also allows the feedback that would facilitate the ongoing development. In the near future, we believe that cancer vaccines will have a significant impact on cancer treatment globally.

## ACKNOWLEDGEMENTS

This study is supported in part by Health and Labor Science Research Grants for Clinical Research and Third Term Comprehensive Control Research for Cancer from the Ministry of Health, Labor, and Welfare, Japan. Y.S. would like to thank the Foundation for Promotion of Cancer Research (Japan) for the Third-Term Comprehensive Control Research for Cancer for the award of a research resident fellowship.

## CONFLICT OF INTEREST

The authors confirm that this chapter contents have no conflict of interest.

# REFERENCES

[1] van der Bruggen P, Traversari C, Chomez P, *et al.* A gene encoding an antigen recognized by cytolytic T lymphocytes on a human melanoma. Science 1991; 254: 1643-7.

[2] Dudley ME, Wunderlich JR, Yang JC, *et al.* A phase 1 study of nonmyeloablative chemotherapy and adoptive transfer of autologous tumor antigen-specific T lymphocytes in patients with metastatic melanoma. J Immunother 2002; 25: 243-51.

[3] Heemskerk B, Kvistborg P, Schumacher NM. The cancer antigenome. EMBO J 2013; 32: 194-203.

[4] Warren RL, Holt RA. A census of predicted mutational epitopes suitable for immunologic cancer control. Human Immunology 2010; 71: 245-54.

[5] Cheever MA, Allison JP, Ferris AS, *et al.* The prioritization of cancer antigens: a national cancer institute pilot project for the acceleration of translational research. Clin Cancer Res 2009; 15: 5323-37.

[6] Marincola FM, Jaffee EM, Hicklin DJ, Ferrone S. Escape of human solid tumors from T-cell recognition: molecular mechanisms and functional significance. Adv Immunol 2000; 74: 181-273.

[7] Valmori D, Fonteneau JF, Lizana CM, *et al.* Enhanced generation of specific tumor-reactive CTL *in vitro* by selected Melan-A/MART-1 immunodominant peptide analogues. J Immunol 1998; 160: 1750-58.

[8] Parkhurst MR, Salgaller ML, Southwood S *et al.* Improved induction of melanoma-reactive CTL with peptides from the melanoma antigen gp100 modified at HLA-A*0201-binding residues. J Immunol 1996; 157: 2539-48.

[9] Fong L, Hou Y, Rivas A, *et al.* Altered peptide ligand vaccination with Flt3 ligand expanded dendritic cells for tumor immunotherapy. Proc Natl Acad Sci USA 2001; 98: 8809-14.

[10] Rosenberg SA, Yang JC, Schwartzentruber DJ, *et al.* Immunologic and therapeutic evaluation of a synthetic peptide vaccine for the treatment of patients with metastatic melanoma. Nat Med 1998; 4: 321-7.

[11] Speiser DE, Lienard D, Rufer N, *et al.* Rapid and strong human CD8+ T cell responses to vaccination with peptide, IFA, and CpG oligodeoxynucleotide 7909. J Clin Invest 2005; 115: 739-46.

[12] Fourcade J, Kudela P, Andrade Filho PA, *et al.* Immunization with analog peptide in combination with CpG and montanide expands tumor antigen-specific CD8+ T cells in melanoma patients. J Immunother 2008; 31: 781-91.

[13] Speiser DE, Baumgaertner P, Voelter V, *et al.* Unmodified self antigen triggers human CD8 T cells with stronger tumor reactivity than altered antigen. Proc Natl Acad Sci USA 2008; 105: 3849-54.

[14] Valmori D, Dutoit V, Ayyoub M, *et al.* Simultaneous CD8+ T cell responses to multiple tumor antigen epitopes in a multipeptide melanoma vaccine. Cancer Immun 2003; 3: 15.

[15] Sampson JH, Heimberger AB, Archer GE, *et al.* Immunologic escape after prolonged progression-free survival with epidermal growth factor receptor variant III peptide vaccination in patients with newly diagnosed glioblastoma. J Clin Oncol 2010; 28: 4722-29.

[16] Schoenberger SP, Toes RE, van der Voort EI, Offringa R, Melief CJ. T-cell help for cytotoxic T lymphocytes is mediated by CD40-CD40L interactions. Nature 1998; 393: 480-3.

[17] Sun JC, Bevan MJ. Defective CD8 T cell memory following acute infection without CD4 T cell help. Science 2003; 300: 339-42.

[18] Fourcade J, Sun Z, Kudela P, *et al.* Human tumor antigen-specific helper and regulatory T cells share common epitope specificity but exhibit distinct T cell repertoire. J Immunol 2010; 184: 6709-18.

[19] Adams S, O'Neill DW, Nonaka D, *et al.* Immunization of malignant melanoma patients with full-length NY-ESO-1 protein using TLR7 agonist imiquimod as vaccine adjuvant. J Immunol 2008; 181: 776-84.

[20] Valmori D, Souleimanian NE, Tosello V, *et al.* Vaccination with NY-ESO-1 protein and CpG in Montanide induces integrated antibody/Th1 responses and CD8 T cells through cross-priming. Proc Natl Acad Sci USA 2007; 104: 8947-52.

[21] Hodi FS, O'Day SJ, McDermott DF, *et al.* Improved survival with ipilimumab in patients with metastatic melanoma. N Engl J Med 2010; 363: 711-723.

[22] Yuan J, Ginsberg B, Page D, *et al.* CTLA-4 blockade increases antigen-specific CD8(+) T cells in prevaccinated patients with melanoma: three cases. Cancer Immunol Immunother 2011; 60: 1137-46.

[23] Sarnaik AA, Yu B, Yu D, *et al.* Extended dose ipilimumab with a peptide vaccine: immune correlates associated with clinical benefit in patients with resected high-risk stage IIIc/IV melanoma. Clin Cancer Res 2011; 17: 896-906.

[24] Villadangos JA, Schnorrer P. Intrinsic and cooperative antigen-presenting functions of dendritic-cell subsets *in vivo*. Nat Rev Immunol 2007; 7: 543-555.

[25] Figdor CG, de Vries IJ, Lesterhuis WJ, Melief CJ. Dendritic cell immunotherapy: mapping the way. Nat Med 2004; 10: 475-80.

[26] Zou W. Regulatory T cells, tumour immunity and immunotherapy. Nat Rev Immunol 2006; 6: 295-307.

[27] Curiel TJ, Coukos G, Zou L, *et al.* Specific recruitment of regulatory T cells in ovarian carcinoma fosters immune privilege and predicts reduced survival. Nat Med 2004; 10: 942-9.

[28] Vieweg J, Su Z, Dahm P, Kusmartsev S. Reversal of tumor-mediated immunosuppression. Clin Cancer Res 2007; 13: 727s-732s.

[29] Muthuswamy R, Urban J, Lee JJ, Reinhart TA, Bartlett D, Kalinski P. Ability of mature dendritic cells to interact with regulatory T cells is imprinted during maturation. Cancer Res 2008; 68: 5972-78.

[30] Kalinski P, Schuitemaker JH, Hilkens CM, Wierenga EA, Kapsenberg ML. Final maturation of dendritic cells is associated with impaired responsiveness to IFN-gamma and to bacterial IL-12 inducers: decreased ability of mature dendritic cells to produce IL-12 during the interaction with Th cells. J Immunol 1999; 162: 3231-36.

[31] Vieira PL, de Jong EC, Wierenga EA, Kapsenberg ML, Kalinski P. Development of Th1-inducing capacity in myeloid dendritic cells requires environmental instruction. J Immunol 2000; 164: 4507-12.

[32] Kalinski P, Schuitemaker JH, Hilkens CM, Kapsenberg ML. Prostaglandin E2 induces the final maturation of IL-12-deficient CD1a+CD83+ dendritic cells: the levels of IL-12 are determined during the final dendritic cell maturation and are resistant to further modulation. J Immunol 1998; 161: 2804-9.

[33] Bender A, Sapp M, Schuler G, Steinman RM, Bhardwaj N. Improved methods for the generation of dendritic cells from nonproliferating progenitors in human blood. J Immunol Methods 1996; 196: 121-35.

[34] Reddy A, Sapp M, Feldman M, Subklewe M, Bhardwaj N. A monocyte conditioned medium is more effective than defined cytokines in mediating the terminal maturation of human dendritic cells. Blood 1997; 90: 3640-6.

[35] Jonuleit H, Kuhn U, Muller G, *et al.* Pro-inflammatory cytokines and prostaglandins induce maturation of potent immunostimulatory dendritic cells under fetal calf serum-free conditions. Eur J Immunol 1997; 27: 3135-42.

[36] Luft T, Jefford M, Luetjens P, *et al.* Functionally distinct dendritic cell (DC) populations induced by physiologic stimuli: prostaglandin E(2) regulates the migratory capacity of specific DC subsets. Blood 2002; 100: 1362-72.

[37] Scandella E, Men Y, Gillessen S, Forster R, Groettrup M. Prostaglandin E2 is a key factor for CCR7 surface expression and migration of monocyte-derived dendritic cells. Blood 2002; 100: 1354-61.

[38] Kalinski P, Vieira PL, Schuitemaker JH, de Jong EC, Kapsenberg ML. Prostaglandin E(2) is a selective inducer of interleukin-12 p40 (IL-12p40) production and an inhibitor of bioactive IL-12p70 heterodimer. Blood 2001; 97: 3466-9.

[39] Trinchieri G. Interleukin-12 and the regulation of innate resistance and adaptive immunity. Nat Rev Immunol 2003; 3: 133-46.

[40] Mitchell MS, Kan-Mitchell J, Morrow PR, Darrah D, Jones VE, Mescher MF. Phase I trial of large multivalent immunogen derived from melanoma lysates in patients with disseminated melanoma. Clin Cancer Res 2004; 10: 76-83.

[41] Sondak VK, Sosman JA. Results of clinical trials with an allogenic melanoma tumor cell lysate vaccine: Melacine. Semin Cancer Biol 2003; 13: 409-15.

[42] El Ansary M, Mogawer S, Elhamid SA, *et al.* Immunotherapy by autologous dendritic cell vaccine in patients with advanced HCC. J Cancer Res Clin Oncol 2013; 139: 39-48.

[43] Quoix E, Ramlau R, Westeel V, *et al.* Therapeutic vaccination with TG4010 and firstline chemotherapy in advanced non-small-cell lung cancer: a controlled phase 2B trial. Lancet Oncol 2011; 12: 1125-33.

[44] Schuetz T, Kaufman H, Marshall J, Safran H, *et al.* Extended survival in second-line pancreatic cancer after therapeutic vaccination. Journal of Clinical Oncology, 2005 ASCO Annual Meeting Proceedings 2005; 23(16S): 2576.

[45] Gulley JL, Arlen PM, Tsang KY, *et al.* Pilot study of vaccination with recombinant CEA-MUC-1-TRICOM poxviral-based vaccines in patients with metastatic carcinoma. Clin. Cancer Res 2008; 14: 3060-69.

[46] Odunsi K, Matsuzaki J, Karbach J, *et al.* Efficacy of vaccination with recombinant vaccinia and fowlpox vectors expressing NY-ESO-1 antigen in ovarian cancer and melanoma patients. Proc Natl Acad Sci USA 2012; 109: 5797-802.

[47] Schwartzentruber DJ, Lawson DH, Richards JM, *et al.* gp100 peptide vaccine and interleukin-2 in patients with advanced melanoma. N Engl J Med 2011; 364: 2119-27.

[48] Prieto PA, Yang JC, Sherry RM, *et al.* CTLA-4 blockade with ipilimumab: long-term follow-up of 177 patients with metastatic melanoma. Clin Cancer Res 2012; 18: 2039-47.

[49] Testori A, Richards J, Whitman E, *et al.* Phase III comparison of vitespen, an autologous tumor-derived heat shock protein gp96 peptide complex vaccine, with physician's choice of treatment for stage IV melanoma: the C-100-21 Study Group. J Clin Oncol 2008; 26: 955-62.

[50] Kantoff PW, Higano CS, Shore ND, *et al.* Sipuleucel-T immunotherapy for castration-resistant prostate cancer. N Engl J Med 2010; 363: 411-22.

[51] Kantoff PW, Schuetz TJ, Blumenstein BA, *et al.* Overall Survival Analysis of a Phase II Randomized Controlled Trial of a Poxviral-Based PSA-Targeted Immunotherapy in Metastatic Castration-Resistant Prostate Cancer. J Clin Oncol 2010; 28: 1099-105.

[52] Noguchi M, Kakuma T, Uemura H, *et al.* A randomized phase II trial of personalized peptide vaccine plus low dose estramustine phosphate (EMP) *versus* standard dose EMP in patients with castration resistant prostate cancer. Cancer Immunol Immunother 2010; 59: 1001-9.

[53] J. Vansteenkiste, M. Zielinski, J. Dahabre, *et al.* Multi-center, double-blind, randomized, placebo-controlled phase II study to assess the efficacy of recombinant MAGE-A3 vaccine as adjuvant therapy in stage IB/II MAGE-A3-positive, completely resected, non-small cell lung cancer (NSCLC). J Clin Oncol(Meeting Abstracts) 2006; 24 Suppl7019.

[54] J. Vansteenkiste, M. Zielinski, A. Linder, *et al.* Final results of a multi-center, double-blind, randomized, placebo-controlled phase II study to assess the efficacy of MAGE-A3 immunotherapeutic as adjuvant therapy in stage IB/II non-small cell lung cancer (NSCLC). J Clin Oncol (Meeting Abstracts) 2007; 25 suppl 7554.

[55] Ho SB, Niehans GA, Lyftogt C, *et al.* Heterogeneity of mucin gene expression in normal and neoplastic tissues. Cancer Res 1993; 53: 641-51.

[56] Butts C, Murray N, Maksymiuk A, *et al.* Randomized phase IIB trial of BLP25 liposome vaccine in stage IIIB and IV non-small-cell lung cancer. J Clin Oncol 2005; 23: 6674-81.

[57] Butts C, Maksymiuk A, Goss G, *et al.* Updated survival analysis in patients with stage IIIB or IV non-small-cell lung cancer receiving BLP25 liposome vaccine (L-BLP25): phase IIB randomized, multicenter, open-label trial. J Cancer Res Clin Oncol 2011; 137: 1337-42.

[58] González G, Crombet T, Catalá M, *et al.* A novel cancer vaccine composed of human-recombinant epidermal growth factor linked to a carrier protein: report of a pilot clinical trial. Ann Oncol 1998; 9: 431-5.

[59] Neninger Vinageras E, de la Torre A, Osorio Rodríguez M, *et al.* Phase II Randomized Controlled Trial of an Epidermal Growth Factor Vaccine in Advanced Non-Small-Cell Lung Cancer. J Clin Oncol 2008; 26: 1452-8.

[60] Walter S, Weinschenk T, Stenzl A, *et al.* Multipeptide immune response to cancer vaccine IMA901 after single-dose cyclophosphamide associates with longer patient survival. Nat Med 2012; 18: 1254-61.

[61] Wood C, Srivastava P, Bukowski R, *et al.* An adjuvant autologous therapeutic vaccine (HSPPC-96; vitespen) *versus* observation alone for patients at high risk of recurrence after nephrectomy for renal cell carcinoma: a multicentre, open-label, randomised phase III trial. Lancet 2008; 372: 145-54.

[62] Llovet JM, Ricci S, Mazzaferro V, *et al.* Sorafenib in advanced hepatocellular carcinoma. N Engl J Med 2008; 359: 378-90.

[63] Greten TF, Manns MP, Korangy F. Immunotherapy of hepatocellular carcinoma. J Hepatol 2006; 45: 868-78.

[64] Sawada Y, Ofuji K, Sakai M, Nakatsura T. Immunotherapy for hepatocellular carcinoma: current status and future perspectives, Liver Tumors - Epidemiology, Diagnosis, Prevention and Treatment, Helen Reeves, Intech, ISBN 978-953-51-1070-5, 2013.

[65] Butterfield LH, Ribas A, Meng WS, *et al.* T-cell responses to HLA-A*0201 immunodominant peptides derived from alpha-fetoprotein in patients with hepatocellular cancer. Clin Cancer Res 2003; 9: 5902-08.

[66] Butterfield LH, Ribas A, Dissette VB, *et al.* A phase I/II trial testing immunization of hepatocellular carcinoma patients with dendritic cells pulsed with four α -fetoprotein peptides. Clin Cancer Res 2006; 12: 2817-25.

[67] Lee WC, Wang HC, Hung CF, Huang PF, Lia CR, Chen MF. Vaccination of advanced hepatocellular carcinoma patients with tumor lysatepulsed dendritic cells: a clinical trial. J Immunother 2005; 28: 496-504.

[68] Palmer DH, Midgley RS, Mirza N, *et al.* A phase II study of adoptive immunotherapy using dendritic cells pulsed with tumor lysate in patients with hepatocellular carcinoma. Hepatology 2009; 49: 124-132.

[69] Kuang M, Peng BG, Lu MD, *et al.* Phase II randomized trial of autologous formalin-fixed tumor vaccine for postsurgical recurrence of hepatocellular carcinoma. Clin Cancer Res 2004; 10: 1574-9.

[70] Peng BG, Liang LJ, He Q, *et al.* Tumor vaccine against recurrence of hepatocellular carcinoma. World J Gastroenterol 2005; 11: 700-4.

[71] Greten TF, Forner A, Korangy F, *et al.* A phase II open trial evaluating safety and efficacy of a telomerase peptide vaccination in patients with advanced hepatocellular carcinoma. BMC cancer 2010; 10: 209.

[72] Nakamoto Y, Mizukoshi E, Tsuji H, *et al.* Combined therapy of transcatheter hepatic arterial embolization with intratumoral dendritic cell infusion for hepatocellular carcinoma: clinical safety. Clin Exp Immunol 2007; 147: 296-305.

[73] Nakatsura T, Yoshitake Y, Senju S, *et al.* Glypican-3, overexpressed specifically in human hepatocellular carcinoma, is a novel tumor marker. BiochemBiophys Res Commun 2003; 306: 16-25.

[74] Capurro MI, Xiang YY, Lobe C, Filmus J. Glypican-3 promotes the growth of hepatocellular carcinoma by stimulating canonical Wnt signaling. Cancer Res 2005; 65 6245-6254.

[75] Feng M, Gao W, Wang R, *et al.* Therapeutically targeting glypican-3 *via* a conformation-specific single-domain antibody in hepatocellular carcinoma. Proc Natl Acad Sci USA 2013; 19: 110(12): E1083-91.

[76] Nakatsura T, Komori H, Kubo T, *et al.* Mouse homologue of a novel human oncofetal antigen, glypican-3, evokes T-cell-mediated tumor rejection without autoimmune reactions in mice. Clin Cancer Res 2004; 10: 8630-40.

[77] Komori H, Nakatsura T, Senju S, *et al.* Identification of HLA-A2- or HLA-A24-restricted CTL epitopes possibly useful for glypican-3-specific immunotherapy of hepatocellular carcinoma. Clin Cancer Res 2006; 12: 2689-97.

[78] Sawada Y, Yoshikawa T, Nobuoka D, *et al.* Phase I trial of a glypican-3-derived peptide vaccine for advanced hepatocellular carcinoma: immunologic evidence and potential for improving overall survival. Clin Cancer Res 2012; 18: 3686-96.

[79] Sawada Y, Sakai M, Yoshikawa T, Ofuji K, Nakatsura T. A glypican-3-derived peptide vaccine against hepatocellular carcinoma. OncoImmunology 2012; 1: 1449-1551.

[80] Nobuoka D,Yoshikawa T, Sawada Y, Fujiwara T, Nakatsura T. Peptide vaccines for hepatocellular carcinoma. Hum Vaccin Immunother 2013; 9: 210-2.

[81] Yoshikawa T, Nakatsugawa M, Suzuki S, *et al.* HLA-A2-restricted glypican-3 peptide-specific CTL clones induced by peptide vaccine show high avidity and antigen-specific killing activity against tumor cells. Cancer Sci 2011; 102(5): 918-25.

[82] Sawada Y, Yoshikawa T, Fujii S, *et al.* Remarkable tumor lysis in a hepatocellular carcinoma patient immediately following glypican-3-derived peptide vaccination. Hum Vaccin Immunother 2013; 9(7): 1228-33.

[83] Nobuoka D, Yoshikawa T, Takahashi, M, *et al.* Intratumoral peptide injection enhances tumor cell antigenicity recognized by cytotoxic T lymphocytes: a potential option for improvement of antigen-specific cancer immunotherapy. Cancer Immunol Immunother 2013; 62: 639-52.

[84] Nobuoka D, Yoshikawa T, Fujiwara T, Nakatsura T. Peptide intra-tumor injection for cancer immunotherapy: Enhancement of tumor cell antigenicity is a novel and attractive strategy. Hum Vaccin Immunother 2013; 9(6): 1234-6.

[85] Zhu Y, Chen L. Cancer therapeutic monoclonal antibodies targeting lymphocyte co-stimulatory pathways. Curr Opin Investig Drugs 2003; 4: 691-5.

[86] Peggs KS, Quezada SA, Korman AJ, Allison JP. Principles and use of anti-CTLA4 antibody in human cancer immunotherapy. Curr Opin Immunol 2006; 18: 206-13.

[87] Mkrtichyan M, Najjar YG, Raulfs EC, *et al.* Anti-PD-1 synergizes with cyclophosphamide to induce potent anti-tumor vaccine effects through novel mechanisms. Eur J immunol 2011; 41: 2977-86.

[88] Attia P, Phan GQ, Maker AV, *et al.* Autoimmunity correlates with tumor regression in patients with metastatic melanoma treated with anti-cytotoxic T-lymphocyte antigen-4. J Clin Oncol 2005; 23: 6043-53.

[89] Jacobs JF, Punt CJ, Lesterhuis WJ, *et al.* Dendritic cell vaccination in combination with anti-CD25 monoclonal antibody treatment: A phase I/II study in metastatic melanoma patients. Clin. Cancer Res 2010; 16: 5067-78.

[90] Pruitt SK, Boczkowski D, de Rosa N, *et al.* Enhancement of anti-tumor immunity through local modulation of CTLA-4 and GITR by dendritic cells. Eur J Immunol 2011; 41: 3553-63.

**CHAPTER 13**

# Summary and Short-Term Outlook

**Jianxun Song***

*Department of Microbiology and Immunology, The Pennsylvania State University College of Medicine, Hershey, PA 17033, USA*

**Abstract:** In this book series, the basis and proceeding of modern cancer immunotherapy have been extensively discussed; however, it is challenging to put all information in one book. It turns out in recent times that combining immunotherapy and targeted therapies are likely to hold the future of cancer treatment. To gain a comprehensive understanding of cancer immunotherapy, readers are encouraged to find other relevant materials. This chapter serves as a summary of this book as well as provided an outlook for the future development of cancer immunotherapy.

**Keywords:** Cancer, immunology, cancer immunotherapy, targeted therapy, immune system, engineered immunotherapy, clinical application, emerging therapeutic approach, summary and outlook.

## SUMMARY

Despite its relatively short history, cancer immunotherapy has drawn a substantial attention from both basic and clinical scientists in treating cancer [1]. Through continuous progressing in understanding the immune system and how it affects tumor development, researchers hypothesized that anti-cancer strategies could be developed by using active components identified by the immune system. Under this guidance, several strategies utilizing immune components have been tested and shown promise for treating cancer in the laboratory. Furthermore, some of them have even been translated from the bench to the bedside to treat cancer patients and have been demonstrated therapeutic efficacy [2].

In general, there are two categories of therapeutic approaches in cancer immunotherapy. One involves indirect enhancement of the host anti-cancer immunity and the other is a more straightforward approach to directly target cancer cells. Prominent examples in the first category are cytokines, vaccines and monoclonal antibodies. They can modulate the host immune system by either

***Corresponding author Jianxun Song:** Department of Microbiology and Immunology, The Pennsylvania State University College of Medicine, Hershey, PA 17033, USA; E-mail: jus35@psu.edu enhancing compromised anti-cancer immunity or suppressing over-activated immunosuppressive mechanisms. The second, more straightforward approach, mainly involves T cells and NK cells that have cytotoxic capabilities. Although both indirect and direct immunotherapies have been tested, effective in treating cancer patients, so far, supplementation of the direct approach such as the use of cytotoxic T cells has been shown to be most effective [3]. However, it is admitted that current cancer immunotherapy is still far away from perfect and a significant amount of work is required to develop more effective treatments for a wide range of cancers.

## Current Update of Cancer Immunotherapy

This concluding chapter serves as a summary of the entire book. In Section 1, the basis of the immune system and anti-tumor immunity is introduced. In the following chapters, different mainstream approaches in current cancer immunotherapy such as T cell-based, NK cell-based and DC-based immunotherapies are described by individual experts in their respective fields.

In Section 2 of this book, a detailed introduction of current cancer immunotherapy in the clinic setting is provided. The three major categories of current clinical focus, T cell-based, antibody-based, and cytokine-based therapies are discussed individually.

Section 3, delves into the potential of novel cancer immunotherapies, which target different aspects of human immune system for the purpose of enhancing anti-tumor immunity or dampening tumor-induced immune system suppression. Development of high efficacy cancer vaccines is also discussed in this section.

Upon completion of this introductory book in cancer immunotherapy, it is recommended that readers shall explore more current literature to understand the most updated proceedings in this field. Also, this book does not and could not include everything in the field of cancer immunotherapy due to the nature of our limited capabilities; readers are highly suggested to use different sources to further satisfy their special interests in understanding cancer immunotherapy.

In the last section of this book, we introduce some promising future directions in cancer immunotherapy. In conclusion, based on current understanding of human immune systems and the progress in the field of cancer immunotherapy, immunotherapy could be a next-generation mainstream cancer treatment approach in near future [4].

## SHORT-TERM OUTLOOK

How to improve current strategies and develop novel concepts in cancer immunotherapy are the focuses of our future studies. Focusing efforts on exploring the immune system and its interaction with tumor should be listed as a high priority. Identifying novel and unique cancer markers could substantially enhance the application of current immunotherapy by providing a better targeting mechanism. In addition, screening of novel immune modulating agents such as cytokines and chemokines in the immune system could aid in a better designing of therapeutic approaches to boost anti-tumor immunity or dampen tumor-induced immunosuppression. Meanwhile, defining a unique fraction of immune cells could also improve tumor management [5, 6]. For instance, in adoptive T cell based cancer immunotherapy, infusion with central memory or stem cell-phenotype T cells could achieve better T cell engraft and persistence in the recipients [7, 8].

Modulating current approaches with bioengineering techniques could also help develop potent and highly effective strategies. For instance, in antibody-based cancer immunotherapy, one approach is to couple antibodies with cytotoxic agents or targeting antibodies for T cell recognition [9, 10]. In T cell-based cancer immunotherapy, two major types of modifications include engineering high-affinity T cell receptor that targets unique tumor markers and generating chimeric antigen receptors that recognize tumor markers [11, 12]. Many improvements could be achieved by these two approaches such as improving antigen-binding affinity, enhancing T cell activation signal transduction and reducing the potential leukemogenesis by using current techniques of gene introduction into T cells [13, 14]. Nevertheless, the FDA designated cancer immunotherapy using CAR gene-transduced T cells as a "Breakthrough Therapy" which resulted in an expedited (60 days) approval process.

At the same time, many new techniques and knowledge developed in recent years could also be adopted in designing novel cancer immunotherapeutic strategies [15, 16]. The most prominent example is the use of induced pluripotent stem cell (iPSC) to differentiate into T cells for adoptive transfer-based cancer immunotherapy [17-20]. From current understanding, iPSC could be a good candidate in future personalized cancer immunotherapy [21]. It has been well known that intrinsic properties related to the differentiation state of adoptively transferred T cell populations affect the success of adoptive immunotherapy. For T cell-based immunotherapy, the *in vitro* generation of naive or central memory T cell-derived effector cells, known as the "right" or *highly reactive* T cells for *in vivo* re-infusion is an optimal approach [22-25]. However, current methodologies are limited in terms of the capacity to generate, isolate and expand a sufficient quantity of such "right" T cells from patients for therapeutic interventions. First, only low numbers of Ag-specific T cells can be harvested from tumor masses and peripheral blood mononuclear cells (PBMC), which contain T cells at different stages of differentiation - naive, early, intermediate and late effector. Current expansion protocols with α-CD3 specific Ab plus recombinant IL-2 (rIL-2) or with specific-Ag plus rIL-2 (the current clinical approach) drive differentiation of Ag-specific T cells in the intermediate and late effector stages, and result in cells with shortened telomeres and diminished lifespan [26]. In addition, many patients have decreased numbers or dysfunctional T cells in the peripheral blood or lesions. In this event, a patient's T cells cannot be used for *in vitro* expansion [27, 28]. In fact, T cell survival *in vivo* is generally short-lived after they have been numerically expanded by *in vitro* culture. As a result, these protocols need to be improved to generate T cells that have adequate functional and survival properties. Second, T cell receptor (TCR) or CAR gene transfer has recently emerged as a method to overcome the obstacles of T cell deletion and dysfunction in the clinic, and introduction of genes into T cells using retroviral vectors has been proven to be safe [29, 30]. In addition, a recent study demonstrated that immune-mobilizing monoclonal TCR (mTCR) against cancer (ImmTAC) overcome immune tolerance to cancer [31], suggesting that CTL with mTCR have potent cytotoxic activity. Gene transduction of T cells from PBMC with Ag-specific TCR [32-35], CAR [36, 37] or mTCR elicits generation of functional CTL and overcomes the challenge of the limited numbers of Ag-specific T cells. Moreover, gene transduction of human PBMC with Ag-specific TCR has been reported to generate functional Ag-specific CTL, which target hepatocellular carcinoma (HCC) expressing viral Ags [32]. However, the engineered T cells express endogenous and exogenous polyclonal TCRs, which reduce their therapeutic potential [38, 39]. Also, TCR mispairing is a concern with regards to the safety of TCR gene-transferred T cells for clinical use, because the formation of new heterodimers of TCR can induce immunopathology, *e.g.*, graft *versus* host disease (GVHD) following ACT [40, 41]. Therefore, there is a need to improve this strategy. Third, the "right" effector T cells from naive or central memory T cells are more attractive for ACT-based immunotherapy than intermediate and later effector T cells [22, 23, 42, 43], because the differentiation state of T cells is inversely related to their capacity to proliferate and persist [44]. The "right" effector T cells resist terminal differentiation, maintain high replicative potential (*e.g.*, expression of common-γ chain - $\gamma_c$, CD132), are less prone to apoptosis (*e.g.*, low expression of PD-1), and have a greater ability to respond to homeostatic cytokines, such as IL-7 and IL-15 [23, 45-48], which facilitate their survival. In addition, the "right" effector T cells express high levels of molecules that facilitate their homing to lymph nodes, such as CD62L and CCR7. Furthermore, after providing an effective immune response, the "right" effector T cells persist in a variety of differentiation states, providing protective immunity. Thus, the "right" effector T cells are the superior subsets for use in adoptive immunotherapy. *Finally*, because there are too few cells, harvesting sufficient numbers of Ag-specific naive or central memory T cells from patients' PBMC for TCR or CAR gene transduction can be problematic. In addition, naive and central memory T cells are usually resistant to gene transduction unless they are activated. Taken together, strong arguments support the development of cell-based therapies using engineered T cells [4, 49]. While clinical trials show the safety, feasibility, and potential therapeutic activity of cell-based therapies using this approach, concerns raised that autoimmunity due to cross-reactivity from mispairing TCR [50, 51] or off-target Ag recognition by non tumor-specific TCR [52] or CAR [53] with healthy tissues is a major safety issue. In addition, genetically modified T cells using current approaches are usually intermediate or later effector T cells (not the "right" effector T cells), which only have short-term persistence *in vivo*. To date, stem cells are the only source available to generate a large number of naive Ag-specific T cells [19, 54-56]. Hematopoietic stem cells (HSC), *e.g.*, $CD34^+$ stem cells, have a greater potential to pass the bone marrow barrier and travel in the blood; the use of HSC for therapeutic purposes has been widely applied clinically, especially in HSC transplantation [57-59]. However, HSC has reduced differentiation and proliferative capacities, and the number of HSC is difficult to expand in cell culture [60-62]. In fact, the ability to expand the number of HSC *in vivo* or *in vitro* would represent a major advance to all current and future medical uses of HSC. In addition, HSC defects have been observed in the aged population and in several disease conditions [63-67]. For pluripotent stem cell (PSC), although the gold standard remains embryonic stem cells (ESC), their acquisition from patients is not feasible. In contrast, iPSC can be easily generated from patients' somatic cells by transduction of various transcription factors and exhibit characteristics identical to those of ESC [68-70]. This approach provides an opportunity to generate patient- or disease-specific PSC [71-73]. Recently, a number of genetic methods as well as protein-based approaches have been developed to produce iPSC with potentially reduced risks, including reduced immunogenicity [74-78]. Furthermore, several laboratories have published results indicating that the programming of Ag-specific iPSC-CTL or iPSC-$T_{regs}$ can be used for cell-based therapies of cancers and autoimmune disorders [17-20, 56, 79, 80]. Collectively, iPSC provides a chance to obtain a renewable source of healthy T cells to treat a wide array of cancers.

In addition to the application of the stem cells, a number of new, innovative approaches in the field of cancer immunotherapy have also been tested, and some of them have shown promising outcomes in either pre-clinical or clinical studies. In particular, laser immunotherapy [81, 82] using local laser irradiation to direct targeted tumor cells and local administration of immunostimulant (immunomodulator) to activate the host immune system has shown promising clinical outcomes [83, 84]. Other methods, such as photodynamic therapy (PDT) in combination with immunomodulation, also showed promising outcomes in pre-clinical studies [85-87]. Of note, combining immunotherapy and targeted therapies is likely to preserve the prospect of cancer treatment [88, 89]. Cancer chemotherapies using compounds to destroy fast dividing cells were grown in the past decades and have remained a mainstay of current treatment, however, this treatment is limited by a restricted therapeutic manifestation, substantial toxicities, and often developed resistance. As a result, more recently targeted approaches aim to restrain molecular signaling pathways that are important to tumor cell growth and survival emerged as a new treatment. Furthermore, targeted therapies also regulate immune responses in addition to inhibiting the molecular pathways, which raises the possibility that combining immunotherapy and targeted therapies is likely to improve clinical outcomes. For example, a Phase I/II clinical trial that combines the mutant B-Raf (V600E) enzyme inhibitor vemurafenib and the blocking Ab ipilimumab (CTLA-4) in patients with metastatic melanoma is being tested (NCT01400451). Take together, the combined treatments by combining two well-established approaches (indirect and direct immunotherapies) or one with new approaches such as photodynamic therapy as well as targeted therapies might be a good strategy for the future cancer treatment.

## ACKNOLEDGEMENTS

We acknowledge all our contributors for their tremendous effort to make this book possible and we appreciate all readers for choosing this book as your reference in cancer immunotherapy.

This work is funded, in part, under grants with the National Institute of Health Grants K18CA151798 and R21AI109239, Breast Cancer Alliance, and the Pennsylvania Department of Health.

# CONFLICT OF INTEREST

The authors confirm that this chapter contents have no conflict of interest.

# REFERENCES


[1] DeVita VT, Jr., Rosenberg SA. Two hundred years of cancer research. N Engl J Med 2012; 366(23): 2207-14.

[2] McNutt M. Cancer immunotherapy. Science 2013; 342(6165): 1417.

[3] Maus MV, Fraietta JA, Levine BL, Kalos M, Zhao Y, June CH. Adoptive immunotherapy for cancer or viruses. Annu Rev Immunol 2014; 32: 189-225.

[4] Couzin-Frankel J. Breakthrough of the year 2013. Cancer immunotherapy. Science 2013; 342(6165): 1432-3.

[5] Darcy PK, Neeson P, Yong CS, Kershaw MH. Manipulating immune cells for adoptive immunotherapy of cancer. Curr Opin Immunol 2014; 27C: 46-52.

[6] Levine BL, June CH. Perspective: assembly line immunotherapy. Nature 2013; 498(7455): S17.

[7] Restifo NP, Dudley ME, Rosenberg SA. Adoptive immunotherapy for cancer: harnessing the T cell response. Nat Rev Immunol 2012; 12(4): 269-81.

[8] Farber DL, Yudanin NA, Restifo NP. Human memory T cells: generation, compartmentalization and homeostasis. Nat Rev Immunol 2014; 14(1): 24-35.

[9] Tse BW, Collins A, Oehler MK, Zippelius A, Heinzelmann-Schwarz VA. Antibody-based immunotherapy for ovarian cancer: where are we at? Ann Oncol 2014; 25(2): 322-31.

[10] Weiner LM, Murray JC, Shuptrine CW. Antibody-based immunotherapy of cancer. Cell 2012; 148(6): 1081-4.

[11] Grupp SA, Kalos M, Barrett D, Aplenc R, Porter DL, Rheingold SR, *et al.* Chimeric antigen receptor-modified T cells for acute lymphoid leukemia. N Engl J Med 2013; 368(16): 1509-18.

[12] Barrett DM, Singh N, Porter DL, Grupp SA, June CH. Chimeric antigen receptor therapy for cancer. Ann Rev Medicine 2014; 65: 333-47.

[13] Gangadhar TC, Vonderheide RH. Mitigating the toxic effects of anticancer immunotherapy. Nat Rev Clin Oncol 2014; 11(2): 91-9.

[14] Blank CU. The perspective of immunotherapy: new molecules and new mechanisms of action in immune modulation. Curr Opin Oncol 2014; 26(2): 204-14.

[15] Dolgin E. Cancer vaccines: Material breach. Nature 2013; 504(7480): S16-7.

[16] Radford KJ, Tullett KM, Lahoud MH. Dendritic cells and cancer immunotherapy. Curr Opin Immunol 2014; 27C: 26-32.

[17] Vizcardo R, Masuda K, Yamada D, Ikawa T, Shimizu K, Fujii S, *et al.* Regeneration of human tumor antigen-specific T cells from iPSCs derived from mature CD8(+) T cells. Cell Stem Cell 2013; 12(1): 31-6.

[18] Themeli M, Kloss CC, Ciriello G, Fedorov VD, Perna F, Gonen M, *et al.* Generation of tumor-targeted human T lymphocytes from induced pluripotent stem cells for cancer therapy. Nat Biotechnol 2013; 31(10): 928-33.

[19] Lei F, Zhao B, Haque R, Xiong X, Budgeon L, Christensen ND, *et al. In vivo* programming of tumor antigen-specific T lymphocytes from pluripotent stem cells to promote cancer immunosurveillance. Cancer Res 2011; 71(14): 4742-7.

[20] Nishimura T, Kaneko S, Kawana-Tachikawa A, Tajima Y, Goto H, Zhu D, *et al.* Generation of rejuvenated antigen-specific T cells by reprogramming to pluripotency and redifferentiation. Cell stem cell 2013; 12(1): 114-26.

[21] Crompton JG, Rao M, Restifo NP. Memoirs of a reincarnated T cell. Cell stem cell 2013; 12(1): 6-8.

[22] Hinrichs CS, Borman ZA, Cassard L, Gattinoni L, Spolski R, Yu Z, *et al.* Adoptively transferred effector cells derived from naive rather than central memory CD8+ T cells mediate superior antitumor immunity. Proc Natl Acad Sci USA 2009; 106(41): 17469-74.

[23] Hinrichs CS, Borman ZA, Gattinoni L, Yu Z, Burns WR, Huang J, *et al.* Human effector CD8+ T cells derived from naive rather than memory subsets possess superior traits for adoptive immunotherapy. Blood 2011; 117(3): 808-14.

[24] Kerkar SP, Sanchez-Perez L, Yang S, Borman ZA, Muranski P, Ji Y, *et al.* Genetic engineering of murine CD8+ and CD4+ T cells for preclinical adoptive immunotherapy studies. J Immunother 2011; 34(4): 343-52.

[25] Fiorenza S, Kenna TJ, Comerford I, McColl S, Steptoe RJ, Leggatt GR, *et al.* A combination of local inflammation and central memory T cells potentiates immunotherapy in the skin. J Immunol 2012; 189(12): 5622-31.

[26] Royer PJ, Bougras G, Ebstein F, Leveque L, Tanguy-Royer S, Simon T, *et al.* Efficient monocyte-derived dendritic cell generation in patients with acute myeloid leukemia after chemotherapy treatment: application to active immunotherapy. Exp Hematol 2008; 36(3): 329-39.

[27] Bargou R, Leo E, Zugmaier G, Klinger M, Goebeler M, Knop S, *et al.* Tumor regression in cancer patients by very low doses of a T cell-engaging antibody. Science 2008; 321(5891): 974-7.

[28] Ramsay AG, Clear AJ, Kelly G, Fatah R, Matthews J, Macdougall F, *et al.* Follicular lymphoma cells induce T-cell immunologic synapse dysfunction that can be repaired with lenalidomide: implications for the tumor microenvironment and immunotherapy. Blood 2009; 114(21): 4713-20.

[29] Newrzela S, Cornils K, Li Z, Baum C, Brugman MH, Hartmann M, *et al.* Resistance of mature T cells to oncogene transformation. Blood 2008; 112(6): 2278-86.

[30] Tebas P, Stein D, Tang WW, Frank I, Wang SQ, Lee G, *et al.* Gene editing of CCR5 in autologous CD4 T cells of persons infected with HIV. N Engl J Med 2014; 370(10): 901-10.

[31] Liddy N, Bossi G, Adams KJ, Lissina A, Mahon TM, Hassan NJ, *et al.* Monoclonal TCR-redirected tumor cell killing. Nat Med 2012; 18(6): 980-7.

[32] Gehring AJ, Xue SA, Ho ZZ, Teoh D, Ruedl C, Chia A, *et al.* Engineering virus-specific T cells that target HBV infected hepatocytes and hepatocellular carcinoma cell lines. J Hepatol 2011; 55(1): 103-10.

[33] Perro M, Tsang J, Xue SA, Escors D, Cesco-Gaspere M, Pospori C, *et al.* Generation of multi-functional antigen-specific human T-cells by lentiviral TCR gene transfer. Gene Therapy 2010; 17(6): 721-32.

[34] Johnson LA, Morgan RA, Dudley ME, Cassard L, Yang JC, Hughes MS, *et al.* Gene therapy with human and mouse T-cell receptors mediates cancer regression and targets normal tissues expressing cognate antigen. Blood 2009; 114(3): 535-46.

[35] Bobisse S, Rondina M, Merlo A, Tisato V, Mandruzzato S, Amendola M, *et al.* Reprogramming T lymphocytes for melanoma adoptive immunotherapy by T-cell receptor gene transfer with lentiviral vectors. Cancer Res 2009; 69(24): 9385-94.

[36] Porter DL, Levine BL, Kalos M, Bagg A, June CH. Chimeric antigen receptor-modified T cells in chronic lymphoid leukemia. N Engl J Med 2011; 365(8): 725-33.

[37] Gill S, Tasian SK, Ruella M, Shestova O, Li Y, Porter DL, *et al.* Preclinical targeting of human acute myeloid leukemia and myeloablation using chimeric antigen receptor-modified T cells. Blood 2014; 123(15): 2343-54.

[38] Hill JA, Feuerer M, Tash K, Haxhinasto S, Perez J, Melamed R, *et al.* Foxp3 transcription-factor-dependent and -independent regulation of the regulatory T cell transcriptional signature. Immunity 2007; 27(5): 786-800.

[39] Stauss HJ, Cesco-Gaspere M, Thomas S, Hart DP, Xue SA, Holler A, *et al.* Monoclonal T-cell receptors: new reagents for cancer therapy. Molecular Ther 2007; 15(10): 1744-50.

[40] Bendle GM, Linnemann C, Hooijkaas AI, Bies L, de Witte MA, Jorritsma A, *et al.* Lethal graft-*versus*-host disease in mouse models of T cell receptor gene therapy. Nat Med 2010; 16(5): 565-70, 1p following 70.

[41] Provasi E, Genovese P, Lombardo A, Magnani Z, Liu PQ, Reik A, *et al.* Editing T cell specificity towards leukemia by zinc finger nucleases and lentiviral gene transfer. Nat Med 2012; 18(5): 807-15.

[42] Sagi Y, Landrigan A, Levy R, Levy S. Complementary costimulation of human T-cell subpopulations by cluster of differentiation 28 (CD28) and CD81. Proc Natl Acad Sci USA 2012; 109(5): 1613-8.

[43] Gattinoni L, Klebanoff CA, Palmer DC, Wrzesinski C, Kerstann K, Yu Z, *et al.* Acquisition of full effector function *in vitro* paradoxically impairs the *in vivo* antitumor efficacy of adoptively transferred CD8+ T cells. J Clin Invest 2005; 115(6): 1616-26.

[44] Chapuis AG, Thompson JA, Margolin KA, Rodmyre R, Lai IP, Dowdy K, *et al.* Transferred melanoma-specific CD8+ T cells persist, mediate tumor regression, and acquire central memory phenotype. Proc Natl Acad Sci USA 2012; 109(12): 4592-7.

[45] Hataye J, Moon JJ, Khoruts A, Reilly C, Jenkins MK. Naive and memory CD4+ T cell survival controlled by clonal abundance. Science 2006; 312(5770): 114-6.

[46] Seki Y, Yang J, Okamoto M, Tanaka S, Goitsuka R, Farrar MA, *et al.* IL-7/STAT5 cytokine signaling pathway is essential but insufficient for maintenance of naive CD4 T cell survival in peripheral lymphoid organs. J Immunol 2007; 178(1): 262-70.

[47] Stemberger C, Huster KM, Koffler M, Anderl F, Schiemann M, Wagner H, *et al.* A single naive CD8+ T cell precursor can develop into diverse effector and memory subsets. Immunity 2007; 27(6): 985-97.

[48] Wang LX, Plautz GE. Tumor-primed, *in vitro*-activated CD4+ effector T cells establish long-term memory without exogenous cytokine support or ongoing antigen exposure. J Immunol 2010; 184(10): 5612-8.

[49] Gravitz L. Cancer immunotherapy. Nature 2013; 504(7480): S1.

[50] Kuball J, Dossett ML, Wolfl M, Ho WY, Voss RH, Fowler C, *et al.* Facilitating matched pairing and expression of TCR chains introduced into human T cells. Blood 2007; 109(6): 2331-8.

[51] van Loenen MM, de Boer R, Amir AL, Hagedoorn RS, Volbeda GL, Willemze R, *et al.* Mixed T cell receptor dimers harbor potentially harmful neoreactivity. Proc Natl Acad Sci USA 2010; 107(24): 10972-7.

[52] Cameron BJ, Gerry AB, Dukes J, Harper JV, Kannan V, Bianchi FC, *et al.* Identification of a Titin-derived HLA-A1-presented peptide as a cross-reactive target for engineered MAGE A3-directed T cells. Sci Transl Med 2013; 5(197): 197ra03.

[53] Fedorov VD, Themeli M, Sadelain M. PD-1- and CTLA-4-based inhibitory chimeric antigen receptors (iCARs) divert off-target immunotherapy responses. Sci Transl Med 2013; 5(215): 215ra172.

[54] Norell H, Zhang Y, McCracken J, Martins da Palma T, Lesher A, Liu Y, *et al.* CD34-based enrichment of genetically engineered human T cells for clinical use results in dramatically enhanced tumor targeting. Cancer Immunol Immunother 2010; 59(6): 851-62.

[55] Zhao Y, Parkhurst MR, Zheng Z, Cohen CJ, Riley JP, Gattinoni L, *et al.* Extrathymic generation of tumor-specific T cells from genetically engineered human hematopoietic stem cells *via* Notch signaling. Cancer Res 2007; 67(6): 2425-9.

[56] Haque R, Lei F, Xiong X, Bian Y, Zhao B, Wu Y, *et al.* Programming of regulatory T cells from pluripotent stem cells and prevention of autoimmunity. J Immunol 2012; 189(3): 1228-36.

[57] Boztug K, Schmidt M, Schwarzer A, Banerjee PP, Diez IA, Dewey RA, *et al.* Stem-cell gene therapy for the Wiskott-Aldrich syndrome. N Engl J Med 2010; 363(20): 1918-27.

[58] Peerani R, Zandstra PW. Enabling stem cell therapies through synthetic stem cell-niche engineering. J Clin Invest 2010; 120(1): 60-70.

[59] Mendez-Ferrer S, Michurina TV, Ferraro F, Mazloom AR, Macarthur BD, Lira SA, *et al.* Mesenchymal and haematopoietic stem cells form a unique bone marrow niche. Nature 2010; 466(7308): 829-34.

[60] Daley GQ. Towards the generation of patient-specific pluripotent stem cells for combined gene and cell therapy of hematologic disorders. Hematology Am Soc Hematol Educ Program. 2007: 17-22.

[61] Boitano AE, Wang J, Romeo R, Bouchez LC, Parker AE, Sutton SE, *et al.* Aryl hydrocarbon receptor antagonists promote the expansion of human hematopoietic stem cells. Science 2010; 329(5997): 1345-8.

[62] Himburg HA, Muramoto GG, Daher P, Meadows SK, Russell JL, Doan P, *et al.* Pleiotrophin regulates the expansion and regeneration of hematopoietic stem cells. Nat Med 2010; 16(4): 475-82.

[63] Kenyon J, Gerson SL. The role of DNA damage repair in aging of adult stem cells. Nucleic Acids Res 2007; 35(22): 7557-65.

[64] Parmar K, Kim J, Sykes SM, Shimamura A, Stuckert P, Zhu K, *et al.* Hematopoietic stem cell defects in mice with deficiency of Fancd2 or Usp1. Stem Cells 2010; 28(7): 1186-95.

[65] Milsom MD, Lee AW, Zheng Y, Cancelas JA. Fanca-/- hematopoietic stem cells demonstrate a mobilization defect which can be overcome by administration of the Rac inhibitor NSC23766. Haematologica 2009; 94(7): 1011-5.

[66] Chen C, Liu Y, Liu Y, Zheng P. Mammalian target of rapamycin activation underlies HSC defects in autoimmune disease and inflammation in mice. J Clin Invest 2010; 120(11): 4091-101.

[67] Beerman I, Bhattacharya D, Zandi S, Sigvardsson M, Weissman IL, Bryder D, *et al.* Functionally distinct hematopoietic stem cells modulate hematopoietic lineage potential during aging by a mechanism of clonal expansion. Proc Natl Acad Sci USA 2010; 107(12): 5465-70.

[68] Nakagawa M, Koyanagi M, Tanabe K, Takahashi K, Ichisaka T, Aoi T, *et al.* Generation of induced pluripotent stem cells without Myc from mouse and human fibroblasts. Nat Biotechnol 2008; 26(1): 101-6.
[69] Okita K, Ichisaka T, Yamanaka S. Generation of germline-competent induced pluripotent stem cells. Nature 2007; 448(7151): 313-7.
[70] Kim JB, Sebastiano V, Wu G, Arauzo-Bravo MJ, Sasse P, Gentile L, *et al.* Oct4-induced pluripotency in adult neural stem cells. Cell 2009; 136(3): 411-9.
[71] Soldner F, Hockemeyer D, Beard C, Gao Q, Bell GW, Cook EG, *et al.* Parkinson's disease patient-derived induced pluripotent stem cells free of viral reprogramming factors. Cell 2009; 136(5): 964-77.
[72] Raya A, Rodriguez-Piza I, Guenechea G, Vassena R, Navarro S, Barrero MJ, *et al.* Disease-corrected haematopoietic progenitors from Fanconi anaemia induced pluripotent stem cells. Nature 2009; 460(7251): 53-9.
[73] Ebert AD, Yu J, Rose FF, Jr., Mattis VB, Lorson CL, Thomson JA, *et al.* Induced pluripotent stem cells from a spinal muscular atrophy patient. Nature 2009; 457(7227): 277-80.
[74] Woltjen K, Michael IP, Mohseni P, Desai R, Mileikovsky M, Hamalainen R, *et al.* piggyBac transposition reprograms fibroblasts to induced pluripotent stem cells. Nature 2009; 458(7239): 766-70.
[75] Yu J, Hu K, Smuga-Otto K, Tian S, Stewart R, Slukvin, II, *et al.* Human induced pluripotent stem cells free of vector and transgene sequences. Science 2009; 324(5928): 797-801.
[76] Jia F, Wilson KD, Sun N, Gupta DM, Huang M, Li Z, *et al.* A nonviral minicircle vector for deriving human iPS cells. Nat Methods 2010; 7(3): 197-9.
[77] Li Z, Yang CS, Nakashima K, Rana TM. Small RNA-mediated regulation of iPS cell generation. EMBO J 2011; 30(5): 823-34.
[78] Zhao T, Zhang ZN, Rong Z, Xu Y. Immunogenicity of induced pluripotent stem cells. Nature 2011; 474(7350): 212-5.
[79] Lei F, Haque R, Weiler L, Vrana KE, Song J. T lineage differentiation from induced pluripotent stem cells. Cellular Immunology 2009; 260(1): 1-5.
[80] Lei F, Haque R, Xiong X, Song J. Directed differentiation of induced pluripotent stem cells towards T lymphocytes. Journal of visualized experiments: JoVE. 2012(63): e3986.
[81] Chen WR, Singhal AK, Liu H, Nordquist RE. Antitumor immunity induced by laser immunotherapy and its adoptive transfer. Cancer Res 2001; 61(2): 459-61.
[82] Chen WR, Liu H, Ritchey JW, Bartels KE, Lucroy MD, Nordquist RE. Effect of different components of laser immunotherapy in treatment of metastatic tumors in rats. Cancer Res 2002; 62(15): 4295-9.
[83] Li X, Naylor MF, Le H, Nordquist RE, Teague TK, Howard CA, *et al.* Clinical effects of *in situ* photoimmunotherapy on late-stage melanoma patients: a preliminary study. Cancer Biol. & Ther 2010; 10(11): 1081-7.
[84] Wang XL, Wang HW, Yuan KH, Li FL, Huang Z. Combination of photodynamic therapy and immunomodulation for skin diseases--update of clinical aspects. Photochem Photobiol Sci 2011; 10(5): 704-11.
[85] Qiang YG, Yow CM, Huang Z. Combination of photodynamic therapy and immunomodulation: current status and future trends. Medicinal Res Rev 2008; 28(4): 632-44.
[86] Tanaka N, Ohata C, Ishii N, Imamura K, Ueda A, Furumura M, *et al.* Comparative study for the effect of photodynamic therapy, imiquimod immunotherapy and combination of both therapies on 40 lesions of actinic keratosis in Japanese patients. The Journal of Dermatol 2013; 40(12): 962-7.
[87] Zheng Y, Yin G, Le V, Zhang A, Lu Y, Yang M, *et al.* Hypericin-based Photodynamic Therapy Induces a Tumor-Specific Immune Response and an Effective DC-based cancer Immunotherapy. Biochemical pharmacology 2014; pii: S0006-2952(14)00075-6.
[88] Vanneman M, Dranoff G. Combining immunotherapy and targeted therapies in cancer treatment. Nat Rev Cancer 2012; 12(4): 237-51.
[89] Miller MJ, Foy KC, Kaumaya PT. Cancer immunotherapy: present status, future perspective, and a new paradigm of peptide immunotherapeutics. Discovery Medicine 2013; 15(82): 166-76.

# Subject Index



**Jianxun Song (Ed)**

## *D*

## *K*



## *L*



## *M*

## *U*



## *V*

Made in the USA
Las Vegas, NV
03 November 2026

57424420R00169